AF680723

This work: "Sepsis Management in Resource-limited Settings", was originally published by Springer Nature and is being sold pursuant to a Creative Commons license permitting commercial use. All rights not granted by the work's license are retained by the author or authors.

Cover Image Credit/Copyright Attribution: IIlerlok_Xolms/Shutterstock

Arjen M. Dondorp
Martin W. Dünser • Marcus J. Schultz
Editors

Sepsis Management in Resource-limited Settings

Editors
Arjen M. Dondorp
Mahidol-Oxford Research Unit (MORU)
Faculty of Tropical Medicine
Mahidol University
Bangkok
Thailand

Department of Intensive Care
Academic Medical Center
University of Amsterdam
Amsterdam
The Netherlands

Marcus J. Schultz
Mahidol-Oxford Research Unit (MORU)
Faculty of Tropical Medicine
Mahidol University
Bangkok
Thailand

Department of Intensive Care
Academic Medical Center
University of Amsterdam
Amsterdam
The Netherlands

Martin W. Dünser
Department of Anesthesiology
and Intensive Care Medicine
Kepler University Hospital
Johannes Kepler University of Linz
Linz
Austria

https://doi.org/10.1007/978-3-030-03143-5

© The Editor(s) (if applicable) and The Author(s) 2019 This book is an open access publication.
Open Access This book is licensed under the terms of the Creative Commons Attribution 4.0 International License (http://creativecommons.org/licenses/by/4.0/), which permits use, sharing, adaptation, distribution and reproduction in any medium or format, as long as you give appropriate credit to the original author(s) and the source, provide a link to the Creative Commons license and indicate if changes were made.
The images or other third party material in this book are included in the book's Creative Commons license, unless indicated otherwise in a credit line to the material. If material is not included in the book's Creative Commons license and your intended use is not permitted by statutory regulation or exceeds the permitted use, you will need to obtain permission directly from the copyright holder.
The use of general descriptive names, registered names, trademarks, service marks, etc. in this publication does not imply, even in the absence of a specific statement, that such names are exempt from the relevant protective laws and regulations and therefore free for general use.
The publisher, the authors, and the editors are safe to assume that the advice and information in this book are believed to be true and accurate at the date of publication. Neither the publisher nor the authors or the editors give a warranty, express or implied, with respect to the material contained herein or for any errors or omissions that may have been made. The publisher remains neutral with regard to jurisdictional claims in published maps and institutional affiliations.

Foreword I

It is a great honour to be writing the foreword for the first edition of *Sepsis Management in Resource-Limited Settings*.

The publication of this book could not be more timely; lives will be saved if the advice and wisdom of the authors of this superb book is translated into everyday clinical care in all settings around the world. Over the last decade, it has become increasingly clear that we can dramatically improve the survival chances of patients with sepsis and other critical care conditions. The key is the earlier identification and initial management and then the continued care of patients and their families. What we do really matters and can make the difference between life and death. It has also become apparent that this is not just the role of doctors, but increasingly paramedics, nurses, pharmacists, other healthcare professionals, and families all have a critical role to play.

This book, authored by people all looking after patients with sepsis today, is inspiring; a brilliant summary of what is known, how to best apply what is known wherever you work; and a pleasure to read whatever your personal experience or qualifications. It will be as useful to someone at the start of their career and will enhance the work of someone with many years of experience. A book for everyone, everywhere.

I cannot commend the authors highly enough, for taking complex, sometimes frightening, issues and making them understandable and accessible. I learnt a huge amount by reading it (after a career of over 30 years) and will make sure to carry it with me. This book will have a tremendous impact on the lives of many people around the world—thank you.

Jeremy J. Farrar
Director of the Wellcome Trust
London, UK

Foreword II

I would like to congratulate and praise all the contributing authors and the Global Intensive Care working group of the European Society of Intensive Care Medicine and the Mahidol Oxford Tropical Medicine Unit in Bangkok for the initiative of writing this book and the result achieved. Sepsis is a very complex syndrome already defined ages ago in various ways. Today, even with advanced medical facilities, the mortality of patients with sepsis remains high. Most of the world's population live in low- and middle-income countries, and they usually have a higher mortality due to sepsis. Next to this, many standard sepsis treatments developed in high-income countries may not be directly applicable in low- and middle-income countries. This could be due to factors such as lack of recognition, medicine, equipment, and access to intensive care and preventive measures. This book provides an in-depth understanding of these issues and applicable treatment alternatives for sepsis patients in low- and middle-income countries.

I feel very privileged to contribute this foreword for this very precious work.

Jozef Kesecioglu
Professor of Intensive Care Medicine
European Society of Intensive Care Medicine, President
Bruxelles, Belgium

Preface

Soon after the concept of sepsis had been described, research unveiled the enormous burden sepsis puts on patients, society, and healthcare services. However, most research came from high-income countries, and it inadvertently suggested that sepsis was primarily a disease condition encountered in emergency departments and intensive care units in North America, Europe, and Australasia. Over time it became apparent that the true epidemic of sepsis had so far gone unnoticed. Annually, millions of deaths due to acute severe infections, and by extension to sepsis, occurred in low- and lower- to middle-income countries without much acknowledgment in the medical literature. Furthermore, this biased view on the topic had falsely shaped our understanding of sepsis. Based on epidemiological studies from high-income countries, sepsis was largely regarded as a life-threatening complication of bacterial and sometimes fungal infection. On a global scale, however, viruses, protozoans, and *Mycobacterium tuberculosis* were, and still are, a major cause of, often fatal, sepsis.

Over the last two decades, the Surviving Sepsis Campaign has summarized contemporary scientific evidence on the management of sepsis and septic shock. However, soon after the first guidelines were published, it became clear that many recommendations were not directly applicable to resource-limited settings where the majority of sepsis mortality resides. Reasons were multiple, ranging from a different epidemiology of sepsis and the lack of trained healthcare staff to the unavailability of key material resources. Prompted by this striking mismatch, several groups took the initiative formulating adapted recommendations for the management of patients with sepsis and septic shock in resource-limited settings. In 2015, the Global Intensive Care Working Group of the European Society of Intensive Care Medicine and the Mahidol Oxford Tropical Medicine Unit in Bangkok launched a large-scale effort to evaluate the “Surviving Sepsis Campaign” recommendations against the latest scientific evidence identified and practical experience collected in resource-limited settings, many of which located in tropical countries. An expert panel of physicians practicing in or with extensive experience working in low- or lower- to middle-income countries was created to review systematically published literature and, when needed, adapt the recommendations on the management of sepsis and septic shock suitable for resource-limited settings. This book summarizes this exercise. Each chapter has been published earlier in a summary format together with extensive online supplementary material.

A constant issue during this exercise was the existing paucity of scientific evidence on the epidemiology, therapy, and outcome of sepsis in low- and lower- to middle-income countries. We sincerely hope this book will benefit the care of those who are so relentlessly affected by sepsis worldwide and that it will inspire new research to improve our understanding and management of this deadly condition in all different settings around the globe.

Bangkok, Thailand — Arjen M. Dondorp
Linz, Austria — Martin W. Dünser
Amsterdam, The Netherlands — Marcus J. Schultz

Contents

Contributors

Neill K.J. Adhikari Sunnybrook Health Sciences Centre, University of Toronto, Toronto, ON, Canada

Derek C. Angus University of Pittsburgh, Pittsburgh, PA, USA

Luciano C. Azevedo Hospital Sírio-Libanês, São Paulo, Brazil

Tim Baker Department of Public Health Sciences, Karolinska Institute, Stockholm, Sweden

Department of Anesthesia, Intensive Care and Surgical Services, Karolinska University Hospital, Stockholm, Sweden

Janet V. Diaz California Pacific Medical Center, San Francisco, CA, USA

World Health Organization, Geneva, Switzerland

Arjen M. Dondorp Mahidol Oxford Tropical Medicine Research Unit, Faculty of Tropical Medicine, Mahidol University, Bangkok, Thailand

Department of Intensive Care, Academic Medical Center, University of Amsterdam, Amsterdam, The Netherlands

Martin W. Dünser Department of Anesthesiology and Intensive Care Medicine, Kepler University and Johannes, Linz, Austria

Emir Festic Mayo Clinic, Jacksonville, FL, USA

Rashan Haniffa Mahidol Oxford Tropical Medicine Research Unit, Faculty of Tropical Medicine, Mahidol University, Bangkok, Thailand

National Intensive Care Surveillance, Ministry of Health, Colombo, Sri Lanka

University of Colombo, Colombo, Sri Lanka

Shivakumar Iyer Bharati Vidyapeeth Deemed University Medical College, Pune, India

Shevin T. Jacob University of Washington School of Medicine, Seattle, WA, USA

Liverpool School of Tropical Medicine, Liverpool, UK

Randeep Jawa Department of Intensive Care, Stony Brook University Medical Center, Stony Brook, NY, USA

Niranjan Kissoon British Columbia Children's Hospital, University of British Columbia, Vancouver, BC, Canada

Arthur Kwizera Makerere University College of Health Sciences, Mulago National Referral Hospital, Kampala, Uganda

Rakesh Lodha All India Institute of Medical Science, Delhi, India

Yoel Lubell Mahidol University, Bangkok, Thailand

Ganbold Lundeg Mongolian National University of Medical Sciences, Ulaanbaatar, Mongolia

Ignacio Martin-Loeches Department of Intensive Care, St. James's University Hospital, Dublin, Ireland

Mervyn Mer Divisions of Critical Care and Pulmonology, Department of Medicine, Faculty of Health Sciences, Charlotte Maxeke Johannesburg Academic Hospital, University of the Witwatersrand, Johannesburg, South Africa

David Misango Department of Anaesthesiology and Critical Care Medicine, Aga Khan University Hospital, Nairobi, Kenya

Sanjib Mohanty Intensive Care Unit, Ispat General Hospital, Rourkela, Sundargarh, Odisha, India

Srinivas Murthy Department of Intensive Care, British Columbia Children's Hospital, University of British Columbia, Vancouver, BC, Canada

Ndidiamaka Musa Seattle Children's Hospital, University of Washington, Seattle, WA, USA

Jane Nakibuuka Department of Intensive Care, Mulago National Referral and University Teaching Hospital, Kampala, Uganda

NT Hoang Mai Oxford University Clinical Research Unit, Hospital for Tropical Diseases, Ho Chi Minh City, District 5, Vietnam

Binh Nguyen Thien Department of Intensive Care, Trung Vuong Hospital, Ho Chi Minh City, Vietnam

Alfred Papali Division of Pulmonary and Critical Care Medicine, Atrium Health, Charlotte, NC, USA

Division of Pulmonary and Critical Care, Institute of Global Health, University of Maryland School of Medicine, Baltimore, MD, USA

Rajyabardhan Pattnaik Department of Intensive Care, Ispat General Hospital, Rourkela, Sundargarh, Odisha, India

Jason Phua National University Hospital, Singapore, Singapore

Luigi Pisani Department of Intensive Care, Academic Medical Center, University of Amsterdam, Amsterdam, The Netherlands

Mahidol-Oxford Research Unit (MORU), Faculty of Tropical Medicine, Mahidol University, Bangkok, Thailand

Pedro Povoa Nova Medical School, CEDOC, New University of Lisbon, Lisbon, Portugal

Hospital de São Francisco Xavier, Centro Hospitalar de Lisboa Ocidental, Lisbon, Portugal

Jacobus Preller Intensive Care Unit, Addenbrooke's Hospital, Cambridge University Hospitals NHS Foundation Trust, Cambridge, UK

Suchitra Ranjit Apollo Hospitals, Chennai, India

Elisabeth D. Riviello Beth Israel Deaconess Medical Center and Harvard Medical School, Boston, MA, USA

Marcus J. Schultz Mahidol-Oxford Research Unit (MORU), Faculty of Tropical Medicine, Mahidol University, Bangkok, Thailand

Department of Intensive Care, Academic Medical Center, University of Amsterdam, Amsterdam, The Netherlands

Ary Serpa Neto Department of Intensive Care, Academic Medical Center, University of Amsterdam, Amsterdam, The Netherlands

Medical Intensive Care Unit, Hospital Israelita Albert Einstein, São Paulo, Brazil

Daniel Talmor Beth Israel Deaconess Medical Center and Harvard Medical School, Boston, MA, USA

Jonarthan Thevanayagam Mzuzu Central Hospital, Mzuzu, Malawi

C. Louise Thwaites Oxford University Clinical Research Unit, Hospital for Tropical Diseases, Ho Chi Min City, Vietnam

Nuffield Department of Medicine, Centre for Tropical Medicine and Global Health, University of Oxford, Oxford, UK

1 Current Challenges in the Management of Sepsis in ICUs in Resource-Poor Settings and Suggestions for the Future

Marcus J. Schultz, Martin W. Dünser, Arjen M. Dondorp, Neill K. J. Adhikari, Shivakumar Iyer, Arthur Kwizera, Yoel Lubell, Alfred Papali, Luigi Pisani, Elisabeth D. Riviello, Derek C. Angus, Luciano C. Azevedo, Timothy Baker, Janet V. Diaz, Emir Festic, Rashan Haniffa, Randeep Jawa, Shevin T. Jacob, Niranjan Kissoon, Rakesh Lodha, Ignacio Martin-Loeches, Ganbold Lundeg, David Misango, Mervyn Mer, Sanjib Mohanty, Srinivas Murthy, Ndidiamaka Musa, Jane Nakibuuka, Ary Serpa Neto, NT Hoang Mai, Binh Nguyen Thien, Rajyabardhan Pattnaik, Jason Phua, Jacobus Preller, Pedro Povoa, Suchitra Ranjit, Daniel Talmor, Jonarthan Thevanayagam, and C. Louise Thwaites

M. J. Schultz (✉) · A. M. Dondorp · L. Pisani
Mahidol University, Bangkok, Thailand

Department of Intensive Care, Academic Medical Center, University of Amsterdam, Amsterdam, The Netherlands

M. W. Dünser
Kepler University Hospital, Johannes Kepler University, Linz, Austria

N. K. J. Adhikari
Sunnybrook Health Sciences Centre, University of Toronto, Toronto, ON, Canada

S. Iyer
Bharati Vidyapeeth Deemed University Medical College, Pune, India

A. Kwizera · J. Nakibuuka
Mulago National Referral Hospital, Kampala, Uganda

© The Author(s) 2019
A. M. Dondorp et al. (eds.), *Sepsis Management in Resource-limited Settings*,
https://doi.org/10.1007/978-3-030-03143-5_1

Y. Lubell
Department of Intensive Care, Academic Medical Center, University of Amsterdam, Amsterdam, The Netherlands

A. Papali
University of Maryland School of Medicine, Baltimore, MD, USA

Division of Pulmonary and Critical Care Medicine, Atrium Health, Charlotte, NC, USA

E. D. Riviello · D. Talmor
Beth Israel Deaconess Medical Center, Harvard Medical School, Boston, MA, USA

D. C. Angus
University of Pittsburgh, Pittsburgh, PA, USA

L. C. Azevedo
Hospital Sirio-Libanes, Saõ Paulo, Brazil

T. Baker
Karolinska Institute, Stockholm, Sweden

J. V. Diaz
California Pacific Medical Center, San Francisco, CA, USA

E. Festic
Mayo Clinic, Jacksonville, FL, USA

R. Haniffa
Mahidol University, Bangkok, Thailand

R. Jawa
Stony Brook University Medical Center, Stony Brook, NY, USA

S. T. Jacob
Liverpool School of Tropical Medicine, Liverpool, UK

N. Kissoon · S. Murthy
British Columbia Children's Hospital, Vancouver, BC, Canada

R. Lodha
All India Institute of Medical Science, Delhi, India

I. Martin-Loeches
St. James's University Hospital, Dublin, Ireland

G. Lundeg
Mongolian National University of Medical Sciences, Ulaanbaatar, Mongolia

D. Misango
Aga Khan University Hospital, Nairobi, Kenya

M. Mer
Johannesburg Hospital, University of the Witwatersrand, Johannesburg, South Africa

S. Mohanty · R. Pattnaik
Ispat General Hospital, Rourkela, Odisha, India

N. Musa
Seattle Children's Hospital, University of Washington, Washington, WA, USA

A. Serpa Neto
Department of Intensive Care, Academic Medical Center, University of Amsterdam, Amsterdam, The Netherlands

Medical Intensive Care Unit, Hospital Israelita Albert Einstein, Sao Paulo, Brazil

NT Hoang Mai
Oxford University Clinical Research Unit, Hospital for Tropical Diseases, Ho Chi Minh City, Vietnam

B. N. Thien
Trung Vuong Hospital, Ho Chi Minh City, Vietnam

J. Phua
National University Hospital, Singapore, Singapore

J. Preller
Addenbrooke's Hospital, Cambridge University Hospitals NHS Foundation Trust, Cambridge, UK

P. Povoa
Nova Medical School, CEDOC, New University of Lisbon, Lisbon, Portugal

Hospital de Sao Francisco Xavier, Centro Hospitalar de Lisboa Ocidental, Lisbon, Portugal

S. Ranjit
Appolo Hospitals, Chennai, India

J. Thevanayagam
Mzuzu Central Hospital, Mzuzu, Malawi

C. L. Thwaites
Nuffield Department of Medicine, Centre for Tropical Medicine and Global Health, University of Oxford, Oxford, UK

1.1 Introduction

In many low- and middle-income countries (LMICs), with improved public health services like sanitation and immunization, the relative importance of curative care to improve health becomes more important. This includes care for sepsis, a major reason for intensive care unit (ICU) admission in LMIC. These patients will currently often be treated in general wards, but basic intensive care facilities are becoming increasingly available. The scope of the current review is limited to the ICU setting. ICUs in resource-restricted settings have to function with important limitations, including both infrastructure and materials and human resources. It is important to address economic aspects around the provision of relatively expensive intensive care in low-income countries. Most LMICs have tropical or subtropical climates, and causes of sepsis will often be different from high-income countries (HICs), where most sepsis guidelines have been developed. Because of the different settings and the different causes of sepsis, existing guidelines will need prudent interpretation. There is a broad research agenda around this, which is currently still hardly addressed. Finally, expansion of setting-adapted training will be important to improve ICU performance in LMICs.

In this review, written by a group of physicians from resource-poor and resource-rich ICUs in LMICs and high-income countries, respectively, who were involved in the development of a series of sets of recommendations for sepsis management in resource-poor settings as recently published [1–4], the estimated burden, pathogens, and pathophysiology of sepsis are compared between resource-poor and resource-rich settings. The availability of critical care and guidelines and costs of critical care in LMICs are compared to that in high-income countries. Suggestions for future directions are provided.

1.2 Burden and Causes of Sepsis and Its Management

1.2.1 Disease Burden

While detailed information has been reported on the epidemiology and outcome of sepsis in HICs [5, 6], only scant systematically collected epidemiological data exist from LMICs [7, 8], despite that these countries carry about 80% of the global mortality caused by infections [9]. At present, the epidemiology of sepsis in LMICs can only be loosely estimated from the epidemiology of acute infectious diseases with a potential to cause sepsis captured in the "Global Burden of Disease" database [10–12]. This database reported important regional differences in the epidemiology of such acute infectious diseases (Fig. 1.1). For instance, while the majority of acute infections in resource-limited settings are acquired in the community [9], the incidence of nosocomial infections such as catheter-related bloodstream infections or ventilator-associated pneumonia is several fold higher in LMICs than in high-income countries like the United States [13]. Similarly, only few data on sepsis mortality in LMICs have so far been published. These suggest that sepsis-related mortality greatly varies among regions and countries according to their income level. The case fatality attributable to sepsis in HICs has been decreasing over the last decades to 30–40% [5, 6], whereas case fatality rates of up to 80% continue to be reported from resource-poor regions of the world [14–17].

1.2.2 Causative Pathogens and Pathogenesis

Although many bacterial pathogens causing sepsis in LMICs are similar to those in high-income countries, resistance patterns to antimicrobial drugs can be very different. It has been suggested that the high prevalence of multidrug-resistant bacteria, including methicillin-resistant *Staphylococcus aureus*, extended spectrum beta-lactamase-producing bacteria, carbapenamase-producing *Enterobacteriaceae*, and *Mycobacterium tuberculosis*, contributes to the excess deaths observed in LMICs caused by invasive infections with these bacteria, particularly among infants [13, 18]. Five countries with the highest burden of under five deaths (China, Nigeria, Pakistan, India, and the Democratic Republic of the Congo) also have the highest neonatal deaths from antimicrobial resistance [19]. The problems with antimicrobial resistance and its implications for the treatment of sepsis in LMICs have been described before [4].

Whereas the majority of severe sepsis in HICs is caused by bacterial infections, in LMICs, many of which are located in the tropics, causes of sepsis also include

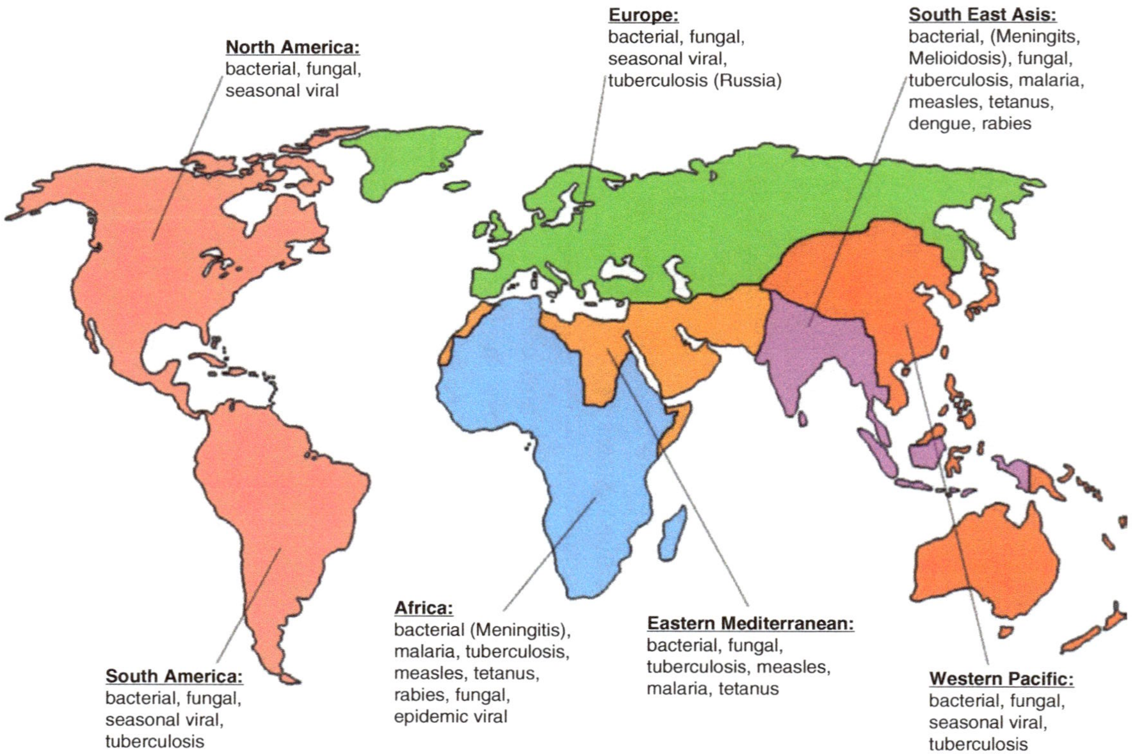

Fig. 1.1 Most relevant infectious diseases as reported by the Global Burden of Disease study stratified by the six World Health Organization regions. From [10, 11]

acute non-bacterial diseases, including protozoal diseases such as malaria, and viral diseases such as measles, dengue, or viral hemorrhagic fevers. The international literature mainly focuses on sepsis caused by invasive bacterial infections and the associated systemic inflammatory response [20, 21]. Therefore, non-bacterial causes are understudied, and the acquired knowledge on the pathophysiology and treatment of sepsis may not be generalizable to these other causes of sepsis [22].

Previous sepsis definitions put a large emphasis on the "dysregulated response of the host's immune system" as the key element of the pathogenesis of sepsis [23, 24]. Although this will be generally correct, it ignores potential direct damaging effects of certain pathogens or pathogen products, which can in particular play a role in tropical diseases. For instance, in severe falciparum malaria, a blocked microcirculation resulting from the sequestered infected red blood cell biomass is a direct cause of vital organ failure [25]; and in dengue shock syndrome, virus proteins are thought to directly damage the glycocalyx lining the endothelium [26, 27]. Intervening in these pathophysiological pathways will obviously require therapeutic approaches different from those in bacterial sepsis.

1.2.3 Poor Availability of Critical Care

There is persisting substantial heterogeneity in ICU capacity around the world. In Europe and Northern America, the ICU capacity is between 5 and 30 beds per 100,000 inhabitants. In LMICs, the scarce data available show ICU capacities that are much lower, albeit quite variable [28]. For instance, in Asia the reported ICU capacity is only 0.3 beds per 100,000 inhabitants in Bangladesh, 2.4 per 100,000 inhabitants in Malaysia, 2.5 per 100.000 inhabitants in Sri Lanka, and 3.9 per 100,000 inhabitants in China [29], but in contrast 11.7 adult and pediatric ICU beds per 100,000 inhabitants in Mongolia [30]. Studies form several countries in sub-Saharan Africa reported as few as 0.1–0.2 ICU beds per 100,000 inhabitants [31, 32]. With the exception of Mongolia [30] and Latin-American countries [33], almost no data on the availability of dedicated pediatric ICU capacities have been published for resource-limited settings [34].

We tend to look at LMICs as if they are "uniform," but this is a too simplistic if not naive approach. Within and between LMICs, there is an important heterogeneity in the availability of intensive care, resourcing of ICUs, quality of services, and case mix [35]. The rapidly expanding urban population in many LMICs will provide a challenge for the current urban ICU capacity because of the associated increase in case load [36].

Another problem in reporting ICU capacity is the lack of a commonly agreed definition of an ICU or ICU bed [37, 38]. The spectrum of how ICUs are staffed and equipped differs vastly between countries and regions. Table 1.1 summarizes published evidence and personal experience of the authors in an attempt to categorize different ICU structures worldwide. As surveys from various countries suggest, the availability of ICU-related material resources directly correlates with the countries' income level and healthcare spendings [7, 31, 32, 39–43]. The shortage of medical

Table 1.1 Proposal for a categorization of intensive care units[a]

Proposed categories	Category I—unrestricted	Category II—moderate restrictions	Category III—severe restrictions	Category IV—no formal ICU structure
Typical setting (not including private settings)	High-income countries	Higher-middle-income countries	Lower-middle and low-income (major cities) countries	Rural areas of low-income countries
Formal ICU structure/service	Yes	Yes	Partly	No
Availability of specifically trained physicians and nurses	Widespread	Irregular	Rare	Unavailable
Availability of ICU equipment (i.e., patient monitor, mechanical ventilator, renal replacement therapy)	Unrestricted	Moderate restrictions (i.e., irregular maintenance of equipment, limited availability of advanced treatment modalities such as RRT)	Severe restrictions (i.e., basic monitoring typically available, limited number of mechanical ventilators, widespread unavailability of advanced treatment modalities such as RRT)	Unavailable
Availability of ICU drugs and disposable materials	Unrestricted	Mild restrictions	Moderate restrictions	Severe restrictions

Abbreviations: *ICU* intensive care unit, *RRT* renal replacement therapy

[a]The categories proposed here should not be seen as definite, but merely should serve as a starting point of future thinking

professionals specifically trained in the care of acutely and critically ill patients is another widespread and serious challenge for ICU services in many LMICs [31, 32, 39–42]. A notable exception to this is well-staffed and well-equipped ICUs in private healthcare facilities. Such services can typically be found in some HICs and LMICs, but these usually remain only accessible for those who can afford it.

The increasing but still low ICU capacity in poorer regions [44] implies that access to ICU services for critically ill patients is usually severely limited. This results in frequent triage decisions [32], which likely increases preventable mortality [45]. Even though costs of care in ICUs of resource-limited settings are only a fraction of those encountered in HICs [46], expenses for ICU care are usually to a large extent covered by the patient's family and relatives in LMICs. Unwanted consequences can be denial or refusal of ICU admission of poor patients, but also the premature withdrawal of lifesaving interventions [47, 48]. In other instances, costs of care for a critically ill patient, who may eventually die, can exceed the limited budget of many families leaving them with high debts or even causing private bankruptcy.

1.2.4 Incomplete and Unadjusted Guidelines

The principle of "evidence-based medicine" is equally important in resource-limited as in resource-rich settings. Development of local evidence is important, since case mix and causes of sepsis, but also available infrastructure and facilities, are essentially different from those in HICs. Resource-limited ICUs are frequently limited in the availability of equipment, laboratory support, and skilled physician and nursing staff. As a result, recommendations on sepsis management in resource-poor settings, such as those developed by the *Global Intensive Care Working Group* of the European Society of Intensive Care Medicine (ESICM) [49], differ in several aspects from the Surviving Sepsis Campaign guidelines, which were developed in high-income settings [50]. Obvious examples include targeting strict blood glucose levels with insulin, which can be safe with frequent and reliable blood glucose monitoring, while it is a dangerous strategy when the effects of insulin titrations are determined infrequently or not at all. Other modifications in recommendations for sepsis management could result from differences in the availability of and indications for fluids in sepsis patients between resource-rich and resource-poor settings, but also the cause of sepsis (see also Box 1.1).

Box 1.1: Availability of and Indications for Fluids in Sepsis Patients Differ Between High-Income Countries and Low- and Middle-Income Countries

Intravenous infusion of fluids is a key intervention in patients with sepsis as this syndrome frequently leads to intravascular hypovolemia from extravasation due to capillary leaking.

RESOURCE-RICH SETTINGS: physicians and nurses, independent from each other, have free and unlimited excess to fluids for intravenous infusion, which may facilitate a "too liberal" fluid approach leading to "overzealous" fluid resuscitation known to be associated with worse outcome of sepsis patients.

RESOURCE-POOR SETTINGS: usually there is a shortage of fluids for intravenous fluids, decision on the amounts of fluids to be given is restricted to attending physicians and not nurses, and the type of fluid chosen may depend on its price (e.g., dextrose-containing fluids, such as 5% dextrose or 10% dextrose, are cheap and thus readily available, opposite to crystalloid solutions); inadequate resuscitation, either because of too low or too late given or wrong fluids infused, may worsen outcome of sepsis patients.

> *FLUID THERAPY IN BACTERIAL SEPSIS*: the recommendations on fluid therapy in sepsis patients are largely built on evidence coming from randomized controlled trials in patients in *RESOURCE-RICH SETTINGS*, where most patients do have *BACTERIAL SEPSIS*.
>
> *FLUID THERAPY IN NON-BACTERIAL SEPSIS*: interestingly, randomized controlled trials including patients with severe falciparum malaria or dengue shock syndrome suggest more restricted fluid therapy than recommended for bacterial sepsis to be better. One major difference between *BACTERIAL SEPSIS* and *NON-BACTERIAL SEPSIS* is that fluid bolus resuscitation is not recommended in hyperlactatemic patients with severe falciparum malaria who are not hypotensive. Also, in dengue shock syndrome, proper fluid management is pivotal to ensure a good outcome; fluid therapy in dengue shock syndrome should ensure adequate circulating volume to support tissue perfusion, but avoid overfilling, which will cause interstitial edema, which is in particular harmful in the lung.

Despite the importance of building "local" evidence, many aspects of existing guidelines and basic principles of good critical care are universal. Access to adequate information has improved massively in this cyber age, and several courses (such as the *BASIC for Developing Healthcare Systems* courses developed by the Chinese University of Hong Kong, Hong Kong, China, and *Médecins Sans Frontières*) are available. Theoretical knowledge of specialist doctors in developing countries is often impressive, but translating this into practical implementation can lag behind, which is an important scope for training. Training should not only be for ICU physicians but also for nurses and other clinical personnel. It will be important that education on sepsis management does not focus only on ICU staff but includes medical schools, nursing schools, and training of other health workers, as many sepsis patients in LMICs receive treatment outside an ICU. "Train-the-trainer" models and fostering local champions for positive change are important to sustain improvements of care.

1.3 Costs of Care in Sepsis

1.3.1 Expensive but Likely Cost-Effective Critical Care

The vast resources consumed by ICUs, up to a staggering 1% of total gross domestic product in the United States [51], demand their subjection to explicit economic cost-benefit considerations [52]. The literature from high-income settings has indeed expanded over the past decade, demonstrating that many critical care interventions offer significant health returns with costs per quality-adjusted life year (QALY) gained well below a threshold of US $50,000, indicative of a cost-effective intervention in this context.

For countries in which more basic services are still relatively undeveloped, it might be questioned whether investment in ICUs should take priority over the strengthening of lower tiers of the healthcare system [53]. Irrespective of these considerations, the reality is that in many growing economies, ICUs are increasing in number [44], with virtually no evidence regarding the cost-effectiveness of their services.

1.3.2 Costs of Critical Care Among Regions

One approach is to consider the evidence from HICs, with a much lower willingness to pay the abovementioned threshold. Applying a threshold of US $4000 per QALY gained [54] suggests that numerous ICU interventions and those for sepsis in particular [55–61] are likely to be cost-effective in ICUs in LMICs (Table 1.2). For several reasons these cost-effectiveness ratios might be conservative in the context of LMICs. First, the cost of ICUs in these countries is much lower than in HICs. The two largest standardized multicountry reviews of critical care costs in high-income settings estimated the cost per ICU day ranging from US $850 to US $3400 in 2015 [63, 64], with labor being the dominant cost driver (61% and 67%, respectively). The proportional difference in labor costs between high-income countries and LMICs will be similar to or higher than that of their respective gross domestic product per capita [65]. This alone implies that the critical care costs in LMICs will be less than a third that in HICs. Other costs, such as laboratory services (10% of total critical care cost [64]), are also likely to be far lower for similar reasons, as well as drug costs and cost-saving practices such as recycling of consumables [66]. In one of the few costing analyses of an ICU from a LMIC, the total cost per ICU admission day in India was estimated at just over US $200 [67], between approximately 5 and 20% that for HICs.

However, also the absolute financial outlay per intervention multiplied by the number of interventions is important to consider, in particular in LMICs. Even in a wealthy country with a high threshold, its tolerance depends exquisitely on the number of times it must spend the money, especially if up-front costs are high. In other words, an intervention might appear cost-effective, but if it would have to be applied to a massive portion of the public, the costs would still be perceived as financially impossible. This also requires there is an effective system of triage in place to see that these interventions are offered to patients who are most likely to benefit, at times a challenge in LMICs.

Finally, we are uncertain whether applying a threshold of US $4000 per QALY gained is one that could be promoted or generalized, as there is a large intra- and inter-region variation in resources. Country- and ideally region-specific currency conversions/purchase power parity comparisons should be made.

Table 1.2 The cost-effectiveness of interventions for the management of severe sepsis

Author, year [Reference]	Cohorts (country)	Intervention	Conventional	Cost/QALY (in 2015 US $)
Huang et al. 2007 [57]	Monte Carlo simulation of patients with sepsis undergoing EGDT beginning either in the ED or ICU (USA)	EGDT in ED or ICU	Standard care	$3506–8953
Talmor et al. 2008 [61]	Prospective cohort study of patients treated with an integrated sepsis protocol compared to controls (USA)	Integrated sepsis protocol	Standard care	$20,265 (2015)
Lehmann et al. 2010 [60]	Monte Carlo simulation of sepsis episodes in ICU patients with use of PCR with cultures to identify the causative organism and initiate tailored antibiotic therapy (EU)	PCR and cultures	Traditional cultures only	$3798
Karlsson et al. 2009 [59]	Prospective cohort study of sepsis patients admitted to the ICU who were followed for 2 years (Finland)	ICU care for severe sepsis	Standard care	$2664
Jones et al. 2011 [58]	Prospective before-after clinical trial to establish the initiation of EGDT in the ED prior to transfer to ICU for newly admitted sepsis patients (USA)	EGDT for sepsis in ED	Standard ED care for sepsis	$6283 (2015)
Suarez et al. 2011 [62]	Prospective before-after clinical trial to assess the impact of an educational program on adherence to "Surviving Sepsis Campaign Guidelines" (Spain)	Surviving sepsis protocol for severe sepsis	Standard care	$7810 (2015)
Assuncao et al. 2014 [55]	Prospective case-control analysis of patients treated with EGDT vs. standard care (Brazil)	EGDT	Standard care	Dominant
Harrison and Collins 2015 [56]	Markov model assessing cost-effectiveness of PCT as a diagnostic tool for bacterial infection in ICU patients (USA)	PCT	Standard diagnostic techniques	Dominant

Abbreviations: *EGDT* early goal-directed therapy, *ED* emergency department, *ICU* intensive care unit, *PCR* polymerase chain reaction, *PCT* procalcitonin

1.3.3 Benefit of Critical Care Among Regions

The mean age of adult patients admitted to ICUs in HICs is consistently higher than those reported in LMICs. For example, in European ICUs, the mean age of adult admissions is typically 55–66 years, much higher than the median age of 34 years in a Rwandan ICU [68], the mean age of 32 years in one of the few ICUs in Uganda [1], and the median age of 37, 51, and 49 years in ICUs in Bangladesh, Nepal, and India [69]. Although not specified for admission diagnoses, it likely also reflects the younger age of sepsis patients. This can be taken as an argument to invest in better intensive care to save these young lives from an in principle treatable disease. Also, in LMICs where social security networks are usually lacking, the loss of an individual's economic activity has far more extensive economic consequences for the families involved.

By generalizing the evidence from HICs and considering the lower costs and higher potential gains, there are strong indications that a wide range of critical care services are likely to be cost-effective in LMICs. Unfortunately, there is a dearth of evidence directly from these settings to confirm this. The only economic evaluation of an ICU in Bosnia and Herzegovina concluded that critical care was highly cost-effective in their setting [46]. A study from Brazil showed that the implementation of a sepsis management protocol was associated with an absolute reduction of 18% in mortality and with cost savings [55].

1.3.4 Impact of Certain Interventions Among Regions

Despite these suggestions that a broad range of ICU services could be cost-effective in LMICs, there is also reason for caution. First, some interventions are likely to have a much lower impact in poorly functioning environments than they might have in resource-rich settings. For example, invasive monitoring in an ICU with poor basic infection control could result in more harm than benefit. For this reason it is imperative that basic standards of care are in place prior to introduction of costly interventions whose effect might otherwise be compromised. Training programs to improve the general quality of care that require no costly interventions have been shown to have beneficial effects [69]. Second, while hypothetically cost-effectiveness should correspond with affordability, in LMICs where health systems are often fragmented and divided between the private and public sector and an abundance of vertically funded health programs, this is often not the case. It is imperative therefore that only interventions with modest budgetary impacts are shortlisted for consideration and those that have the greatest beneficial effects, with the lowest incremental costs, are selected for implementation. Some such low-cost approaches have been identified and should be prioritized for evaluation. Better surveillance systems for local etiologies of sepsis and antimicrobial susceptibility patterns have been recognized as a key requirement for improving the management of sepsis and critical care [4], and a modeling-based economic evaluation supported the notion that this is likely to be highly cost-effective [70].

Likewise, the development and adaptation of LMIC-specific risk prediction models have been shown to potentially outperform models widely used in high-income settings like the frequently used Acute Physiology and Chronic Health Evaluation Score and the Simplified Acute Physiology Score [68], which might not even be feasible in many ICUs in LMICs. The same is true for scoring systems in children, and scoring systems that are context relevant should also be explored because the Predicted Risk of Mortality may underpredict mortality [71].

Critical care in general and a subset of specific interventions can be an efficient use of scarce resources in LMICs. But despite the aforementioned lower costs, an ICU admission, e.g., in India, would most likely represent a catastrophic expenditure consuming over half the mean annual household income [44, 67] (see also: Box 1.2). As such facilities expand in LMICs and inevitably consume increasing resources, it is imperative for health authorities to ensure these offer affordable and cost-effective services while monitoring and continuing to seek opportunities to improve the quality of critical care and their efficiency at low cost. This was exemplified by the United Kingdom in the late 1990s, where a countrywide initiative to transform and modernize critical care was associated with a 10% reduction in mortality at lower cost increases than would otherwise be expected [72].

Box 1.2: Critical Care Expenditure in Indian Hospitals

In India critical care services are offered in four broad types of hospitals, with variable reimbursements. Variable reimbursements potentially lead to a great diversity in care of the critically ill, especially those who tend to have an extended ICU stay (i.e., longer than just a view days).

GOVERNMENTAL hospitals: the ICU bed, ventilation, and basic medications may be free of costs, but patient will need to spend out of pocket for expensive medications like certain antibiotics and disposables and for the family to stay in a distinct place (far) away from their homes. Often in a few days, they will exhaust their meager finances after which their care will be compromised.

PUBLIC CHARITY TRUST hospitals, including hospitals of private medical colleges: these hospitals have a mandate to provide free treatment to patients below the poverty line. In addition, these hospitals also offer concessional treatment under various governmental insurance schemes for poor patients that, however, are mainly utilized for surgical patients and short-stay patients like myocardial infarction and stroke. The insurance offered for sepsis is very meager and cannot cover more than the first few days in ICU. Patients thus will need to spend out of pocket for expensive medications like certain antibiotics and disposables and for the family to stay in a distinct place (far) away from their homes.

PRIVATE CORPORATE hospitals: these will treat affording patients either paying out of pocket or through some form of insurance. Except for the rich and very rich, in a week or two, such patient will exhaust their finances and will then either be transferred to *GOVERNMENTAL* hospitals or *PUBLIC CHARITY TRUST* hospitals. These transfers however are not easy given scarcity of beds. Public charitable hospitals will generally have an admission policy that will discourage patients that are deemed unsalvageable or may require some form of limitation of therapy. *GOVERNMENTAL* hospitals have to accept such patients, but here the bed crunch is often more severe. This leaves patient and caregivers in a very difficult position and may lead to withdrawal of care or discharge against medical advice.

Smaller *PRIVATE NURSING HOMES*: these may offer critical services for selected patients, but this too follows a similar trajectory as that of the *PRIVATE CORPORATE* hospitals, i.e., once patients' finances are exhausted, they need to be transferred.

1.4 Sepsis Research in Resource-Limited Settings

1.4.1 A Yet Largely Untouched Research Agenda

With only 1.7% of all biomedical research publications originating in LMICs [73], and a likely even greater disparity in critical care [44], both the needs and the opportunities for critical care research are vast. Recent rigorous attempts to quantify the global burdens of sepsis, infection, and respiratory failure confirm a profound lack of epidemiologic critical illness data from LMICs, with the only reliable data limited to single-center descriptions [68, 74–77]. The *International Severe Acute Respiratory and Emerging Infection Consortium* (ISARIC), the *Global Intensive Care Working Group* of the ESICM, and the Mahidol Oxford Research Unit in Bangkok, Thailand, are three examples of groups working to create the infrastructure for global epidemiologic data on critical illness, for use both as baseline data at regular intervals and in preparation for disease outbreaks [78].

Research on infectious diseases that lead to critical illness are perhaps the most successful areas of investigation thus far, with impressive scientific advancements in diseases such as malaria, tuberculosis, and melioidosis [79–81]. Defining and testing quality metrics are an area prioritized in both critical care and global public health [82], but quality improvement in resource-limited ICUs remains largely unexplored [44, 83]. The latter requires some ability to benchmark ICUs with severity of illness scores, also a nascent area of study [68]. Research into medical education models like the *Human Resources for Health* program in Rwanda [84], decision support tools like the *Checklist for Early Recognition and Treatment of Acute IllNess* (CERTAIN) [85], and *Vital Signs Directed Therapy* [86] could help in better defining how to optimize knowledge acquisition and application for providers in resource-limited settings.

1.4.2 Challenges with Research in Resource-Restricted Settings

The realities of restriction in resources interact to create complex challenges to producing quality critical care research. Many short-term multisite epidemiologic studies depend on individual sites to participate without funding for the perceived minimal data collection burden. However, staff at resource-constrained sites often cannot spare even the short-term investment required to participate, and "standard" clinical data such as arterial blood gas analyses and chest radiographs are often not available at these sites [76, 78]. Likewise, multicenter clinical trials are significantly more expensive to perform in resource-limited settings since baseline clinical or analytic infrastructure of any sort cannot be assumed. Efforts to build resource capacity in research and to ensure fair authorship opportunities also mean that research has two resource-intensive and sometimes competing goals: that of developing local researchers without prior training and that of producing high-quality research. An unintended consequence of (appropriate) increasing involvement by local institutional review boards is that lack of staffing and experience may lead to unnecessary delays in research approvals. These resource barriers to collecting epidemiologic data are exacerbated by the fact that "critical illness" is not a laboratory-defined condition but rather one that is often defined by the expensive resources used to treat it [28, 87].

Ethical considerations are complex as well. All participants in resource-limited settings must be considered potentially "vulnerable" populations due to extreme need and lack of health or research literacy. Deciding where equipoise exists for interventions proven to work in high-resource settings in settings of low resources is difficult. Asking the question, "How do we do this better given limited resources?" uncomfortably raises the question "How do we increase resources and to what extent are we obligated to do so?" Ethical considerations also include relationships between local and foreign researchers, the latter who often bring financial and experiential resources leading to unequal power dynamics and potential for abuse [88]. Allowing lower standards for publication for research originating in low-resource settings has been considered in order to decrease some of the publication bias toward resource-rich settings; however, it is not at all clear that publishing poor-quality research that could impact clinical care is ethical or advisable.

1.5 Suggestions for the Future

1.5.1 Better Definition of Sepsis

The latest sepsis definition [89], which refers to sepsis as life-threatening organ dysfunction caused by a dysregulated host response to infection, better reflects the fact that sepsis can complicate any serious acute infection. As pointed out earlier, direct damaging effects of the pathogen itself or its products can sometimes be the main process. Consequently, research on sepsis treatment should not focus only on immunomodulating strategies in bacterial sepsis but also on faster illumination of the pathogen and its products, which could be in particular relevant in certain non-bacterial causes of sepsis like falciparum malaria, cryptococcal, and various viral infections.

Another unmet need is to validate the various definitions for sepsis in more varied populations, like children in LMICs, adults in LMICs, and areas where the causative pathogens of sepsis differ from Western countries where the present definitions have been developed.

1.5.2 Better Research Infrastructures and Planning

Experience, resources, and human power are critical for building evidence, which are not routinely available in resource-poor settings. The global critical care community should help building local clinical research capacities and contribute to obtaining adequate funding. Engagement of a variety of stakeholders, including local intensive care societies, healthcare authorities (e.g., ministries of health), and universities, will be crucial in this respect [90]. There are large funding bodies, such as the Wellcome Trust, that support several efforts, but additional funds are clearly needed. Teaming up of researchers from established groups in HICs with local groups in resource-limited settings has proven a good model, provided equal and reciprocal relationships are guaranteed. Formulating essential topics for research will be important and could benefit from increased networking between critical care physicians from developing countries. This would also foster research networks needed to perform adequately powered clinical trials. Requirements for quality clinical research are not necessarily available in many LMICs, with often little research infrastructure or human resources for research available. Hospitals and their doctors can be overburdened by their service delivery tasks, leaving little room for research. Offering a career path to clinical research physicians could free up manpower for this important aspect of improving evidence-based critical care. Priority settings and governance regarding financial resources for research and implementation projects will become extremely important. Also, local institutions, including ethical review boards, should help create an enabling environment for research benefiting the local population, and not promote unnecessary barriers, which is now at times the case.

1.5.3 Obtaining Relevant Evidence and Adapting Guidelines

Obtaining local intelligence on the most important causes of sepsis and the resistance patterns of the infecting microorganisms is crucial to guide local empirical antimicrobial treatment. Since microbiological capacity is often lacking in hospitals in LMICs, research collaborations could help obtaining this evidence from strategically located sentinel study sites.

We need additional recommendations for those interventions not yet covered in the published guidelines. Multicenter trials assessing clinical efficacy and effectiveness of new interventions and interventions known to be effective in resource-rich settings are sorely needed, given differences in epidemiologic and treatment contexts [44]. The Fluid Expansion As Supportive Therapy (FEAST) trial on fluid resuscitation in febrile African children with shock demonstrates that these trials are feasible and may yield unexpected results [91]. Networks of critical care researchers are increasingly established in more resource-limited areas of the world, which could lead to additional studies of this kind [44]. Beyond these broad areas of research, specific subtypes deserve special attention in resource-limited settings. Social determinants of disease and barriers to care are of particular relevance to all research in resource-limited settings including intensive care [82]. While cost-effectiveness analyses are arguably important in all environments without infinite resources, their need is more acute in places with fewer resources to allocate [92]. Locally adapted prediction models can help ensure that interventions are targeted in a cost-effective manner.

Another important area for critical care research is on developing templates for expanding urban ICU capacity in fast-growing cities [36]. Setting-specific guidance, instead of country-specific guidance on how to build and equip an ICU probably, is an additional and substantial area of research.

Finally, research on the process whereby scientific knowledge is translated into improved quality of care, "global health delivery science," gets at the immediate challenge in patient care in resource-poor settings, the fact that so much of what is known is not implemented effectively [82].

1.5.4 Opportunities

While the challenges are daunting, the opportunities are similarly impressive. Outbreaks like Ebola have increased the drive for intensive care research in resource-limited settings both by demonstrating how critical illness in these settings impacts people in resource-rich settings and by highlighting the need for improved critical care capacity in all areas of the world [93]. Interest in and funding for global health have increased steadily over the last few decades, such that career path and funding opportunities for HIC researchers are better than ever before. Researchers from resource-limited settings now also have opportunities for high-quality training and mentorship through programs, for example, through the Wellcome Trust or the UK "Medical Research Council" schemes and the American Thoracic Society's "Methods in Epidemiologic, Clinical, and Operations Research" (MECOR) program [94].

An example of building a research structure is one from India, where the Indian Society of Critical Care Medicine initiated a "cloud-based database" called "Customized, Health in Intensive care, Trainable Research, and Analysis (CHITRA)" (http://www.isccm.org/chitra.aspx).

Finally, LMICs and HICs could mutually benefit from their research agendas; HICs also gain from more LMIC research. For example, LMIC considerations about direct pathogen effects could, in turn, generate better critical thinking about sepsis, from which both HICs and LMICs gain. Similarly, technologic innovation under resource constraints can yield gains for all. Critical care could be ripe for this at times called "frugal innovation" or "reverse innovation" concept [95]. Also, in our personal experience [69], nurses from HICs who have worked in LMICs, and even for a short time, are more cost-conscious than their colleagues.

1.6 Conclusions

Strategies to improve the quality of sepsis management in resource-poor settings require consideration of disease-specific and setting-specific factors and meticulous evaluation of the best way to adapt and deploy quality improvement initiatives. Critical care, including sepsis management, is expensive but likely cost-effective in LMICs, but we need to better understand what the true financial impact of critical care is, both at a macro- and micro-economy level. Sepsis management in resource-limited settings is a largely unexplored frontier with a clear mandate and exciting opportunities for impact.

Acknowledgments All authors of this chapter are members of the Global Intensive Care Working Group of the European Society of Intensive Care Medicine. The authors thank the Working Group and the Society for their support.

References

1. Kwizera A, Festic E, Dunser MW. What's new in sepsis recognition in resource-limited settings? Intensive Care Med. 2016;42(12):2030–3.
2. Musa N, Murthy S, Kissoon N. Pediatric sepsis and septic shock management in resource-limited settings. Intensive Care Med. 2016;42(12):2037–9.
3. Serpa Neto A, Schultz MJ, Festic E. Ventilatory support of patients with sepsis or septic shock in resource-limited settings. Intensive Care Med. 2016;42:100–3.
4. Thwaites CL, Lundeg G, Dondorp AM, sepsis in resource-limited settings-expert consensus recommendations group of the European Society of Intensive Care Medicine, the Mahidol-Oxford Research Unit in Bangkok, Thailand. Recommendations for infection management in patients with sepsis and septic shock in resource-limited settings. Intensive Care Med. 2016;42(12):2040–2.
5. Martin GS, Mannino DM, Eaton S, Moss M. The epidemiology of sepsis in the United States from 1979 through 2000. N Engl J Med. 2003;348:1546–54.
6. Vincent JL, Sakr Y, Sprung CL, Ranieri VM, Reinhart K, Gerlach H, Moreno R, Carlet J, Le Gall JR, Payen D, Sepsis Occurrence in Acutely Ill Patients Investigators. Sepsis in European intensive care units: results of the SOAP study. Crit Care Med. 2006;34:344–53.
7. Phua J, Koh Y, Du B, Tang YQ, Divatia JV, Tan CC, Gomersall CD, Faruq MO, Shrestha BR, Gia Binh N, Arabi YM, Salahuddin N, Wahyuprajitno B, Tu ML, Wahab AY, Hameed AA, Nishimura M, Procyshyn M, Chan YH, MOSAICS Study Group. Management of severe sepsis in patients admitted to Asian intensive care units: prospective cohort study. BMJ. 2011;342:d3245.
8. Murthy S, Leligdowicz A, Adhikari NK. Intensive care unit capacity in low-income countries: a systematic review. PLoS One. 2015;10:e0116949.
9. Cheng AC, West TE, Limmathurotsakul D, Peacock SJ. Strategies to reduce mortality from bacterial sepsis in adults in developing countries. PLoS Med. 2008;5:e175.

10. GBD 2013 Mortality and Causes of Death Collaborators. Global, regional, and national age-sex specific all-cause and cause-specific mortality for 240 causes of death, 1990–2013: a systematic analysis for the Global Burden of Disease Study 2013. Lancet. 2015;385:117–71.
11. Global Burden of Disease Study 2013 Collaborators. Global, regional, and national incidence, prevalence, and years lived with disability for 301 acute and chronic diseases and injuries in 188 countries, 1990–2013: a systematic analysis for the Global Burden of Disease Study 2013. Lancet. 2015;386:743–800.
12. GBD 2015 Mortality and Causes of Death Collaborators. Global, regional, and national life expectancy, all-cause mortality, and cause-specific mortality for 249 causes of death, 1980–2015: a systematic analysis for the Global Burden of Disease Study 2015. Lancet. 2016;388:1459–544.
13. Rosenthal VD, Bijie H, Maki DG, Mehta Y, Apisarnthanarak A, Medeiros EA, Leblebicioglu H, Fisher D, Alvarez-Moreno C, Khader IA, Del Rocio Gonzalez Martinez M, Cuellar LE, Navoa-Ng JA, Abouqal R, Guanche Garcell H, Mitrev Z, Pirez Garcia MC, Hamdi A, Duenas L, Cancel E, Gurskis V, Rasslan O, Ahmed A, Kanj SS, Ugalde OC, Mapp T, Raka L, Yuet Meng C, le Thu TA, Ghazal S, Gikas A, Narvaez LP, Mejia N, Hadjieva N, Gamar Elanbya MO, Guzman Siritt ME, Jayatilleke K, INICC members. International Nosocomial Infection Control Consortium (INICC) report, data summary of 36 countries, for 2004–2009. Am J Infect Control. 2012;40:396–407.
14. Frikha N, Mebazaa M, Mnif L, El Euch N, Abassi M, Ben Ammar MS. Septic shock in a Tunisian intensive care unit: mortality and predictive factors. 100 cases. Tunis Med. 2005;83:320–5.
15. Jacob ST, Moore CC, Banura P, Pinkerton R, Meya D, Opendi P, Reynolds SJ, Kenya-Mugisha N, Mayanja-Kizza H, Scheld WM, Promoting Resource-Limited Interventions for Sepsis Management in Uganda Study Group. Severe sepsis in two Ugandan hospitals: a prospective observational study of management and outcomes in a predominantly HIV-1 infected population. PLoS One. 2009;4:e7782.
16. Siddiqui S. Not "surviving sepsis" in the developing countries. J Indian Med Assoc. 2007;105:221.
17. Dunser MW, Bataar O, Tsenddorj G, Lundeg G, Torgersen C, Romand JA, Hasibeder WR, Helfen Beruhrt Study Team. Differences in critical care practice between an industrialized and a developing country. Wien Klin Wochenschr. 2008;120:600–7.
18. Vernet G, Mary C, Altmann DM, Doumbo O, Morpeth S, Bhutta ZA, Klugman KP. Surveillance for antimicrobial drug resistance in under-resourced countries. Emerg Infect Dis. 2014;20:434–41.
19. Laxminarayan R, Matsoso P, Pant S, Brower C, Rottingen JA, Klugman K, Davies S. Access to effective antimicrobials: a worldwide challenge. Lancet. 2016;387:168–75.
20. Bone RC, Balk RA, Cerra FB, Dellinger RP, Fein AM, Knaus WA, Schein RM, Sibbald WJ. Definitions for sepsis and organ failure and guidelines for the use of innovative therapies in sepsis. The ACCP/SCCM Consensus Conference Committee. American College of Chest Physicians/Society of Critical Care Medicine. Chest. 1992;101:1644–55.
21. Levy MM, Fink MP, Marshall JC, Abraham E, Angus D, Cook D, Cohen J, Opal SM, Vincent JL, Ramsay G, International Sepsis Definitions Conference. 2001 SCCM/ESICM/ACCP/ATS/SIS International Sepsis Definitions Conference. Intensive Care Med. 2003;29:530–8.
22. Kissoon N, Daniels R, van der Poll T, Finfer S, Reinhart K. Sepsis-the final common pathway to death from multiple organ failure in infection. Crit Care Med. 2016;44:e446.
23. Auma MA, Siedner MJ, Nyehangane D, Nalusaji A, Nakaye M, Mwanga-Amumpaire J, Muhindo R, Wilson LA, Boum Y II, Moore CC. Malaria is an uncommon cause of adult sepsis in south-western Uganda. Malar J. 2013;12:146.
24. White NJ, Pukrittayakamee S, Hien TT, Faiz MA, Mokuolu OA, Dondorp AM. Malaria. Lancet. 2014;383:723–35.
25. White NJ, Turner GD, Day NP, Dondorp AM. Lethal malaria: Marchiafava and Bignami were right. J Infect Dis. 2013;208:192–8.

26. Chen Y, Maguire T, Hileman RE, Fromm JR, Esko JD, Linhardt RJ, Marks RM. Dengue virus infectivity depends on envelope protein binding to target cell heparan sulfate. Nat Med. 1997;3:866–71.
27. Avirutnan P, Zhang L, Punyadee N, Manuyakorn A, Puttikhunt C, Kasinrerk W, Malasit P, Atkinson JP, Diamond MS. Secreted NS1 of dengue virus attaches to the surface of cells via interactions with heparan sulfate and chondroitin sulfate E. PLoS Pathog. 2007;3:e183.
28. Adhikari NK, Fowler RA, Bhagwanjee S, Rubenfeld GD. Critical care and the global burden of critical illness in adults. Lancet. 2010;376:1339–46.
29. Haniffa R, De Silva AP, Iddagoda S, Batawalage H, De Silva ST, Mahipala PG, Dondorp A, de Keizer N, Jayasinghe S. A cross-sectional survey of critical care services in Sri Lanka: a lower middle-income country. J Crit Care. 2014;29:764–8.
30. Mendsaikhan N, Begzjav T, Lundeg G, Brunauer A, Dunser MW. A nationwide census of ICU capacity and admissions in Mongolia. PLoS One. 2016;11:e0160921.
31. Jochberger S, Ismailova F, Lederer W, Mayr VD, Luckner G, Wenzel V, Ulmer H, Hasibeder WR, Dunser MW; "Helfen Beruhrt" Study Team. Anesthesia and its allied disciplines in the developing world: a nationwide survey of the Republic of Zambia. Anesth Analg. 2008;106:942–948, table of contents
32. Kwizera A, Dunser M, Nakibuuka J. National intensive care unit bed capacity and ICU patient characteristics in a low income country. BMC Res Notes. 2012;5:475.
33. Campos-Mino S, Sasbon JS, von Dessauer B. Pediatric intensive care in Latin America. Med Intensiva. 2012;36:3–10.
34. Kissoon N. Sepsis care differences unlike beauty are not skin deep. Pediatr Crit Care Med. 2016;17:568–9.
35. Divatia JV, Amin PR, Ramakrishnan N, Kapadia FN, Todi S, Sahu S, Govil D, Chawla R, Kulkarni AP, Samavedam S, Jani CK, Rungta N, Samaddar DP, Mehta S, Venkataraman R, Hegde A, Bande BD, Dhanuka S, Singh V, Tewari R, Zirpe K, Sathe P, INDICAPS Study Investigators. Intensive care in India: the Indian intensive care case mix and practice patterns study. Indian J Crit Care Med. 2016;20:216–25.
36. Austin S, Murthy S, Wunsch H, Adhikari NK, Karir V, Rowan K, Jacob ST, Salluh J, Bozza FA, Du B, An Y, Lee B, Wu F, Nguyen YL, Oppong C, Venkataraman R, Velayutham V, Duenas C, Angus DC, International Forum of Acute Care Trialists. Access to urban acute care services in high- vs. middle-income countries: an analysis of seven cities. Intensive Care Med. 2014;40:342–52.
37. Marshall JC, Bosco L, Adhikari NK, Connolly B, Diaz JV, Dorman T, Fowler RA, Meyfroidt G, Nakagawa S, Pelosi P, Vincent JL, Vollman K, Zimmerman J. What is an intensive care unit? A report of the task force of the World Federation of Societies of Intensive and Critical Care Medicine. J Crit Care. 2017;37:270–6.
38. Rhodes A, Ferdinande P, Flaatten H, Guidet B, Metnitz PG, Moreno RP. The variability of critical care bed numbers in Europe. Intensive Care Med. 2012;38:1647–53.
39. Baelani I, Jochberger S, Laimer T, Otieno D, Kabutu J, Wilson I, Baker T, Dunser MW. Availability of critical care resources to treat patients with severe sepsis or septic shock in Africa: a self-reported, continent-wide survey of anaesthesia providers. Crit Care. 2011;15:R10.
40. Baker T, Lugazia E, Eriksen J, Mwafongo V, Irestedt L, Konrad D. Emergency and critical care services in Tanzania: a survey of ten hospitals. BMC Health Serv Res. 2013;13:140.
41. Bataar O, Lundeg G, Tsenddorj G, Jochberger S, Grander W, Baelani I, Wilson I, Baker T, Dunser MW, Helfen Beruhrt Study Team. Nationwide survey on resource availability for implementing current sepsis guidelines in Mongolia. Bull World Health Organ. 2010;88:839–46.
42. Hsia RY, Mbembati NA, Macfarlane S, Kruk ME. Access to emergency and surgical care in sub-Saharan Africa: the infrastructure gap. Health Policy Plan. 2012;27:234–44.
43. Arabi YM, Phua J, Koh Y, Du B, Faruq MO, Nishimura M, Fang WF, Gomersall C, Al Rahma HN, Tamim H, Al-Dorzi HM, Al-Hameed FM, Adhikari NK, Sadat M, Asian Critical Care Clinical Trials Group. Structure, organization, and delivery of critical care in Asian ICUs. Crit Care Med. 2016;44:e940–8.

44. Dondorp AM, Iyer SS, Schultz MJ. Critical care in resource-restricted settings. JAMA. 2016;315:753–4.
45. Mendsaikhan N, Begzjav T, Lundeg G, Dünser MW. Potentially preventable deaths by intensive care medicine in Mongolian hospitals. Crit Care Res Pract. 2016; https://doi.org/10.1155/2016/8624035.
46. Cubro H, Somun-Kapetanovic R, Thiery G, Talmor D, Gajic O. Cost effectiveness of intensive care in a low resource setting: a prospective cohort of medical critically ill patients. World J Crit Care Med. 2016;5:150–64.
47. Phua J, Joynt GM, Nishimura M, Deng Y, Myatra SN, Chan YH, Binh NG, Tan CC, Faruq MO, Arabi YM, Wahjuprajitno B, Liu SF, Hashemian SM, Kashif W, Staworn D, Palo JE, Koh Y, ACME Study Investigators; Asian Critical Care Clinical Trials Group. Withholding and withdrawal of life-sustaining treatments in low-middle-income versus high-income Asian countries and regions. Intensive Care Med. 2016;42:1118–27.
48. Kissoon N. Healthcare costs to poor families: an agonising burden. Indian J Pediatr. 2016;83:1063–4.
49. Dunser MW, Festic E, Dondorp A, Kissoon N, Ganbat T, Kwizera A, Haniffa R, Baker T, Schultz MJ, Global Intensive Care Working Group of European Society of Intensive Care Medicine. Recommendations for sepsis management in resource-limited settings. Intensive Care Med. 2012;38:557–74.
50. Dellinger RP, Levy MM, Rhodes A, Annane D, Gerlach H, Opal SM, Sevransky JE, Sprung CL, Douglas IS, Jaeschke R, Osborn TM, Nunnally ME, Townsend SR, Reinhart K, Kleinpell RM, Angus DC, Deutschman CS, Machado FR, Rubenfeld GD, Webb SA, Beale RJ, Vincent JL, Moreno R, Surviving Sepsis Campaign Guidelines Committee including the Pediatric Subgroup. Surviving sepsis campaign: international guidelines for management of severe sepsis and septic shock: 2012. Crit Care Med. 2013;41:580–637.
51. Halpern NA, Pastores SM, Greenstein RJ. Critical care medicine in the United States 1985–2000: an analysis of bed numbers, use, and costs. Crit Care Med. 2004;32:1254–9.
52. Pinsky MR. Understanding costs and cost-effectiveness in critical care: report from the second American Thoracic Society workshop on outcomes research. Am J Respir Crit Care Med. 2002;165:540–50.
53. Shann F. Role of intensive care in countries with a high child mortality rate. Pediatr Crit Care Med. 2011;12:114–5.
54. Approximating the GNI per capita used to differentiate between a lower-middle and upper-middle income country by the World Bank. https://datahelpdesk.worldbank.org/knowledgebase/articles/906519-worldbank-country-and-lending-groups. Accessed 14 Mar 2017.
55. Assuncao MS, Teich V, Shiramizo SC, Araujo DV, Carrera RM, Serpa Neto A, Silva E. The cost-effectiveness ratio of a managed protocol for severe sepsis. J Crit Care. 2014;29(692):e691–6.
56. Harrison M, Collins CD. Is procalcitonin-guided antimicrobial use cost-effective in adult patients with suspected bacterial infection and sepsis? Infect Control Hosp Epidemiol. 2015;36:265–72.
57. Huang DT, Clermont G, Dremsizov TT, Angus DC, Pro CI. Implementation of early goal-directed therapy for severe sepsis and septic shock: a decision analysis. Crit Care Med. 2007;35:2090–100.
58. Jones AE, Troyer JL, Kline JA. Cost-effectiveness of an emergency department-based early sepsis resuscitation protocol. Crit Care Med. 2011;39:1306–12.
59. Karlsson S, Ruokonen E, Varpula T, Ala-Kokko TI, Pettila V, Finnsepsis Study Group. Long-term outcome and quality-adjusted life years after severe sepsis. Crit Care Med. 2009;37:1268–74.
60. Lehmann LE, Herpichboehm B, Kost GJ, Kollef MH, Stuber F. Cost and mortality prediction using polymerase chain reaction pathogen detection in sepsis: evidence from three observational trials. Crit Care. 2010;14:R186.
61. Talmor D, Greenberg D, Howell MD, Lisbon A, Novack V, Shapiro N. The costs and cost-effectiveness of an integrated sepsis treatment protocol. Crit Care Med. 2008;36:1168–74.

62. Suarez D, Ferrer R, Artigas A, Azkarate I, Garnacho-Montero J, Goma G, Levy MM, Ruiz JC, Edusepsis Study Group. Cost-effectiveness of the Surviving Sepsis Campaign protocol for severe sepsis: a prospective nation-wide study in Spain. Intensive Care Med. 2011;37:444–52.
63. Negrini D, Sheppard L, Mills GH, Jacobs P, Rapoport J, Bourne RS, Guidet B, Csomos A, Prien T, Anderson G, Edbrooke DL. International Programme for Resource Use in Critical Care (IPOC)—a methodology and initial results of cost and provision in four European countries. Acta Anaesthesiol Scand. 2006;50:72–9.
64. Tan SS, Bakker J, Hoogendoorn ME, Kapila A, Martin J, Pezzi A, Pittoni G, Spronk PE, Welte R, Hakkaart-van Roijen L. Direct cost analysis of intensive care unit stay in four European countries: applying a standardized costing methodology. Value Health. 2012;15:81–6.
65. Dräger S, Dal Poz MR, Evans DB. Health workers wages: an overview from selected countries. Geneva: WHO; 2006.
66. Parikh CR, Karnad DR. Quality, cost, and outcome of intensive care in a public hospital in Bombay, India. Crit Care Med. 1999;27:1754–9.
67. Kulkarni AP, Divatia JV. A prospective audit of costs of intensive care in cancer patients in India. Indian J Crit Care Med. 2013;17:292–7.
68. Riviello ED, Kiviri W, Fowler RA, Mueller A, Novack V, Banner-Goodspeed VM, Weinkauf JL, Talmor DS, Twagirumugabe T. Predicting mortality in low-income country ICUs: the Rwanda Mortality Probability Model (R-MPM). PLoS One. 2016;11:e0155858.
69. Haniffa R, Lubell Y, Cooper BS, Mohanty S, Shamsul A, Karki A, Pattnaik R, Maswood A, Pangeni R, Schultz MJ, Dondorp AM. Impact of a structured ICU training programme in resource-limited settings in Asia. PLoS One. 2017; https://doi.org/10.1371/journal.pone.0173483.
70. Penno EC, Baird SJ, Crump JA. Cost-effectiveness of surveillance for bloodstream infections for sepsis management in low-resource settings. Am J Trop Med Hyg. 2015;93:850–60.
71. Thukral A, Lodha R, Irshad M, Arora NK. Performance of Pediatric Risk of Mortality (PRISM), Pediatric Index of Mortality (PIM), and PIM2 in a pediatric intensive care unit in a developing country. Pediatr Crit Care Med. 2006;7:356–61.
72. Hutchings A, Durand MA, Grieve R, Harrison D, Rowan K, Green J, Cairns J, Black N. Evaluation of modernisation of adult critical care services in England: time series and cost effectiveness analysis. BMJ. 2009;339:b4353.
73. Rahman M, Fukui T. Biomedical publication—global profile and trend. Public Health. 2003;117:274–80.
74. Bellani G, Laffey JG, Pham T, Fan E, Brochard L, Esteban A, Gattinoni L, van Haren F, Larsson A, McAuley DF, Ranieri M, Rubenfeld G, Thompson BT, Wrigge H, Slutsky AS, Pesenti A, LUNG SAFE Investigators; ESICM Trials Group. Epidemiology, patterns of care, and mortality for patients with acute respiratory distress syndrome in intensive care units in 50 countries. JAMA. 2016;315:788–800.
75. Fleischmann C, Scherag A, Adhikari NK, Hartog CS, Tsaganos T, Schlattmann P, Angus DC, Reinhart K, International Forum of Acute Care Tialists. Assessment of global incidence and mortality of hospital-treated sepsis. Current estimates and limitations. Am J Respir Crit Care Med. 2016;193:259–72.
76. Vincent JL, Marshall JC, Namendys-Silva SA, Francois B, Martin-Loeches I, Lipman J, Reinhart K, Antonelli M, Pickkers P, Njimi H, Jimenez E, Sakr Y, ICON investigators. Assessment of the worldwide burden of critical illness: the intensive care over nations (ICON) audit. Lancet Respir Med. 2014;2:380–6.
77. Kang KT, Chandler HK, Espinosa V, Kissoon N. Systems for paediatric sepsis: a global survey. West Indian Med J. 2014;63:703–10.
78. ISARIC. International Severe Acute Respiratory and Emerging Infection Consortium. 2016. https://isaric.tghn.org/about/
79. Ashley EA, Dhorda M, Fairhurst RM, Amaratunga C, Lim P, Suon S, Sreng S, Anderson JM, Mao S, Sam B, Sopha C, Chuor CM, Nguon C, Sovannaroth S, Pukrittayakamee S, Jittamala P, Chotivanich K, Chutasmit K, Suchatsoonthorn C, Runcharoen R, Hien TT, Thuy-Nhien NT, Thanh NV, Phu NH, Htut Y, Han KT, Aye KH, Mokuolu OA, Olaosebikan RR, Folaranmi OO,

Mayxay M, Khanthavong M, Hongvanthong B, Newton PN, Onyamboko MA, Fanello CI, Tshefu AK, Mishra N, Valecha N, Phyo AP, Nosten F, Yi P, Tripura R, Borrmann S, Bashraheil M, Peshu J, Faiz MA, Ghose A, Hossain MA, Samad R, Rahman MR, Hasan MM, Islam A, Miotto O, Amato R, MacInnis B, Stalker J, Kwiatkowski DP, Bozdech Z, Jeeyapant A, Cheah PY, Sakulthaew T, Chalk J, Intharabut B, Silamut K, Lee SJ, Vihokhern B, Kunasol C, Imwong M, Tarning J, Taylor WJ, Yeung S, Woodrow CJ, Flegg JA, Das D, Smith J, Venkatesan M, Plowe CV, Stepniewska K, Guerin PJ, Dondorp AM, Day NP, White NJ, Tracking Resistance to Artemisinin Collaboration. Spread of artemisinin resistance in Plasmodium falciparum malaria. N Engl J Med. 2014;371:411–23.

80. Chantratita N, Tandhavanant S, Myers ND, Seal S, Arayawichanont A, Kliangsa-Ad A, Hittle LE, Ernst RK, Emond MJ, Wurfel MM, Day NP, Peacock SJ, West TE. Survey of innate immune responses to Burkholderia pseudomallei in human blood identifies a central role for lipopolysaccharide. PLoS One. 2013;8:e81617.
81. Desjardins CA, Cohen KA, Munsamy V, Abeel T, Maharaj K, Walker BJ, Shea TP, Almeida DV, Manson AL, Salazar A, Padayatchi N, O'Donnell MR, Mlisana KP, Wortman J, Birren BW, Grosset J, Earl AM, Pym AS. Genomic and functional analyses of Mycobacterium tuberculosis strains implicate ald in D-cycloserine resistance. Nat Genet. 2016;48:544–51.
82. Kim JY, Farmer P, Porter ME. Redefining global health-care delivery. Lancet. 2013;382:1060–9.
83. Scott KW, Jha AK. Putting quality on the global health agenda. N Engl J Med. 2014;371:3–5.
84. Binagwaho A, Kyamanywa P, Farmer PE, Nuthulaganti T, Umubyeyi B, Nyemazi JP, Mugeni SD, Asiimwe A, Ndagijimana U, Lamphere McPherson H, Ngirabega Jde D, Sliney A, Uwayezu A, Rusanganwa V, Wagner CM, Nutt CT, Eldon-Edington M, Cancedda C, Magaziner IC, Goosby E. The human resources for health program in Rwanda—new partnership. N Engl J Med. 2013;369:2054–9.
85. Vukoja M, Kashyap R, Gavrilovic S, Dong Y, Kilickaya O, Gajic O. Checklist for early recognition and treatment of acute illness: international collaboration to improve critical care practice. World J Crit Care Med. 2015;4:55–61.
86. Baker T, Schell CO, Lugazia E, Blixt J, Mulungu M, Castegren M, Eriksen J, Konrad D. Vital signs directed therapy: improving care in an intensive care unit in a low-income country. PLoS One. 2015;10:e0144801.
87. Riviello ED, Kiviri W, Twagirumugabe T, Mueller A, Banner-Goodspeed VM, Officer L, Novack V, Mutumwinka M, Talmor DS, Fowler RA. Hospital incidence and outcomes of the acute respiratory distress syndrome using the Kigali modification of the Berlin definition. Am J Respir Crit Care Med. 2016;193:52–9.
88. Chu KM, Jayaraman S, Kyamanywa P, Ntakiyiruta G. Building research capacity in Africa: equity and global health collaborations. PLoS Med. 2014;11:e1001612.
89. Singer M, Deutschman CS, Seymour CW, Shankar-Hari M, Annane D, Bauer M, Bellomo R, Bernard GR, Chiche JD, Coopersmith CM, Hotchkiss RS, Levy MM, Marshall JC, Martin GS, Opal SM, Rubenfeld GD, van der Poll T, Vincent JL, Angus DC. The third international consensus definitions for sepsis and septic shock (Sepsis-3). JAMA. 2016;315:801–10.
90. Arabi YM, Schultz MJ, Salluh JI. Intensive care medicine in 2050: global perspectives. Intensive Care Med. 2016;43(11):1695–9.
91. Maitland K, Kiguli S, Opoka RO, Engoru C, Olupot-Olupot P, Akech SO, Nyeko R, Mtove G, Reyburn H, Lang T, Brent B, Evans JA, Tibenderana JK, Crawley J, Russell EC, Levin M, Babiker AG, Gibb DM, FEAST Trial Group. Mortality after fluid bolus in African children with severe infection. N Engl J Med. 2011;364:2483–95.
92. Riviello ED, Letchford S, Cook EF, Waxman AB, Gaziano T. Improving decision making for massive transfusions in a resource poor setting: a preliminary study in Kenya. PLoS One. 2015;10:e0127987.
93. Leligdowicz A, Fischer WA II, Uyeki TM, Fletcher TE, Adhikari NK, Portella G, Lamontagne F, Clement C, Jacob ST, Rubinson L, Vanderschuren A, Hajek J, Murthy S, Ferri M, Crozier I, Ibrahima E, Lamah MC, Schieffelin JS, Brett-Major D, Bausch DG, Shindo N, Chan AK,

O'Dempsey T, Mishra S, Jacobs M, Dickson S, Lyon GM III, Fowler RA. Ebola virus disease and critical illness. Crit Care. 2016;20:217.

94. Buist AS, Parry V. The American Thoracic Society methods in epidemiologic, clinical, and operations research program. A research capacity-building program in low- and middle-income countries. Ann Am Thorac Soc. 2013;10:281–9.
95. Howitt P, Darzi A, Yang GZ, Ashrafian H, Atun R, Barlow J, Blakemore A, Bull AM, Car J, Conteh L, Cooke GS, Ford N, Gregson SA, Kerr K, King D, Kulendran M, Malkin RA, Majeed A, Matlin S, Merrifield R, Penfold HA, Reid SD, Smith PC, Stevens MM, Templeton MR, Vincent C, Wilson E. Technologies for global health. Lancet. 2012;380:507–35.

Open Access This chapter is licensed under the terms of the Creative Commons Attribution 4.0 International License (http://creativecommons.org/licenses/by/4.0/), which permits use, sharing, adaptation, distribution and reproduction in any medium or format, as long as you give appropriate credit to the original author(s) and the source, provide a link to the Creative Commons license and indicate if changes were made.

The images or other third party material in this chapter are included in the chapter's Creative Commons license, unless indicated otherwise in a credit line to the material. If material is not included in the chapter's Creative Commons license and your intended use is not permitted by statutory regulation or exceeds the permitted use, you will need to obtain permission directly from the copyright holder.

2 Development of the Guidelines: Focus on Availability, Feasibility, Affordability, and Safety of Interventions in Resource-Limited Settings

Marcus J. Schultz, Martin W. Dünser, and Arjen M. Dondorp

2.1 Introduction

In 2014, the "Global Intensive Care Working Group" of the "European Society of Intensive Care Medicine" (ESICM) and the "Mahidol Oxford Tropical Medicine Research Unit" (MORU) in Bangkok, Thailand, decided to refine and rewrite the guidelines for sepsis treatment in resource-limited settings as published in 2012 [1]. This chapter describes the development of eight sets of recommendations for care of septic patients in resource-limited settings as published in *Intensive Care Medicine* [2–8] and the *Transactions of Royal Society of Tropical Medicine and Hygiene* [9] in 2016 and 2017.

M. J. Schultz (✉)
Department of Intensive Care, Academic Medical Center, University of Amsterdam, Amsterdam, The Netherlands

Laboratory of Experimental Intensive Care and Anesthesiology (L.E.I.C.A), Academic Medical Center, University of Amsterdam, Amsterdam, The Netherlands

Mahidol–Oxford Research Unit (MORU), Faculty of Tropical Medicine, Mahidol University, Bangkok, Thailand

M. W. Dünser
Department of Anesthesiology and Intensive Care Medicine, Kepler University Hospital, Johannes Kepler University Linz, Linz, Austria

A. M. Dondorp
Mahidol–Oxford Research Unit (MORU), Faculty of Tropical Medicine, Mahidol University, Bangkok, Thailand

© The Author(s) 2019

A. M. Dondorp et al. (eds.), *Sepsis Management in Resource-limited Settings*,
https://doi.org/10.1007/978-3-030-03143-5_2

2.2 Heads and Subheads

The chairmen of the newly formed "Sepsis in Resource-Limited Settings" guidelines group, Marcus J. Schultz, Martin W. Dünser, and Arjen M. Dondorp, contacted potential subgroup chairs (Table 2.1) for the development of eight sets of recommendations focusing on (1) intensive care unit (ICU) organization and structure, (2) sepsis recognition, (3) infection management, (4) tropical sepsis, (5) hemodynamic monitoring and support, (6) ventilatory support, (7) general supportive care, and (8) pediatric sepsis. The selection of subgroup chairs was based on interest in specific aspects of sepsis and hands-on experience in ICUs in resource-limited settings. In total, three subgroup chairs per set of recommendations were contacted. Marcus J. Schultz, Martin W. Dünser, and Arjen M. Dondorp set out a protocol for the appraisal of various aspects within each set of recommendations and discussed this with the subgroup chairs.

2.3 Other Subgroup Members

The chairs of each subgroup recruited additional members for each set of recommendations (Table 2.1). Alike selection of subgroup chairs, recruitment of group members was based on interest in specific aspects of sepsis and hands-on experience in ICUs in resource-limited settings. Additional group members were appointed by the group heads to address content needs for the development process. Several group members had experience in "Grading of Recommendations, Assessment, Development and Evaluation" (GRADE) process and the use of the GRADEpro Guideline Development Tool [10].

2.4 Meetings

Initial Internet subgroup chair meetings established the procedures for literature review and drafting of tables for evidence analysis. Subgroup chairs continued work remotely via the Internet. Several meetings occurred at major international meetings, teleconferences, and electronic-based discussions among subgroup chairs and members from other subgroups.

In the first meetings, up to 10 clearly defined questions regarding specific aspects of care for sepsis patients were formulated, using the GRADEpro Guideline Development Tool [10]. These were reviewed for content and clarity by all subgroup members. After the approval by the subgroup members, the subgroup chairs split up, each one to seek for evidence for recommendations regarding three or four of the specific questions posed, seeking help from the subgroup members in identifying relevant publications where necessary. During this process, questions could be combined or adjusted—in some cases extra questions were added. The subgroup chairs summarized the evidence and formulated the recommendations after

Table 2.1 Group chairs, subgroup chairs, and subgroup members

Group chairs							
Marcus J. Schultz, Martin W. Dünser, and Arjen M. Dondorp							
Group 1 ICU organization and structure	*Group 2* Sepsis recognition	*Group 3* Infection management	*Group 4* Tropical sepsis	*Group 5* Hemodynamic monitoring and support	*Group 6* Ventilatory support	*Group 7* General supportive care	*Group 8* Pediatric sepsis
Subgroup chairs							
Alfred Papali	Arthur Kwizera	Ganbold Lundeg	Mai Nguyen Thi Hoang	David Misango	Ary Serpa Neto	Mervyn Mer	Srinivas Murthy
Marcus J. Schultz	Emir Festic	Louise Thwaites	Arjen M. Dondorp	Timothy Baker	Marcus J. Schultz	Marcus J. Schultz	Ndidiamaka Musa
Martin W. Dünser	Martin W. Dünser	Arjen M. Dondorp	Mervyn Mer	Rajyabardhan Pattnaik	Emir Festic	Neill Adhikari	Niranjan Kissoon
Other members							
Neill Adhikari	Rashan Haniffa	Arthur Kwizera	Sanjib Mohanty	Martin W. Dünser	Neill Adhikari	Arthur Kwizera	Rakesh Lodha
Janet Diaz	Neill Adhikari	Mervyn Mer	Marcus J. Schultz	Marcus J. Schultz	Arjen M. Dondorp	David Misango	Suchitra Ranjit
Arjen M. Dondorp	Ganbold Lundeg	Neill Adhikari	Louise Thwaites	Arjen M. Dondorp	Rajyabardhan Pattnaik	Sanjib Mohanty	
Shevin Jacob	Arjen M. Dondorp	Marcus J. Schultz	Martin W. Dünser		Louise Thwaites	Arjen M. Dondorp	
Jason Phua	Derek Angus	Randeep Jawa	Jane Nakibuuka		Pedro Povoa	Ary Serpa Neto	
Marc Romain	Ignacio Martin Loeches	Jane Nakibuuka			Ignacio Martin Loeches	Kobus Preller	
	Niranjan Kissoon	Srinivas Murthy			Luigi Pisani		
		Binh Nguyen Thien					

interactive telephone conferences. These were communicated among subgroup members. After their approval, the subgroup chairs summarized the evidence in a report, which was then sent for approval to all members of all eight subgroups.

2.5 Search Process

The search for literature followed the same methods as described for the development of the Surviving Sepsis Campaign guidelines [11]. In case a question was identical to one in those guidelines, the subgroup chairs searched for additional articles, specifically (new) investigations or meta-analyses related to the questions, in a minimum of one general database (i.e., MEDLINE, EMBASE) and the Cochrane Libraries. Furthermore, subgroup members paid specific attention to identify publication originating in low- and middle-income countries.

2.6 Grading of Recommendations

The subgroup chairs followed the principles of the GRADE process as described for the development of the Surviving Sepsis Campaign guidelines [11]. In short, GRADE classifies the quality of evidence as high (grade A), moderate (grade B), low (grade C), or very low (grade D) and recommendations as strong (grade 1) or weak (grade 2). The factors influencing this classification are presented in Table 2.2.

Different from the grading of recommendations in the Surviving Sepsis Campaign guidelines [11], the subgroup chairs paid extensive attention to several other factors as used before, but now focusing on resource-limited settings, i.e., availability and feasibility in resource-limited ICUs, affordability for low-resource ICUs, and last but not the least its safety in resource-limited ICUs (Table 2.3).

A strong recommendation was worded as "we recommend" and a weak recommendation as "we suggest." Some recommendations remained as ungraded best practice statements, when in the opinion of the subgroup members, such

Table 2.2 Quality of evidence

A	Randomized controlled trials	High
B	Downgraded randomized controlled trial(s) or upgraded observational studies	Moderate
C	Observational studies	Low
D	Downgraded observational studies or expert opinion	Very low

Factors that may decrease the strength of evidence: poor quality of planning and implementation of available RCTs, suggesting high likelihood of bias; inconsistency of results, including problems with subgroup analyses; indirectness of evidence (differing population, intervention, control, outcomes, comparison); imprecision of results; and high likelihood of reporting bias
Factors that may increase the strength of evidence: large magnitude of effect (direct evidence, relative risk >2 with no plausible confounders); very large magnitude of effect with relative risk >5 and no threats to validity (by two levels); and dose-response gradient

Table 2.3 Strong versus weak recommendations[a]

What should be considered	Recommended process
High or moderate evidence	The higher the quality of evidence, the more likely a strong recommendation
Certainty about the balance of benefits vs. harms and burdens	The larger/smaller the difference between the desirable and undesirable consequences and the certainty around that difference, the more likely a strong/weak recommendation
Certainty in or similar values	The more certainty or similarity in values and preferences, the more likely a strong recommendation
Resource implications	The lower/higher the cost of an intervention compared to the alternative, the more likely a strong/weak recommendation
Availability and feasibility in LMICs	The less available, the more likely a weak recommendation
Affordability for LMICs	The less affordable, the more likely a weak recommendation
Safety of the intervention in LMICs	The less safe in an LMIC, the more likely a weak recommendation

[a]In case of a strong recommendation, we use "we recommend ..."; in case of a weak recommendation, we use "we suggest ..."

recommendations were clear, clinically relevant, likely to result in benefit, supported by indirect evidence, and unsuitable for a formal evidence generation and review process (opportunity cost) [12].

2.7 Reporting

Each report was edited for style and form, with final approval by subgroup heads and then by the entire "Sepsis in Resource-Limited Settings" guidelines group.

Acknowledgments All authors of this chapter are members of the "European Society of Intensive Care Medicine (ESICM) Global Intensive Care" Working Group and the Mahidol–Oxford Research Unit (MORU) in Bangkok, Thailand.

Conflicts of interest Group chairs, subgroup chairs, and subgroup members did not represent industry, and there was no industry input into the development of the recommendations. Group chairs, subgroup chairs, and subgroup members did not receive honoraria for any role in the guideline development process. Group chairs, subgroup chairs, and subgroup members provided a standard conflict of interest form, to be uploaded through the GRADEpro Guideline Development Tool website—none reported conflicts of interest.

References

1. Dunser MW, Festic E, Dondorp A, Kissoon N, Ganbat T, Kwizera A, Haniffa R, Baker T, Schultz MJ, Global Intensive Care Working Group of European Society of Intensive Care M. Recommendations for sepsis management in resource-limited settings. Intensive Care Med. 2012;38:557–74.
2. Papali A, Schultz MJ, Dunser MW, European Society of Intensive Care Medicine Global Intensive Care working g, The Mahidol-Oxford Research Unit in Bangkok T. Recommendations

on infrastructure and organization of adult ICUs in resource-limited settings. Intensive Care Med. 2017;44(7):1133–7.

3. Mer M, Schultz MJ, Adhikari NK, European Society of Intensive Care Medicine Global Intensive Care Working G, the Mahidol-Oxford Research Unit BT. Core elements of general supportive care for patients with sepsis and septic shock in resource-limited settings. Intensive Care Med. 2017;43:1690–4.
4. Dondorp AM, Hoang MNT, Mer M, Sepsis in Resource-Limited Settings-Expert Consensus Recommendations Group of the European Society of Intensive Care M, the Mahidol-Oxford Research Unit in Bangkok T. Recommendations for the management of severe malaria and severe dengue in resource-limited settings. Intensive Care Med. 2017;43:1683–5.
5. Thwaites CL, Lundeg G, Dondorp AM, sepsis in resource-limited settings-expert consensus recommendations group of the European Society of Intensive Care M, the Mahidol-Oxford Research Unit in Bangkok T. Recommendations for infection management in patients with sepsis and septic shock in resource-limited settings. Intensive Care Med. 2016;42:2040–2.
6. Serpa Neto A, Schultz MJ, Festic E. Ventilatory support of patients with sepsis or septic shock in resource-limited settings. Intensive Care Med. 2016;42:100–3.
7. Musa N, Murthy S, Kissoon N. Pediatric sepsis and septic shock management in resource-limited settings. Intensive Care Med. 2016;42:2037–9.
8. Kwizera A, Festic E, Dunser MW. What's new in sepsis recognition in resource-limited settings? Intensive Care Med. 2016;42:2030–3.
9. Misango D, Pattnaik R, Baker T, Dunser MW, Dondorp AM, Schultz MJ, Global Intensive Care Working G, of the European Society of Intensive Care M, the Mahidol Oxford Tropical Medicine Research Unit in Bangkok T. Haemodynamic assessment and support in sepsis and septic shock in resource-limited settings. Trans R Soc Trop Med Hyg. 2017;111:483–9.
10. GRADE handbook for grading quality of evidence and strength of recommendations. 2013. https://gdt.gradepro.org/app/handbook/handbook.html. Accessed Oct 2013.
11. Dellinger RP, Levy MM, Rhodes A, Annane D, Gerlach H, Opal SM, Sevransky JE, Sprung CL, Douglas IS, Jaeschke R, Osborn TM, Nunnally ME, Townsend SR, Reinhart K, Kleinpell RM, Angus DC, Deutschman CS, Machado FR, Rubenfeld GD, Webb SA, Beale RJ, Vincent JL, Moreno R, Surviving Sepsis Campaign Guidelines Committee including the Pediatric S. Surviving sepsis campaign: international guidelines for management of severe sepsis and septic shock: 2012. Crit Care Med. 2013;41:580–637.
12. Guyatt GH, Alonso-Coello P, Schunemann HJ, Djulbegovic B, Nothacker M, Lange S, Murad MH, Akl EA. Guideline panels should seldom make good practice statements: guidance from the GRADE Working Group. J Clin Epidemiol. 2016;80:3–7.

Open Access This chapter is licensed under the terms of the Creative Commons Attribution 4.0 International License (http://creativecommons.org/licenses/by/4.0/), which permits use, sharing, adaptation, distribution and reproduction in any medium or format, as long as you give appropriate credit to the original author(s) and the source, provide a link to the Creative Commons license and indicate if changes were made.

The images or other third party material in this chapter are included in the chapter's Creative Commons license, unless indicated otherwise in a credit line to the material. If material is not included in the chapter's Creative Commons license and your intended use is not permitted by statutory regulation or exceeds the permitted use, you will need to obtain permission directly from the copyright holder.

Infrastructure and Organization of Adult Intensive Care Units in Resource-Limited Settings

3

Alfred Papali, Neill K. J. Adhikari, Janet V. Diaz, Arjen M. Dondorp, Martin W. Dünser, Shevin T. Jacob, Jason Phua, Marc Romain, and Marcus J. Schultz

3.1 Introduction

Published guidelines regarding optimal infrastructure and organization of intensive care units (ICUs) are based on evidence primarily from resource-rich settings [1]. These guidelines may be less applicable to resource-limited settings [2]. ICUs

A. Papali
Division of Pulmonary and Critical Care Medicine, Atrium Health, Charlotte, NC, USA

Division of Pulmonary and Critical Care, Institute of Global Health, University of Maryland School of Medicine, Baltimore, MD, USA

N. K. J. Adhikari
Sunnybrook Health Sciences Centre, University of Toronto, Toronto, ON, Canada

J. V. Diaz
Pacific Medical Center, San Francisco, CA, USA

World Health Organization, Geneva, Switzerland

A. M. Dondorp
Faculty of Tropical Medicine, Mahidol University, Bangkok, Thailand

Academic Medical Center, University of Amsterdam, Amsterdam, The Netherlands

Nuffield Department of Clinical Medicine, Oxford Centre for Tropical Medicine and Global Health, University of Oxford, Oxford, UK

M. W. Dünser (✉)
Department of Anesthesia and Intensive Care Medicine, Kepler University Hospital, Johannes Kepler University Linz, Linz, Austria

S. T. Jacob
World Health Organization, Geneva, Switzerland

University of Washington School of Medicine, Seattle, WA, USA

Liverpool School of Tropical Medicine, Liverpool, UK

© The Author(s) 2019

A. M. Dondorp et al. (eds.), *Sepsis Management in Resource-limited Settings*,
https://doi.org/10.1007/978-3-030-03143-5_3

J. Phua
National University Hospital, Singapore, Singapore

M. Romain
Hadassah–Hebrew University Medical Center, Jerusalem, Israel

M. J. Schultz
Faculty of Tropical Medicine, Mahidol University, Bangkok, Thailand

Department of Intensive Care, Academic Medical Center, Amsterdam, The Netherlands

Laboratory of Experimental Intensive Care and Anesthesiology (L·E·I·C·A), Academic Medical Center, Amsterdam, The Netherlands

around the world differ in available resources, and our working group [2] and others [1] have different definitions what an ICU entails. In this chapter, we aim to answer seven questions basic prerequisites for quality intensive care in resource-limited settings: (1) Which healthcare professionals should provide care in ICUs in resource-limited settings? (2) How should these healthcare professionals be trained? (3) How should electricity be supplied to ICUs in resource-limited settings? (4) How should oxygen be supplied to ICUs in resource-limited settings? (5) Which hygienic facilities are fundamental in ICUs in resource-limited settings? (6) Which technical equipment should be available in ICUs in resource-limited settings? (7) Which quality measures to improve care should be implemented in ICUs in resource-limited settings? We provide a series of simple, pragmatic recommendations for optimizing ICU infrastructure and organization in resource-limited settings, with a focus on adult ICUs (Table 3.1). Understanding the great variability of technical, material, and human resources within and between these environments, each institution must determine the utility of implementing these recommendations based on local capabilities.

3.2 Staffing

In resource rich settings, intensive care medicine has evolved into a multidisciplinary and team-based approach. Involvement of ICU physicians and other healthcare professionals results in better outcomes and reduces costs of care [3, 4]. Postgraduate training in the specialty of intensive care medicine is becoming more commonplace for ICU physicians, ICU nurses, and even allied healthcare professionals in most high-income countries [5, 6]; training in intensive care medicine is commonly available for physicians from different medical specialties. Most training programs last at least 1 year and end with a national or international examination [6]. Accreditation and certification in different sub-specialties (e.g., neuro-intensive care) or examination techniques (e.g., echocardiography, lung ultrasound) can be achieved in some countries [6].

Studies in resource-rich settings show that the physician–staffing model in use affects outcomes of critically ill patients [7–9]. In comparison to a so-called open ICU model, in which physicians from outside the ICU remain directly responsible

Table 3.1 Recommendations for ICU infrastructure and organization in resource-limited settings (with grading)

1	Staffing	We *suggest* that, if possible, ICUs use a closed-format model where physicians specifically trained or experienced in intensive care medicine direct patient care (2B). We further *suggest* that ICUs be staffed with nurses who are trained in intensive care nursing (2C). Wherever available, allied healthcare professionals (e.g., pharmacists) should be part of an ICU team (UG). Currently, no recommendation on ICU telemedicine in resource-limited settings can be made
2	Training	We suggest that all healthcare professionals working in ICUs be specifically trained in the care of the critically ill patient (2C). Unless national or regional specialty training programs in intensive care medicine are available, we suggest that training of ICU physicians, nurses, and allied healthcare professionals occurs through longitudinal, multimodal programs coordinated by partnerships between Ministries of Health, national and international professional societies, nongovernmental organizations, as well as institutions with well-established programs in ICU training (2D). We recommend that such ICU training programs adhere to validated, international standards of intensive care medicine, but that they be adapted to local needs and resources (1C)
3	Electricity	A stable electricity supply is an essential infrastructural component of an ICU (UG). We recommend that ICUs use voltage stabilizers in case voltage fluctuations endanger the function of electrical medical equipment (1D). We recommend that adequate backup electrical sources be available to bridge power cuts (1C). We suggest that these backup electrical sources take over electricity supply automatically allowing for (near) continuous functioning of life-sustaining medical equipment (2D). We recommend that ICUs with no adequate backup electrical source have protocols in place guiding ICU staff how to bridge life-sustaining therapies during power cuts (1D)
4	Oxygen	Oxygen therapy is an essential provision for critically ill patients, and an adequate oxygen supply is a crucial infrastructural component of an ICU (UG). We recommend that ICUs choose the type of oxygen supply (concentrators, cylinders, centralized system) based on site-specific conditions and requirements (1B). We suggest that, if feasible, oxygen be supplied by centralized, piped systems to ICUs when mechanical ventilators are used (2D)
5	Hygiene	We recommend that ICUs have available an adequate number of and easily accessible facilities for handwashing/hand hygiene (1A). We recommend hand hygiene after each patient contact with an alcohol-based solution (1A). Exception are hand hygiene in the context of Ebola virus disease requiring chlorine-based solutions (1C) and *Clostridium difficile* requiring water and soap. In case alcohol-based solutions are unavailable, we recommend using soap and water for handwashing (1A). Alcohol hand rub solutions may be produced locally and carried in small bottles by each healthcare worker (UG). We recommend that non-sterile, clean examination gloves for self-protection of medical staff be available (1C). Importantly, gloved hands can equally transmit infectious pathogens; use of gloves does not replace the need for subsequent hand hygiene (UG). We recommend the availability of masks, caps, sterile gowns, sterile drapes, and sterile gloves for invasive procedures, such as insertion of central venous catheters (1A). We recommend that ICUs and hospitals in areas where highly contagious infectious diseases (e.g., tuberculosis, Ebola virus disease) are endemic have rapid access to adequate quantities of personal protective equipment as recommended by the World Health Organization and the Centers for Disease Control and Prevention (1C). We suggest that hospitals develop individual policies and procedures for reuse of disposable personal protective and other medical equipment (2C). When ICUs are renovated or newly built, we suggest compliance with national and international best-practice recommendations on ICU architectural design (2D)

(continued)

Table 3.1 (continued)

6	Equipment	Acquisition of technical equipment should be guided by local availability and feasibility of routine maintenance (UG). We recommend basic vital signs monitors (including electrocardiogram, respiratory rate, oscillometric blood pressure, and pulse oximetry) available for each ICU bed (1C). We recommend that ICUs have one or more mechanical ventilators available (1C). These mechanical ventilators should also deliver noninvasive ventilatory modes, measure tidal volume and airway pressures, and support oxygen delivery (1B). We suggest that ICUs providing invasive ventilatory support have the ability to measure end-tidal carbon dioxide (2C) and to perform blood gas analysis (2C). We recommend that ICUs have point-of-care capabilities for measuring blood glucose (e.g., glucometers) (1B). We recommend that ICUs have capabilities for measuring blood lactate levels (1B). We suggest that ICUs have available point-of-care ultrasound devices (2C) and that key clinical staff undergo formal ultrasound training (2C)
7	Quality	We recommend maintaining patient records and ICU documentation in accordance with national regulations and requirements (1D). We suggest that ICUs develop locally applicable bundles, protocols, and checklists to improve quality of care (2C). We suggest that ICUs systematically collect quality and performance indicators and participate in national/international benchmarking projects (2C)

Abbreviations: *ICU* intensive care unit, *UG* ungraded

for the care of their patients, a so-called closed ICU model, in which one or more physicians, usually trained in intensive care medicine, and exclusively based within the ICU, become responsible for the critically ill patients, results in lower mortality rates, shorter length of stay, and reduced costs of care [7].

Studies in resource-rich settings also show that the nurse–staffing model affects outcomes of critically ill patients [10]. More nurses available per ICU bed improves survival rates, particularly for patients at a high risk of dying [11], reduces postoperative [12] and infectious complications like ventilator-associated pneumonia [13], and prevents medication errors [14]. A higher nurse-to-patient ratio is also independently associated with a better compliance with, for example, sepsis care bundles [15]. Notably, a higher nurse-to-patient ratio prevents burnout of nurses [16]. Studies in resource-rich settings also suggest that the presence of allied healthcare professionals like pharmacists [17], respiratory or physical therapists [18], and dieticians [19] within a multidisciplinary ICU team improves patient outcomes [3]. Furthermore, proactive communications with infectious disease specialists or microbiologists favorably affect antibiotic use and costs [20].

Finally, so-called telemedicine in ICUs in resource-rich settings, mainly to solve the problem of physician shortages during nighttime hours and in some ICUs with low-intensity staffing [21], has been shown to improve early identification of patients who deteriorate [22] and increases the number of interventions [23], but the effect on ICU outcomes remains controversial [24] and costs of required technological infrastructure are high [25].

There is minimal evidence from resource-limited settings that ICU outcomes improve after changing from an “open ICU model” to a “closed ICU model.” One before–after study from Thailand showed a 4% absolute mortality reduction (from 27.4 to 23.4%, $p = 0.03$) and shortening of length of stay of 0.8 days (−1.3 to −0.25, $p < 0.01$) in a surgical ICU [26]. The reduction in mortality was greatest in patients with a length of stay >48 h (22.7 vs. 13.9%, $p < 0.01$). A prospective before–after study in a large university hospital in Turkey demonstrated a 4.5-fold reduction of in-hospital mortality after introduction of the "closed ICU model" [27]. The survival effects were most prominent in patients requiring mechanical ventilation. Postgraduate training programs in intensive care medicine for physicians have been established in selected resource-limited settings such as India [28], Ethiopia [29], Brazil [30], China [31], and South Africa [32], but the literature fails to report on outcome changes after its establishment.

No studies have been published from resource-limited settings evaluating patient outcomes related to nurse-to-patient ratios. Evidence from resource-limited settings confirms the benefits of including pharmacists into the multidisciplinary ICU team on patient outcomes [17]. Studies from China, Thailand, Jordan, Egypt, and Vietnam demonstrated consistent reductions in medication costs [33–35] and adverse events [36] after involvement of a pharmacist in daily ICU practice. No studies on the effects of including physicians from other backgrounds (e.g., infectious disease specialists) or allied healthcare professionals (e.g., psychologists, case managers, social workers, respiratory therapists, dieticians, or physical therapists) into ICU teams in resource-limited settings were identified by our search.

Data on implementation of telemedicine in resource-limited ICUs is minimal despite reports of successful implementation in areas with a scarcity of specialists [37]. Only one study, performed in India in patients with acute myocardial infarction, showed a reduction in mortality following implementation of telemedicine [38].

Despite the trends indicating that a "closed ICU model" improves patient outcomes in resource-limited ICUs, human resources are inconsistently available in most of these settings. The number of physicians per 1000 inhabitants is substantially lower in low- and middle- than high-income countries [39]. This leaves many hospitals in resource-limited areas with a critical shortage of physicians, particularly during off-hours, weekends, and holidays. From the authors' experience, in some hospitals, a physician is completely absent during nighttime. Patient care is then, for example, overseen by mid-level providers, such as clinical officers.

No systematic data on the availability of physicians specialized in intensive care medicine have been published for resource-limited settings. There also are no studies detailing the relevance of ICU training methods typically found in resource-rich settings amid the different cultural and disease pattern contexts of resource-limited settings. Despite the availability of specialty training programs in selected countries, regional data and the experience of the authors suggest that intensive care specialists are unavailable in many ICUs in resource-limited settings [40]. Some ICUs in sub-Saharan Africa are, for example, run and staffed by "anesthetic officers" (non-physicians with specific training in certain elements of anesthesia) in close cooperation with surgeons, internal medicine specialists, and pediatricians [41–44].

The number of nurses per 1000 inhabitants is substantially lower in low- and middle- than in high-income countries [45]. Consequently, the number of nursing staff is limited in many ICUs in resource-limited settings [46]. Limited availability of nursing staff in resource-limited ICUs naturally leads to low nurse-to-patient ratios of often 1:4 or higher, particularly during off-hours and weekends. It can be assumed that similar associations between nurse-to-patient ratios and outcomes exist in resource-limited and resource-rich settings. However, given the general shortage of nursing staff, especially those trained in intensive care nursing, it is highly questionable whether cutoff values for nurse-to-patient ratios established in resource-rich setting specific guidelines (e.g., 1:2) can be extrapolated to ICUs in resource-limited settings. Allied healthcare professionals, such as physiotherapists and dieticians, are usually unavailable in many, if not most, resource-limited ICUs [40]. If these healthcare professionals are available in the hospital or even the ICU, they are, in the experience of the authors, often not trained or experienced in caring for the critically ill patient. Accordingly, dedicated critical care pharmacists are uncommon in many resource-limited ICUs [47], and even if available, their presence during ICU rounds, where benefits are strongest [48], is limited [49]. In addition, high staff-related costs may strain or exceed tight budgets of hospitals and be another reason why a multidisciplinary ICU model appears less feasible in resource-limited than in resource-rich settings. In the absence of dedicated ICU staff, family members often assume an important role in caring for the patient.

Increasing global Internet connectivity and the ubiquity of mobile phones could facilitate low-cost ICU telemedicine and translate to rapid and accessible ICU consultative services in some resource-limited settings [50]. However, related implementation and maintenance costs, unavailability of stable Internet coverage in many rural or remote areas, and questions of credentialing and accountability for out-of-country-based telemedicine providers remain ongoing challenges. Author experience suggests that telemedicine links between "sister hospitals," one in a resource-limited setting and one in a resource-rich setting, may provide meaningful collaboration and educational opportunities on both sides. Finally, we could not identify any safety considerations to the implementation of a multidisciplinary team approach in ICUs in resource-limited settings.

We *suggest* that, if possible, ICUs use a closed-format model where physicians specifically trained or experienced in intensive care medicine direct patient care (2B). We further *suggest* that ICUs be staffed with nurses who are trained in intensive care nursing (2C). Wherever available, allied healthcare professionals (e.g., pharmacists) should be part of an ICU team (ungraded). Currently, no recommendation on ICU telemedicine in resource-limited settings can be made.

3.3 Training

The care of the critically ill patient substantially differs from noncritically ill patients and thus requires specific training of all healthcare professionals involved due to the complex care requirements. High-performing ICUs are typically staffed with ICU physicians and nurses and allied health professionals who, in addition to general training, have pursued further training in intensive care. Regulatory bodies in these settings frequently consider specialty certification as a prerequisite to permanently work in an ICU. However, formal intensive care specialty training programs are rare or nonexistent in resource-limited settings. This lack of specialty education is likely to translate into limited knowledge about the pathophysiology and diagnostic and therapeutic management of critically ill patients [51]. It remains unclear how healthcare professionals working in ICUs in resource-limited settings, where no established regional or national specialty education programs in intensive care medicine exist, should be trained.

The majority of studies from resource-limited settings describe small-scale, focused training courses in individual institutions and pre- and post-course tests of knowledge. Four investigations, one in Ghana [52] and three in Sri Lanka [53–55], were about regional or national training programs for physicians, ICU nurses, and physical therapists. Dedicated courses in trauma and intensive care- and emergency medicine-related procedures improve knowledge in "best clinical practice" of healthcare professionals working in ICUs in resource-limited settings [56, 57]. Focused training programs that use well-established training models, such as the "Fundamental Critical Care Support" course, facilitated immediate knowledge gain, especially in junior clinicians or those with limited practical experience taking care of critically ill patients [57]. However, data on influences on patient care and long-term knowledge retention are limited. Intensive care-specific courses also demonstrated benefit in allied health professionals in resource-limited settings [55].

A national train-the-trainers program for critical care nursing in Sri Lanka was structured as seven educational blocks over a period of 18 months [53]. Using didactics, simulation, and small group learning, by 2014, this program trained 584 nurses and 29 faculty and allowed local trainers eventually to take command of course directorship. In Ghana, a countrywide continuing medical education course in acute trauma management was developed, and targeting general practitioners in rural hospitals showed significant knowledge retention and critical procedural skills improvement even 1 year after course completion [52].

In locations where institutional, regional, or national courses are unavailable, the use of mobile health technology to facilitate intensive care education and training is of great interest. A pilot study in Haiti showed that non-physician ultrasound learners, linked to ultrasound instructors in the United States via mobile phone video chat technology, can learn how to obtain clinically useful ultrasound images [58]. Validated e-learning methodologies are also in use to enhance critical care education and capacity in Cambodia, although specific outcomes have yet to be declared [59].

Among nearly all available studies from resource-limited settings, a universal theme is partnerships between an institution based in a resource-limited and one in a resource-rich setting. These partnerships, when successful, can evolve from simple facility-to-facility ventures [60] to more longitudinal, systems-based programs [61]. Whether approached vertically (institution-based) or horizontally (systems-based), partnerships also permit local personnel in resource-limited settings to advance knowledge or develop specific skill sets while remaining in their setting. In many cases, the goal is for the resource-limited settings partner to administer the program independently. One successful example of such a horizontally integrated program is the East African Training Initiative, a pulmonary/critical care fellowship training program in Addis Ababa, Ethiopia [29]. In partnership with the Ethiopian Ministry of Health, international professional societies, nongovernmental organizations, and a consortium of universities in Europe and North America, a growing cadre of domestically trained intensive care physicians is now assuming leadership roles in ICU education and clinical care in the country, where only a few years ago no such opportunities existed. A similar project has been established successfully to train nurses in emergency and critical care medicine in Ethiopia [62].

Dedicated and sustainable partnerships at national and international levels incorporating both vertical and horizontal planning, such as the East Africa Training Initiative, require funding, enormous coordination, and sustained buy-in from numerous parties with diverse interests. Consequently, such partnerships are likely less feasible and more expensive to establish; however, they are more likely to have lasting success. Partnerships between individual institutions in resource-limited settings and professional societies in high-income countries are also possible but may lack sustainability. A serious risk to such partnerships is "brain drain," the emigration of well-trained and specialized healthcare workers from resource-limited to resource-rich settings or from low- and middle-income to high-income countries [40]. Solutions to the "brain drain" are complex and must involve systematic national programs to facilitate return of well-educated emigrated healthcare professionals to their home countries.

Small-scale initiatives, such as intermittent, institution-level ICU training courses like the "Fundamental Critical Care Support" course and others, are least likely to provide long-term benefit given their temporary nature. The teaching content may be difficult to implement in some resource-limited settings. Furthermore, start-up costs for formal courses, especially the ones developed in high-income countries, may exceed local budgets [52]. Focused critical care teaching courses, such as BASIC for Developing Health Systems, which is free and nonproprietary, have been developed and adjusted to resource-limited healthcare systems [63, 64]. Remote education via telemedicine may play a role in the future to reduce costs and improve availability of training options. We could not identify any published safety concerns to the implementation of educational interventions in ICUs in resource-limited settings.

We *suggest* that all healthcare professionals working in ICUs be specifically trained in the care of the critically ill patient (2C). Unless national or regional specialty training programs in intensive care medicine are available, we *suggest* that training of ICU physicians, nurses, and allied healthcare professionals occurs through longitudinal, multimodal programs coordinated by partnerships between Ministries of Health, national and international professional societies, nongovernmental organizations, as well as institutions with well-established programs in ICU training (2D). We *recommend* that such ICU training programs adhere to validated, international standards of intensive care medicine, but that they be adapted to local needs and resources (1C).

3.4 Electricity

Modern ICUs provide around-the-clock, life-sustaining therapies often by the use of electricity-driven machines such as mechanical ventilators, syringe pumps, or extracorporeal therapies. Unexpected power cuts interrupt these therapies and may result in significant harm to or death of critically ill patients. Consistent and reliable electrical power supply is therefore a key logistical requirement of every ICU. However, electricity supply in resource-limited settings is often inconsistent. Major challenges include wide voltage fluctuations, which are deleterious to electricity-driven medical equipment. In many resource-limited settings, electrical power cuts occur on a regular basis and backup electrical sources are frequently absent. In a survey of 231 health centers in 12 African countries, only 35.1% of facilities were reported to have a reliable electricity supply and 56.7% had a backup power source such as a generator. The same survey showed that 16.5% of healthcare facilities did not have any electricity supply [65]. From personal experiences of one of the authors (AP) in 2011, the national public hospital in South Sudan sometimes had to function without electricity for days, limiting hospital services to dispensing medications and making already hot inpatient wards unbearable since fans were not working. Basic clinical services during these periods were performed by flashlight in the evening and not at all at night. Ensuring continuous electric supply is therefore imperative for ICUs to function effectively.

Voltage surges can be attenuated by installing voltage stabilizers into the main electrical supply line(s) of the ICU. Power cuts can be bridged by backup electrical sources, including batteries. Although multiple technical options exist (including solar power sources), fuel- or diesel-driven generators are the most commonly available technical solution in resource-limited settings. It is important to install an electrical backup source that provides adequate electrical power to supply essential medical apparatus in the ICU (e.g., mechanical ventilators, oxygen concentrators, syringe pumps delivering catecholamine agents) and other important machines (e.g., air compressor supporting the pressurized air system). Even when such backup power supplies are available, the time delay between mains power cut and startup of the backup supplies can be a limiting factor. Since even brief power cuts cause electrical equipment to shut down, backup sources that start automatically and immediately are crucial. Using battery-equipped equipment with short (30–60 min) automatic emergency electrical supply can help to mitigate patient harm. If backup sources must be started manually, protocols must be in place to guide ICU workers how to act in response to abrupt interruptions of life-sustaining therapies. Such protocols should ideally focus on three steps in a descending priority: (a) compensation of stopped mechanical ventilators (e.g., by manual bagging), (b) compensation of stopped catecholamine infusions (e.g., by injecting adrenaline into gravity infusions with titration of drops per minute), and (c) compensation of interrupted oxygen supply if oxygen concentrators are used for oxygen supply (e.g., by activating backup oxygen cylinders). It is important that these protocols can be implemented during daylight and nighttime (e.g., availability of functioning flashlights is essential) and that the ICU staff, particularly the nurses and nurse assistants, is adequately trained to implement them. Periodic mock "drills" may help to ensure smooth implementation in the event of an actual event.

Solar power has great potential for ICUs in resource-limited settings, especially given that many of these settings are located in tropical, sunny environments. Solar panel installation was associated with a significant reduction in mean inpatient pediatric mortality in a single-center, retrospective, before-and-after observational study in Sierra Leone [66]. An observational, proof-of-concept study in Uganda also demonstrated improvements in physiologic variables related to respiratory failure after solar panels were installed to power oxygen concentrators in a pediatric ICU [67]. These improvements were consistent even on cloudy days.

The greatest barrier to ensure adequate electrical supply to an ICU in a resource-limited setting is financial. While voltage stabilizers are not costly and are readily available even in resource-limited settings, generators and other backup power sources are expensive, especially with automatic bridging functions. Diesel generators large enough to function through sustained power cuts require steady supply of fuel, which itself can be cost-prohibitive or in short supply. Another commonly faced challenge is maintenance of these systems, which requires technical expertise. Particularly during nighttime when technicians are not readily available, the ICU/hospital staff needs to be familiar with activation of the available backup power source if activation does not occur automatically, a situation that poses logistical and safety challenges when the primary concern is stabilization of critically ill patients. When exposed to extreme weather conditions, generator malfunctions can occur and require skilled local technicians for repair.

A stable electricity supply is an essential infrastructural component of an ICU (ungraded). We *recommend* that ICUs use voltage stabilizers in case voltage fluctuations endanger the function of electrical medical equipment (1D). We *recommend* that adequate backup electrical sources be available to bridge power cuts (1C). We *suggest* that these backup electrical sources take over electricity supply automatically allowing for (near) continuous functioning of life-sustaining medical equipment (2D). We *recommend* that ICUs with no adequate backup electrical source have protocols in place guiding ICU staff how to bridge life-sustaining therapies during power cuts (1D).

3.5 Oxygen

The World Health Organization considers oxygen fundamentally important and lists it on page one of the Essential Medication List [67]. In 2015, the Lancet Commission on Global Surgery revealed that approximately one quarter of hospitals surveyed in resource-limited countries lack sufficient oxygen supply [68]. This analysis reinforced previous data reporting similar deficiencies in multiple resource-limited settings across the world [65, 69, 70]. Since severity of hypoxemia correlates with mortality [71] and often goes undiagnosed in resource-limited settings [72], ensuring adequate oxygen supply to ICUs in resource-limited settings is of critical importance.

There are three commonly used methods to supply ICUs in resource-limited settings with oxygen: oxygen cylinders, oxygen concentrators, and centralized, piped oxygen systems [73]. Oxygen cylinders provide pressurized oxygen at variably high flow rates but—depending on their size—only do so for a limited period. They do not require electrical power supply but do require pressure regulators and flowmeters to deliver oxygen safely to the patient. Oxygen cylinders are purchased or rented from supply companies and refilled at central distribution points, often making long transportation times to (remote) healthcare facilities necessary. They are generally easy to use, but problems include oxygen leakage from the adaptors (varying from 10 to 70% of the entire cylinder oxygen content), difficulty moving due to size and weight, and sometimes confusion with the local color coding system [74]. Oxygen concentrators are devices which purify oxygen (>90%) from ambient air by absorbing nitrogen onto zeolite membranes. Most concentrators deliver oxygen flow rates of up to 6 L/min. While this is typically enough to deliver oxygen noninvasively to (one to three) moderately unwell neonates or small children, it may not be enough in critically ill older children or adult patients. In contrast to oxygen cylinders, oxygen concentrators depend on a continuous electrical power supply. They also require technical maintenance including regular filter changes. Not all models of oxygen concentrators are technically suitable for sustained use in a tropical environment [75]. Centralized, piped oxygen systems typically deliver pressurized oxygen through wall outlets to bed spaces in the ICU. These systems are supplied by either a liquid oxygen tank, an oxygen concentrator, or several large oxygen cylinders. Proper functioning of centralized oxygen systems depends on adequate engineering expertise and technical maintenance. Specifically, pipeline conditions (presence and severity of gas leak) and diameter (to ensure adequate gas flow), compatible wall outlets, and the presence of shutoff valves must be considered. All three modes of oxygen supply to an ICU require the presence of a backup oxygen source in case of premature emptying (e.g., oxygen cylinders, centralized oxygen system supported by oxygen cylinders), electrical power cuts (e.g., oxygen concentrators), or technical defects (e.g., oxygen concentrators, centralized oxygen system). In many resource-limited settings, oxygen cylinders are used as backup oxygen systems.

Most modern mechanical ventilators depend on pressurized air and oxygen supply. Although oxygen cylinders may be used, doing so may require frequent exchange, particularly at high minute volumes or inspiratory oxygen concentrations. Therefore, centralized, pressurized oxygen and air systems appear most practical to run these types of ventilators. Selected types of mechanical ventilators and the majority of noninvasive (home) ventilators generate their driving pressure by internal air compressors and do not depend on a pressurized gas supply. When using these ventilators, oxygen can be delivered to the Y-piece or the inspiration tubing using either an oxygen cylinder or an oxygen concentrator. Oxygen concentrators are unable to serve as a pressurized oxygen source to run mechanical ventilators but can be used to enrich the oxygen concentration of inspiratory breaths delivered by compressor-driven ventilators. Although the latter practice results in unclear inspiratory oxygen concentrations, the oxygen flow of the oxygen concentrator can be titrated to achieve a desired blood oxygen saturation.

Taking the aforementioned conditions into account, the choice of the most appropriate method to supply an ICU with oxygen depends on site-specific requirements and conditions. A non-ICU study from The Gambia found that cylinders were better than concentrators due to local factors at 10 out of 12 hospitals studied. The authors suggested that concentrators are most advantageous when electrical power is reliable; cylinders may be preferable when power supply is erratic but only when weighed against substantial transportation and delivery costs [76]. Additionally, oxygen concentrators cannot be used to run mechanical ventilators that depend on a pressurized oxygen source as they generate insufficient oxygen flows and pressures.

Installation and maintenance of oxygen systems in an ICU in a resource-limited setting face multiple challenges. While oxygen cylinders are commonly available, also in remote areas, oxygen concentrators are often not locally available and can only be purchased in metropolitan areas or from overseas. Although some materials to set up centralized oxygen systems are ubiquitously available (e.g., copper pipes), key parts, such as wall outlets or liquid oxygen tanks, are not. Copper pipes are also prone to theft [77]. Maintenance of all oxygen supply systems is frequently impeded by financial constraints and a shortage of workers with sufficient training, equipment, and technical experience [76].

A before–after study evaluated the feasibility and outcome effects of improved oxygen delivery on case fatality rates of children with pneumonia admitted to five hospitals in Papua New Guinea. After introduction of pulse oximeters to detect hypoxemia and installation of oxygen concentrators, the risk of death for a child with pneumonia was reduced by 35% [risk ratio 0.65 (CI 95%, 0.52–0.78) compared to the time period before oximeters and oxygen concentrators were made available]. The implementation costs were estimated to be USD $51 per patient treated, USD $1673 per life saved, and USD $50 per disability-adjusted life year averted [78]. Multiple studies from resource-limited settings demonstrated greater cost reductions with oxygen concentrator systems compared to cylinders and generators. In Papua New Guinea, the overall 2-year cost estimate for cylinders, capable of producing 35,000 L/day, was approximately USD $205,000 when compared to three oxygen concentrators (USD $82,400) and an oxygen generator system (USD $390,000), both capable of producing 60,000 L/day, [73]. In The Gambia, annual costs for cylinders at one hospital were USD $152,747 vs. USD $18,742 for concentrators with 24 h availability of grid power [76]. A different 8-year, single-center analysis from The Gambia estimated that installation of oxygen concentrators with a reliable backup power supply saved 51% on oxygen supply costs compared to cylinders (assuming 2 L/min flow rate). When accounting for air leaks and the estimated costs of backup power supply maintenance, the authors estimated total savings of USD $45,000 over 8 years [74]. Given regional variations in supply chains, local engineering and maintenance capabilities, electrical power supply, and other factors, these cost analyses cannot be applied uniformly to other resource-limited settings. A decision support algorithm to determine the best mode of oxygen supply to an individual ICU in a resource-limited setting has been suggested by some authors [76].

Oxygen is an essential medication for critically ill patients, and an adequate oxygen supply is a crucial infrastructural component of an ICU (ungraded). We *recommend* that ICUs in resource-limited settings choose the type of oxygen supply (concentrators, cylinders, centralized system) based on site-specific conditions and requirements (1B). We *suggest* that, when feasible, oxygen be supplied by centralized, piped systems to ICUs when mechanical ventilators are used (2D).

3.6 Hygiene

While healthcare-acquired infections are prevalent throughout the world, the burden is highest in resource-limited settings. The World Health Organization estimates that healthcare-associated infection rates are roughly 20 times higher in low- and middle-income countries compared to high-income countries [79]. In ICUs specifically, a meta-analysis reported an overall incidence of ICU-associated infections of 47.9 per 1000 patient days in developing countries. This was three times greater than the prevalence reported from the United States. Surgical site infections were most common, but device-associated infections were highly prevalent as well [80]. Healthcare-associated infections can be transmitted via myriad mechanisms. Many, if not most, can be prevented easily with simple measures. However, lack of hygienic facilities, insufficient training of staff, and lack of administrative oversight (e.g., by hospital-level and national-level infection control measures) are likely to contribute to the deleteriously high rates of nosocomial infection rates in ICUs in resource-limited settings [81].

In line with findings from resource-rich settings, several studies originating in resource-limited settings suggest that hand hygiene is the most effective method of reducing healthcare-acquired infections. Healthcare workers can contaminate hands and medical devices with even a single contact with the patient or his/her immediate surroundings. Contaminant transfer to other patients and healthcare workers is common if hand hygiene is inadequate or not performed [82]. Innumerable challenges to improving hand hygiene in resource-limited settings have been identified, but reasons vary from location to location [83]. Convincing evidence indicates that implementation of multimodal hand hygiene programs can not only improve hand hygiene compliance but also reduce ICU-acquired infection rates. A prospective observational study involving 99 ICUs in 19 resource-limited countries demonstrated a significant 23.1% overall increase in hand hygiene compliance after implementation of a multidimensional hand hygiene program involving administrative support, supply availability, education and training, workplace reminders, process surveillance, and performance feedback [84]. These findings have been replicated in geographically diverse locations including India [85], China [86], and Mexico [87]. A prospective study in six Colombian ICUs demonstrated a significant reduction (12.7% annually during the 4-year study period) in central line-associated bloodstream infections after introduction of a targeted hand hygiene program that included installation of alcohol-based hand rub dispensers adjacent to each ICU bed and regular feedback to healthcare workers [88]. In a Vietnamese tertiary ICU, the combination of hand hygiene and antimicrobial mixing reduced MRSA infections significantly, but not the incidence of the four hospital-acquired gram-negative infections studied.

Several large studies from resource-limited and resource-rich countries reported superior efficacy of hand rubbing with alcohol-based solutions over handwashing with antiseptic soap to reduce hand contamination. A study including three Egyptian ICUs and a renal dialysis unit found that hand rubbing with alcohol-based liquids or gels resulted in a higher reduction of bacterial counts on the hands of ICU staff compared to handwashing with soap and water (77–99% vs. 30%, $p < 0.001$) [89]. These results are in line with the findings of a randomized controlled trial conducted in French ICUs that observed a 26% reduction in bacterial hand contamination when using alcohol-based hand rub compared to soap and water [90].

During the West African Ebola virus disease outbreak, chlorine-based hand hygiene was commonly used following patient encounters in Ebola treatment centers and in affected communities. This practice is supported by an observational study conducted in Ebola treatment centers in Sierra Leone demonstrating elimination of Ebola virus RNA from contaminated personal protective equipment following treatment with locally produced chlorine solutions [91]. Although this study did not determine whether detection of Ebola RNA on personal protective equipment translated to an increased risk of infection, it can be inferred that reducing contamination is likely to decrease the risk of iatrogenic infection. Although frequent hand hygiene with chlorine-based solution may increase skin irritation, the severity of irritation is little different than with use of soap and water and alcohol-based solutions based on a randomized trial comparing different handwash regimens [92].

Non-sterile, clean examination gloves function as a protective barrier for medical staff who potentially encounter blood, body fluids, or other possibly infectious material. The bacterial bioburden of non-sterile examination gloves is very low [93] and does not differ between newly opened and nearly empty boxes [94]. A randomized controlled trial performed in US ICUs reported that the total bacterial colony counts of gloved hands were not different if hand hygiene was performed before non-sterile examination gloves were donned or not, suggesting that hand hygiene before donning non-sterile gloves is unnecessary [95]. Several studies, however, indicate that contaminated examination gloves can spread bacterial pathogens from healthcare workers to patients [96]. Furthermore, examination gloves do not avoid bacterial contamination of healthcare workers' hands due to microlesions [97]. Based on these results, the WHO emphasizes that wearing gloves does not replace the need for subsequent hand hygiene [83]. Reuse of medical examination or surgical gloves is commonplace in many resource-limited settings [ref], but the limited studies available suggest that reprocessing and reuse of disposable gloves may be harmful to patients and healthcare professionals. A laboratory-based study from Kenya comparing sterility and physical integrity of reprocessed plastic surgical gloves compared to new, sterilized surgical gloves demonstrated alarmingly reduced physical integrity and sterility of the reprocessed gloves [98].

A before–after study from Pakistan found that the use of (plastic) shoe covers by medical staff and visitors was not helpful in preventing infections with common ICU pathogens or improving the outcome of critically ill patients [99]. Further infection control measures such as fogging and spraying of disinfectants, the use of disinfection or sticky mats, and routine use of face masks or caps by ICU staff or visitors have not been shown to influence infection rates in ICUs [100]. No trials from resource-limited settings on the routine use of gloves, gowns, and aprons to prevent nosocomial or cross infection in critically ill patients were identified. Three large randomized trials from the United States concluded that the universal use of gloves and gowns for all patient contact compared with usual care (adequate hand hygiene and use of gloves in case of contact with blood, body fluids, or other contaminants) did not reduce adverse events or the transmission rate of multiresistant bacteria [101–103]. Similarly, a Cochrane meta-analysis primarily consisting of studies from resource-rich settings could not identify evidence that overgowns used by staff or visitors are effective in limiting death, infection, or bacterial colonization in infants admitted to neonatal wards or intensive care units [104].

Critically ill patients with known or suspected airborne, droplet, or contact infections require specific hygienic precautions. Although no randomized controlled trials were identified by our literature search, (cohort) isolation of patients with airborne (e.g., *Mycobacterium tuberculosis*) or droplet infections (e.g., influenza virus, measles, varicella zoster virus, *Neisseria meningitidis*, coronavirus) in separate rooms is recommended by international and national guidelines both in resource-rich and resource-limited settings [105, 106]. In addition to standard hygienic measures, adequate hand hygiene in particular, the use of masks has been recommended to protect healthcare workers caring for (critically ill) patients with acute respiratory infections. Despite surrogate exposure studies indicating that N95 respirators are associated with less filter penetration and inward leakage than surgical masks, large clinical trials and meta-analyses failed to show that N95 respirators are superior to surgical masks in protecting healthcare workers against influenza during routine care [107–109]. The Centers for Disease Control and Prevention recommends use of N95 disposable, powered air-purifying, or self-contained breathing apparatus respirators for healthcare workers caring for patients with tuberculosis [110]. In addition to isolation, patients with highly contagious infectious diseases, such as viral hemorrhagic fever or smallpox infection, require specific hygienic precautions. In its latest guidelines on personal protective equipment for use in a filovirus disease outbreak, the World Health Organization recommends the use of face shields or goggles, a fluid-resistant head cover and surgical mask, double gloves, and protective body wear, as well as waterproof aprons and boots, in addition to regular on-duty clothing [111].

A large before–after study in North America showed that the use of full-barrier precautions during insertion of central venous catheters, in addition to adequate hand hygiene when handling catheters, significantly reduced the risk of central venous catheter-related bloodstream infections by up to 66% over the 18-month study period [112]. Full sterile barrier precautions include the use of a cap, mask, sterile drapes, a sterile gown, and sterile gloves following adequate skin preparation and hand hygiene; these components have not been studied separately. Other observational studies confirmed these findings and suggest that the rate of central venous catheter-related bloodstream or other device-related infections can be minimized with the use of appropriate hygienic precautions [113–117].

No randomized controlled trials from resource-limited or resource-rich settings on the architectural design of ICUs to prevent transmission of microbial pathogens were identified by our search and a previous review of the literature [118]. A prospective study from the United Kingdom reported that isolation of patients colonized or infected with methicillin-resistant *Staphylococcus aureus* in single rooms or cohorted bays did not reduce cross infection as long as adequate hand hygiene measures were maintained [119]. In contrast, studies suggest that isolation of critically ill patients in rooms that are poorly visualized by staff is likely related to a higher risk of death [120].

National and international guidelines recommend isolation of patients with highly contagious infectious diseases (e.g., tuberculosis, influenza, measles, rubeola infection, varicella zoster infection, hemorrhagic virus disease) or severe immune suppression (e.g., neutropenia, burns, transplant) [106, 110]. Atmospheric pressure in isolation rooms should be controllable to target negative pressure when isolating patients with airborne infections and positive pressure when caring for patients who require protective isolation [106, 110]. A survey-based study of 83 ICUs in resource-limited Asian countries (Bangladesh, India, Nepal, Pakistan, and the Philippines) found that 34 did not have single rooms and 64 did not have negative pressure rooms [121]. A study from Peru reported that upper-room ultraviolet lights and negative air ionization prevented most airborne tuberculosis transmission detectable by guinea pig air sampling [122]. These observations have recently been confirmed by a study from South Africa suggesting that upper-room ultraviolet light is an effective, low-cost intervention for use in tuberculosis infection control in high-risk clinical settings [123]. Regarding the architectural design of new or newly renovated ICUs, consensus-based guidelines published by the Indian Society of Critical Care Medicine recommend the installation of filter-containing central air-conditioning systems with a minimum of six total air changes per room per hour (filter efficiency 99% down to 5 μm); clearly demarcated routes of traffic flow through the ICU; adequate space around and between beds; an adequate number of washbasins; a separate medication preparation area; separate areas for clean, soiled, and waste storage/disposal; and adequate toilet facilities [124]. Alcohol hand rub dispensers are recommended to be placed at the ICU entry and exits and at every bed space and workstation [124].

Despite the clear evidence that the use of alcohol-based hand rub solutions reduces the risk of infection transmission [83], commercial alcohol-based hand rubs are often unavailable in resource-limited settings [82]. A study from Egypt suggests that locally prepared alcohol-based hand rubs are similarly effective to commercial products [89], so local preparation of these products may be feasible and potentially more affordable than purchase of foreign-made products, with recipes readily available [125]. Locally produced chlorine-based handwashing solutions are also effective for decontamination in Ebola virus disease [92], but careful attention must be paid to varying shelf lives among solutions of differing chemical composition, especially in hot environments [126]. Hand hygiene dispensers are commonly used to supply ICU workers in resource-rich countries with alcohol-based hand rub solutions. These dispensers are, however, often unavailable or restricted to the operating theaters in hospitals in resource-limited settings. In addition, they depend on regular refilling by dedicated staff, which may be problematic in understaffed ICUs. In the absence of adequate hand hygiene dispensers, small pocket bottles containing alcohol-based hand rub solutions can be carried, used, and refilled by each ICU worker (Fig. 3.1). A multifaceted hand hygiene program (including upgrading hand hygiene facilities, provision of alcohol-based hand rub at point of care, hand hygiene campaigns, continuous hand hygiene education) not only reduced the incidence of hospital-acquired infections in 17 Vietnamese ICUs but also proved to be cost-effective [127]. Although a cluster-randomized, crossover trial in rural Kenya failed to show differences in surgical site infections between handwashing with alcohol or soap and water (8.3 vs. 8%) in 3133 patients undergoing clean or clean-contaminated surgery, the use of alcohol-based hand rubbing solutions was as feasible and affordable (€4.6 vs. €3.3 per week) as handwashing with soap and water [128]. Religious beliefs do not influence the use of alcohol-based hand rub solutions for hand hygiene but may impact implementation effectiveness [129].

Respirator masks are often unavailable and underused in resource-limited settings where acute respiratory infections are highly prevalent. Given cost concerns and the unclear scientific benefit of using N95 respirators compared with surgical masks [107], it appears advisable that if N95 respirators are in short supply they should be reserved to protect healthcare workers caring for patients with tuberculosis or other airborne infectious diseases or when caring for patients with droplet-spread infections during aerosol-generating procedures or when caring for patients in very hot and humid environments for long periods when surgical masks may become wet and ineffective (e.g., during the Ebola epidemic). Importantly, cloth

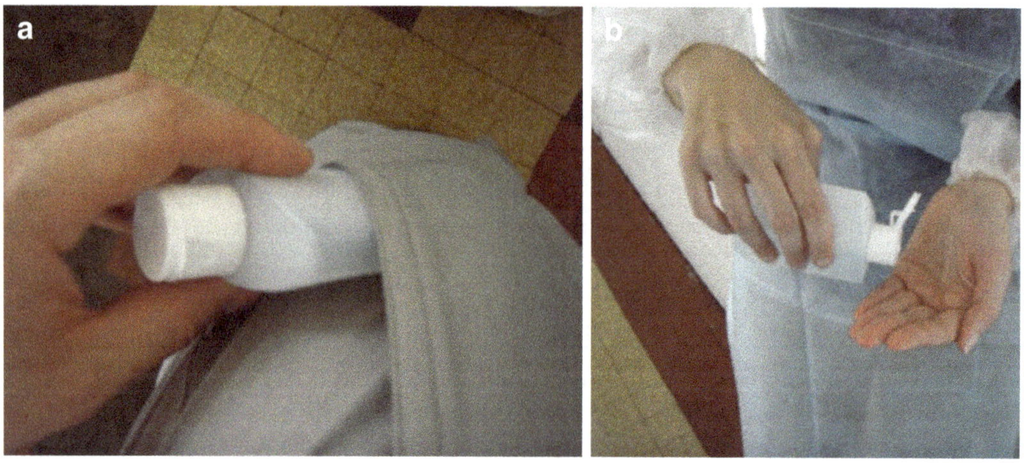

Fig. 3.1 Pocket bottles filled with alcohol-based hand rub for hand hygiene in ICUs in resource-limited settings (Courtesy of Martin W. Dünser, MD)

masks are prone to moisture retention and poor filtration when reused [130]. As suggested by a randomized controlled trial, they should not replace surgical masks in high-risk situations [131]. One striking challenge during the most recent Ebola virus disease epidemic was the shortage of personal protective equipment faced by healthcare workers caring for diseased patients in West Africa, as global fears of a disease spread rose and resource-rich countries filled their stocks with protective body suits. Since single-use, disposable sterile gowns and drapes, commonly used for invasive procedures in ICUs in resource-rich settings, are expensive and mostly unavailable in resource-limited countries, autoclavable gowns and cloths may be used instead for the majority of common ICU illnesses. For Ebola virus disease, the WHO emphasizes use of disposable personal protective equipment [132].

We *recommend* that ICUs have available an adequate number of and easily accessible facilities for handwashing/hand hygiene (1A). We *recommend* hand hygiene after each patient contact with an alcohol-based solution (1A) or, for Ebola virus disease specifically, with chlorine-based solution (1C). In case alcohol-based solutions are unavailable, we *recommend* using soap and water for handwashing (1A). Alcohol hand rub solutions may be produced locally and carried in small bottles by each healthcare worker (ungraded). We *recommend* that non-sterile, clean examination gloves for self-protection of medical staff be available (1C). Importantly, gloved hands can equally transmit infectious pathogens and that the use of gloves does not replace the need for subsequent hand hygiene (ungraded). We *recommend* the availability of masks, caps, sterile gowns, sterile drapes, and sterile gloves for invasive procedures such as insertion of central venous catheters (1A). We r*ecommend* that ICUs and hospitals in areas where highly contagious infectious diseases (e.g., tuberculosis, Ebola virus disease) are endemic have rapid access to adequate quantities of personal protective equipment as recommended by the World Health Organization and the Centers for Disease Control and Prevention (1C). We *suggest* that hospitals develop individual policies and procedures for reuse of disposable personal protective and other medical equipment (2C). When ICUs are renovated or newly built, we *suggest* compliance with national and international best-practice recommendations on ICU architectural design (2D).

3.7 Equipment

The very nature of an ICU warrants a higher reliance on technical equipment, devices, and other technologies compared to the general medical ward. Irrespective of the geographic location or level of resource limitation, technical equipment constitutes an essential component of ICU-level patient care. What specific types of technical equipment are essential, however, remains undetermined. In resource-limited settings, multiple challenges in terms of equipment procurement and maintenance exist [133]. For example, can the technical equipment run with frequent electric current interruptions? How reliable are the supply chains to obtain or replace the equipment and are local technicians available for repairs? Is donated equipment relevant in the local context and are clinicians educated on how to use it [134]?

Given these considerations, resource-limited hospitals and health systems must find and fund equipment purchase or donation sustainably and in the most targeted manner possible.

No large clinical trial has so far shown a reproducible survival benefit related to the use of a single monitoring device in critically ill patients. Monitors improve the care of the critically ill only if healthcare staff make timely and appropriate changes in the therapeutic management based on data from monitors. In view of the fact that pathologic deviations of vital signs such as heart rate, respiratory rate, arterial blood pressure, and arterial oxygen saturation are associated with an increased risk of organ dysfunction and death [135–138], especially in settings where artificial life support is inconsistently available [139–145], it appears sensible to measure these parameters continuously or at regular intervals. A prospective, before-and-after interventional study including 447 ICU patients in a Tanzanian university hospital reported that a vital signs-directed therapy improved the acute management of patients with abnormal vital signs. While overall in-hospital mortality was unchanged before and after the intervention, critically ill patients with arterial hypotension experienced a lower post-implementation mortality (69.2 vs. 92.3%, $p = 0.02$; number needed to treat 4.3) [146].

No conclusive evidence—either from resource-limited or resource-rich settings—was identified to answer the question whether noninvasive or invasive blood pressure measurement is superior in critically ill patients. While a study performed in critically ill patients in an emergency department in a resource-rich country reported inaccuracy of oscillometric blood pressure measurements at hypotensive blood pressure ranges [147], a prospective multicenter study from France found a good discriminative power of noninvasive blood pressure measurements to identify arterial hypotension (mean arterial blood pressure < 65 mmHg) and track arterial blood pressure in 111 patients with shock [148]. A survey among US intensivists observed that 73% and 47% of respondents reported using noninvasive blood pressure measurements in hypotensive patients and patients on vasopressor support, respectively [149].

A recent Cochrane meta-analysis could not identify convincing evidence that the use of pulse oximetry conveys a significant survival benefit in perioperative patients [150]. However, a large, multicenter, before-and-after intervention study from Papua New Guinea observed a survival benefit associated with the systematic use of pulse oximetry to monitor and treat children with pneumonia, when coupled with a reliable oxygen supply [78]. In settings where blood gas analyzers are unavailable, the plethysmographic oxygen saturation relative to the inspiratory oxygen concentration (SpO_2/FiO_2 ratio) can be used for decision-making and continuous monitoring [151, 152].

A systematic review of the literature evaluated the benefit associated with the use of portable ultrasound devices in low- and middle-income countries [153]. Although several reports were identified describing the successful diagnosis, triage, and management of patients with complex, life-threatening conditions with the use of point-of-care ultrasound, no randomized controlled trial has so far evaluated the impact of ultrasound-guided diagnosis and treatment in resource-limited settings. A Haitian–US study demonstrated that tele-mentoring of non-physicians performing ultrasound in a resource-limited setting was feasible and adequate to make clinical decisions in the majority (89%) of cases [58].

Our literature search did not identify any randomized controlled trials evaluating the effects of mechanical ventilators on mortality in critically ill patients both in resource-limited and resource-rich settings. However, mortality of patients with hypoxemia who do not receive mechanical ventilatory support is extremely high, suggesting that mechanical ventilation associates with a survival benefit [152]. Observational evidence from ICUs in Vietnam suggest that general intensive care measures, including mechanical ventilation, can improve clinical outcomes [154, 155]. A structured ICU training program that included modules on mechanical ventilation improved overall ICU mortality in two of three ICUs in India, Nepal, and Bangladesh [156].

Reports from India and Africa confirm the feasibility of noninvasive ventilation in resource-limited settings [157, 158]. A randomized controlled trial including four rural hospitals in Ghana found that continuous positive airway pressure application by local nurses significantly reduced respiratory rate and was not associated with complications in 70 children with respiratory distress [159]. A randomized controlled trial that was stopped early including 225 Bangladeshi children with severe pneumonia and hypoxemia found that the use of bubble continuous positive airway pressure reduced the risk of treatment failure and death compared with standard low-flow oxygen therapy [160]. These results were confirmed by studies from India and Malawi [161, 162]. No randomized controlled trials on the use of end-tidal carbon dioxide monitoring in resource-limited settings were identified. Studies from both resource-limited and resource-rich settings prove that end-tidal carbon dioxide measurement is a reliable technique to verify endotracheal tube placement and an adequate tool to monitor mechanical ventilation [163–165]. Although differences between arterial and end-tidal carbon dioxide values are common and vary individually [166, 167], the trends over time appear helpful to guide mechanical ventilation, particularly when arterial blood gas analyzers are unavailable [168–170].

Renal replacement therapy improves short- and long-term survival of patients with severe acute renal injury [171, 172]. Recommendations regarding renal replacement therapy for critically ill patients in resource-limited settings are discussed in another chapter in this book [173].

Abnormal blood glucose levels and increased blood lactate levels have both been associated with increased mortality in the critically ill in resource-limited and resource-rich settings [174–184]. A Ugandan multicenter study recorded an incidence of hypoglycemia of 16.3% among 532 sepsis patients. In this study, hypoglycemia was an independent risk factor for in-hospital mortality and could not be adequately predicted by clinical examination [185]. Hypoglycemia is a well-known complication of malaria, particularly in children [186] and those treated with quinine [187]. Although our literature search did not reveal a randomized controlled trial showing that measurement of blood glucose is associated with improved outcome, it is sensible to assume that detection of dysglycemic episodes is associated with improved care. While studies from resource-limited settings suggest that results of point-of-care methods to measure blood glucose levels are closely correlated with those of laboratory measurements [188, 189], some studies from resource-rich settings have highlighted inaccuracies of point-of-care devices in lower blood glucose ranges [190]. A recent international multicenter study, however, demonstrated that bedside blood glucose monitoring systems were acceptable for use in critically ill patient settings when compared to a central laboratory reference method [191]. Similarly, lactate levels as measured by a point-of-care blood lactate analyzer reliably predicted mortality in Ugandan sepsis patients [179], as well as febrile children in Tanzania [180]. No randomized controlled trials from resource-limited settings were identified evaluating the outcome effects of lactate measurements or lactate-guided interventions in critically ill patients. Although limited by insufficient information size, a meta-analysis with sequential analysis of randomized controlled trials originating in resource-rich countries suggested that the use of lactate clearance as a goal to guide resuscitation was associated with a reduction in the risk of death in adult patients with sepsis [192].

Similar to glucose and lactate measurement, our literature search failed to find studies demonstrating improved outcomes for arterial or venous blood gas measurement. A Swiss prospective observational study demonstrated that lower pH was an independent predictor of 12-month mortality in emergency department patients presenting with dyspnea, but arterial blood gas analysis itself had very limited diagnostic value [193]. According to international consensus definitions developed in high-income countries, measurement of the partial pressure of oxygen is required to diagnose the acute respiratory distress syndrome (ARDS) [194]. Similar recommendations have been made for sepsis-induced ARDS diagnosis in resource-limited settings [152], supported by observational evidence to show that patients with increasing severity of ARDS as determined by the arterial partial pressure of oxygen to fraction of inspired oxygen ratio have higher mortality and higher noninvasive ventilation failure rates [195].

The availability of vital signs monitors, mechanical ventilators, renal replacement devices, and point-of-care tools in ICUs varies substantially between resource-limited regions [196–204]. Several studies suggest that hospitals in middle-income countries and metropolitan areas of low-income countries have more technical equipment available than healthcare facilities in low-income countries and rural areas [200–204]. Except for remote areas [202, 205], the availability of vital signs monitors and glucometers appears consistently high; point-of-care laboratory facilities and renal replacement equipment are strikingly unavailable in certain areas [202–204]. Common challenges of installing and maintaining technical equipment in ICUs in resource-limited settings are high investment costs depending on the regional availability of medical retailers, the need for reliable electrical power supply, disposable materials (e.g., ECG electrodes, printer paper), as well as technical maintenance and repair in case of device malfunction or breakdown [206]. A mathematical model based on cost-effectiveness threshold and the results of previous studies concluded that the perioperative use of pulse oximeters is cost-effective in resource-limited settings [207].

In addition to challenges faced with installation and maintenance of vital signs monitors and as previously described, mechanical ventilators additionally require a reliable oxygen and/or (pressurized) gas supply as well as structured training of healthcare staff. In contrast to invasive mechanical ventilation, noninvasive mechanical ventilation appears to be feasible and safe in resource-limited settings after short, structured education of ICU staff [159, 208]. A study from India even reported that the use of noninvasive mechanical ventilation to treat patients with acute exacerbations of chronic obstructive pulmonary disease in non-ICU wards was both feasible and cost-effective [209]. Although continuous positive airway pressure and/or high-flow oxygen devices may be implemented in clinical practice with relatively low implementation costs and a concise staff training, its maintenance may consume high amounts of oxygen, particularly when used at high inspiratory oxygen concentrations in adults. Oxygen requirements in children are substantially lower due to lower minute ventilation.

Whereas both the implementation and maintenance costs to run point-of-care glucometers in the ICU are low, other point-of-care laboratory facilities (e.g., blood gas analyzers, including lactate measurements) critically depend on the local availability of (costly) supply materials (e.g., reactive agents), reliable electrical supply, as well as regular maintenance by skilled laboratory or medical technicians. Although cassette-based blood gas analyzers show a comparable accuracy to traditional blood gas analyzers [210] and require less technical maintenance, they are associated with much higher costs, particularly when large amounts of blood samples are analyzed. Separate point-of-care devices measuring blood lactate levels have been suggested as cheaper alternatives to blood gas analyzers in resource-limited settings [189, 211]. Moreover, availability of blood gas analyzers is severely limited [212], and contemporary evidence from resource-rich and resource-limited settings suggest that arterial blood gas measurement may not be necessary to diagnose and to improve outcomes for ARDS [137, 213].

Acquisition of technical equipment should be guided by local availability and feasibility of routine maintenance (ungraded). We *recommend* that ICUs have basic vital signs monitors (including electrocardiogram, respiratory rate, oscillometric blood pressure, and pulse oximetry) available for each ICU bed (1C). We *recommend* that ICUs have one or more mechanical ventilators available (1C). These mechanical ventilators should also deliver noninvasive ventilatory modes, measure tidal volume and airway pressures, and support oxygen delivery (1B). We *suggest* that ICUs that provide invasive ventilatory support have facilities available to measure end-tidal carbon dioxide (2C) and to perform blood gas analysis (2C). We *recommend* that ICUs have point-of-care capabilities for measuring blood glucose (e.g., glucometers) (1B). We *recommend* that ICUs have capabilities for measuring blood lactate levels (1B). We *suggest* that ICUs have available point-of-care ultrasound devices (2C) and that key clinical staff undergo formal ultrasound training (2C).

3.8 Quality

The sepsis and intensive care literature is replete with examples of poor quality care [51]. The great challenge is how best to improve quality of care for critically ill patients in resource-limited settings when faced with countless financial, resource, and administrative constraints. A significant limitation is that sparse epidemiologic data detailing sepsis presentation and management in resource-limited settings have been published [214]. Without these data, it is difficult, if not impossible, to identify effective interventions that work at the population level. Various authors have developed general roadmaps for the future [215], but specific interventions demonstrating convincing improvements in intensive care in resource-limited settings are still lacking.

Regular documentation of the patient's history of care is a medicolegal requirement in almost all healthcare systems. Medical records are the integral repository of the patient's disease course, healthcare planning, and documentation of communications with other healthcare providers, the patient, and his/her family. Furthermore, medical records are used to assess compliance of care with institutional, national, or international guidelines and regulations. Although electronic data documentation has become commonplace in many ICUs in resource-rich settings and resulted in improved accuracy and legibility of documents, a meta-analysis failed to show that implementation of electronic medical records has a substantial effect on relevant ICU outcomes such as mortality, length of stay, or costs of care [216]. Although introduction of a daily goal form can improve communication between ICU healthcare professionals and possibly reduce ICU length of stay [217–221], a large, randomized, controlled, multicenter trial from a resource-limited setting failed to reproduce beneficial effects of a multifaceted quality improvement intervention with daily checklists, goal setting, and clinician prompting on in-hospital mortality of critically ill patients [222].

A multitude of quality improvement methods to implement and translate scientific evidence into clinical care have been published. Education, audit and feedback, protocols, bundles of care, and checklists are common tools studied to improve the quality of ICU and sepsis care. Most reports originate in resource-rich settings. A large nationwide educational effort to implement international sepsis guidelines using two care bundles was associated with improved guideline compliance and lower hospital mortality in Spain [223]. These results were confirmed by several other reports [224, 225], indicating that a higher compliance with international sepsis guidelines was directly and significantly associated with improved survival [226–228]. A large prospective interventional study in Uganda found that a bundled protocol to implement early monitored sepsis management improved survival of patients with severe sepsis in two hospitals [229]. A small observational cohort study in Haiti demonstrated improved process measures in septic care after implementation of a simplified sepsis protocol developed by the World Health Organization, although there was no mortality effect [230]. Similarly, two hospital-wide, protocol-based quality improvement programs significantly reduced the rate of catheter-associated urinary tract and catheter-associated bloodstream infections in Thailand [231, 232]. Checklists have been implemented successfully to optimize sepsis care [233] and high-risk procedures [234] in critically ill patients in resource-rich settings. A large international quality improvement project based on checklists to minimize preventable deaths, disability, and complications in critically ill patients is underway and includes several ICUs based in resource-limited settings [235].

Benchmarking is another accepted quality improvement concept in healthcare to identify performance gaps and to improve the quality of care based on anonymous comparison of quality indicators with other institutions and services. Although multiple benchmarking projects and ICU registries exist in resource-rich countries, no evidence currently supports that they translate into improved patient outcomes. A reduction in the standardized mortality ratio in Dutch ICUs occurring concurrently with the Dutch national benchmarking activities suggests that benchmarking of ICU performance indicators is a promising tool to improve quality of ICU care [236]. Quality and performance indicators of ICUs have been published by national and international societies in both resource-rich and resource-limited settings [237–239]. While several national and international ICU registries and benchmarking projects exist in resource-rich countries [240], only a few national ICU registries exist in resource-limited settings, such as Sri Lanka [241] and Malaysia [242]. Similarly, internal and external clinical audits have been suggested as promising methods to improve quality of ICU care in resource-rich countries [243, 244], but consistent data from resource-limited settings are lacking.

Although implementation of protocols, bundles, and checklists into clinical practice requires a variable amount of funding, preliminary results of studies from resource-limited settings suggest that these interventions may prevent adverse events and complications [231, 232]. A delicate and important challenge of implementing protocols, care bundles, and checklists into clinical practice in ICUs in resource-limited settings is the lack of safety data. Different disease pathologies, as well as absent treatment options (e.g., airway protection and mechanical ventilation), could well explain why certain interventions that were shown to improve patient outcome in resource-rich settings increased morbidity and mortality in resource-limited settings [215, 245–247]. This underlines the urgent need to test the efficacy and safety of adjusted care bundles and protocols to improve care of critically ill and sepsis patients in settings where resources are constrained [215, 248]. Another consideration is that quality control measure implementation may divert financial resources from clinical care. Although long-term reduction savings may occur due to avoidance of adverse events, the up-front expenditure may prove burdensome.

We *recommend* maintaining patient records and ICU documentation in accordance with national regulations and requirements (1D). We suggest that ICUs develop locally applicable bundles, protocols, and checklists to improve quality of care (2C). We *suggest* that ICUs systematically collect quality and performance indicators and participate in national/international benchmarking projects (2C).

3.9 Conclusions

We provide a series of simple, pragmatic recommendations for optimizing ICU infrastructure and organization in resource-limited settings. Understanding the great variability of technical, material, and human resources within and between these environments, each institution must determine the utility of implementing these recommendations based on local capabilities. Given the paucity of evidence, there remains a clear need for additional studies from resource-limited settings.

References

1. Marshall JC, Bosco L, Adhikari NK, Connolly B, Diaz JV, Dorman T, et al. What is an intensive care unit? A report of the task force of the World Federation of Societies of Intensive and Critical Care Medicine. J Crit Care. 2017;37:270–6. https://doi.org/10.1016/j.jcrc.2016.07.015.
2. Schultz MJ, Dunser MW, Dondorp AM, Adhikari NK, Iyer S, Kwizera A, et al. Global Intensive Care Working Group of the European Society of Intensive Care Medicine. Current challenges in the management of sepsis in ICUs in resource-poor settings and suggestions for the future. Intensive Care Med. 2017;43:612–624. https://doi.org/10.1007/s00134-017-4750-z.
3. Yoo EJ, Edwards JD, Dean ML, Dudley RA. Multidisciplinary critical care and intensivist staffing: results of a statewide survey and association with mortality. J Intensive Care Med. 2016;31:325–32. https://doi.org/10.1177/0885066614534605.
4. Wilcox ME, Chong CA, Niven DJ, Rubenfeld GD, Rowan KM, Wunsch H, et al. Do intensivist staffing patterns influence hospital mortality following ICU admission? A systematic review and meta-analyses. Crit Care Med. 2013;41(10):2253–74. https://doi.org/10.1097/CCM.0b013e318292313a.
5. Barrett H, Bion JF. An international survey of training in adult intensive care medicine. Intensive Care Med. 2005;31(4):553–61. https://doi.org/10.1007/s00134-005-2583-7.
6. CoBaTrICE Collaboration. The educational environment for training in intensive care medicine: structures, processes, outcomes and challenges in the European region. Intensive Care Med. 2009;35(9):1575–83.
7. van der Sluis FJ, Slagt C, Liebman B, Beute J, Mulder JW, Engel AF. The impact of open versus closed format ICU admission practices on the outcome of high risk surgical patients: a cohort analysis. BMC Surg. 2011;11:18.
8. Kerlin MP, Adhikari NK, Rose L, Wilcox ME, Bellamy CJ, Costa DK, et al. ATS Ad Hoc Committee on ICU Organization. An official American Thoracic Society Systematic review: the effect of nighttime intensivist staffing on mortality and length of stay among intensive care unit patients. Am J Respir Crit Care Med. 2017;195(3):383–93.
9. Banerjee R, Naessens JM, Seferian EG, Gajic O, Moriarty JP, Johnson MG, et al. Economic implications of nighttime attending intensivist coverage in a medical intensive care unit. Crit Care Med. 2011;39(6):1257–62.
10. Bray K, Wren I, Baldwin A, St Ledger U, Gibson V, Goodman S, et al. Standards for nurse staffing in critical care units determined by: The British Association of Critical Care Nurses, The Critical Care Networks National Nurse Leads, Royal College of Nursing Critical Care and In-flight Forum. Nurs Crit Care. 2010;15(3):109–11.
11. West E, Barron DN, Harrison D, Rafferty AM, Rowan K, Sanderson C. Nurse staffing, medical staffing and mortality in intensive care: an observational study. Int J Nurs Stud. 2014;51(5):781–94.
12. Dang D, Johantgen ME, Pronovost PJ, Jenckes MW, Bass EB. Postoperative complications: does intensive care unit staff nursing make a difference? Heart Lung. 2002;31(3):219–28.
13. Hugonnet S, Uçkay I, Pittet D. Staffing level: a determinant of late-onset ventilator-associated pneumonia. Crit Care. 2007;11(4):R80.
14. Valentin A, Capuzzo M, Guidet B, Moreno R, Metnitz B, Bauer P, et al. Research Group on Quality Improvement of the European Society of Intensive Care Medicine (ESICM); Sentinel Events Evaluation (SEE) Study Investigators. Errors in administration of parenteral drugs in intensive care units: multinational prospective study. BMJ. 2009;338:b814.
15. Kim JH, Hong SK, Kim KC, Lee MG, Lee KM, Jung SS, et al. Influence of full-time intensivist and the nurse-to-patient ratio on the implementation of severe sepsis bundles in Korean intensive care units. J Crit Care. 2012;27(4):414.e11–21.
16. Cho SH, Yun SC. Bed-to-nurse ratios, provision of basic nursing care, and in-hospital and 30-day mortality among acute stroke patients admitted to an intensive care unit: cross-sectional analysis of survey and administrative data. Int J Nurs Stud. 2009;46(8):1092–101.

17. Chant C, Dewhurst NF, Friedrich JO. Do we need a pharmacist in the ICU? Intensive Care Med. 2015;41(7):1314–20.
18. Engel HJ, Tatebe S, Alonzo PB, Mustille RL, Rivera MJ. Physical therapist-established intensive care unit early mobilization program: quality improvement project for critical care at the University of California San Francisco Medical Center. Phys Ther. 2013;93(7):975–85.
19. Braga JM, Hunt A, Pope J, Molaison E. Implementation of dietitian recommendations for enteral nutrition results in improved outcomes. J Am Diet Assoc. 2006;106(2):281–4.
20. Rimawi RH, Mazer MA, Siraj DS, Gooch M, Cook PP. Impact of regular collaboration between infectious diseases and critical care practitioners on antimicrobial utilization and patient outcome. Crit Care Med. 2013;41(9):2099–107.
21. Pronovost PJ, Angus DC, Dorman T, Robinson KA, Dremsizov TT, Young TL. Physician staffing patterns and clinical outcomes in critically ill patients: a systematic review. JAMA. 2002;288(17):2151–62.
22. Siebig S, Kuhls S, Imhoff M, Langgartner J, Reng M, Schölmerich J, et al. Collection of annotated data in a clinical validation study for alarm algorithms in intensive care—a methodologic framework. J Crit Care. 2010;25(1):128–35.
23. Weiss CH, Moazed F, McEvoy CA, Singer BD, Szleifer I, Amaral LA. Prompting physicians to address a daily checklist and process of care and clinical outcomes: a single-site study. Am J Respir Crit Care Med. 2011;184(6):680–6.
24. Wilcox ME, Adhikari NK. The effect of telemedicine in critically ill patients: systematic review and meta-analysis. Crit Care. 2012;16(4):R127.
25. Berenson RA, Grossman JM, November EA. Does telemonitoring of patients—the eICU—improve intensive care? Health Aff (Millwood). 2009;28(5):w937–47.
26. Chittawatanarat K, Pamorsinlapathum T. The impact of closed ICU model on mortality in general surgical intensive care unit. J Med Assoc Thail. 2009;92(12):1627–34.
27. Topeli A, Laghi F, Tobin MJ. Effect of closed unit policy and appointing an intensivist in a developing country. Crit Care Med. 2005;33(2):299–306.
28. Prayag S. ICUs worldwide: critical care in India. Crit Care. 2002;6(6):479–80.
29. Sherman CB, Carter EJ, Braendli O, Getaneh A, Schluger NW. The East African Training Initiative. A model training program in pulmonary and critical care medicine for low-income countries. Ann Am Thorac Soc. 2016;13(4):451–5.
30. Livianu J, Orlando JM, Giannini A, Terzi RG, Moock M, Marcos C, et al. Organization and staffing of intensive care units in Brazil. Crit Care. 2000;4(1):P219.
31. Du B, Xi X, Chen D, Peng J, China Critical Care Clinical Trial Group (CCCCTG). Clinical review: critical care medicine in mainland China. Crit Care. 2010;14(1):206.
32. Mathivha LR. ICUs worldwide: an overview of critical care medicine in South Africa. Crit Care. 2002;6(1):22–3.
33. Jiang SP, Zheng X, Li X, Lu XY. Effectiveness of pharmaceutical care in an intensive care unit from China. A pre- and post-intervention study. Saudi Med J. 2012;33(7):756–62.
34. Saokaew S, Maphanta S, Thangsomboon P. Impact of pharmacist's interventions on cost of drug therapy in intensive care unit. Pharm Pract (Granada). 2009;7(2):81–7.
35. Aljbouri TM, Alkhawaldeh MS, Abu-Rumman AE, Hasan TA, Khattar HM, Abu-Oliem AS. Impact of clinical pharmacist on cost of drug therapy in the ICU. Saudi Pharm J. 2013;21(4):371–4.
36. Wang T, Benedict N, Olsen KM, Luan R, Zhu X, Zhou N, et al. Effect of critical care pharmacist's intervention on medication errors: a systematic review and meta-analysis of observational studies. J Crit Care. 2015;30(5):1101–6.
37. Hassibian MR, Hassibian S. Telemedicine acceptance and implementation in developing countries: benefits, categories, and barriers. Razavi Int J Med. 2016;4(3).
38. Gupta S, Dewan S, Kaushal A, Seth A, Narula J, Varma A. eICU reduces mortality in STEMI patients in resource-limited areas. Glob Heart. 2014;9(4):425–7.
39. The World Bank. https://data.worldbank.org/indicator/SH.MED.PHYS.ZS?view=chart. Accessed 15 July 2017.
40. Crisp N, Chen L. Global supply of health professionals. N Engl J Med. 2014;370(10):950–7.

41. Rice B, Periyanayagam U, Chamberlain S, Dreifuss B, Hammerstedt H, Nelson S, et al. Mortality in children under five receiving nonphysician clinician emergency care in Uganda. Pediatrics. 2016;137(3):e20153201.
42. Chamberlain S, Stolz U, Dreifuss B, Nelson SW, Hammerstedt H, Andinda J, et al. Mortality related to acute illness and injury in rural Uganda: task shifting to improve outcomes. PLoS One. 2015;10(4):e0122559.
43. Baker T, Lugazia E, Eriksen J, Mwafongo V, Irestedt L, Konrad D. Emergency and critical care services in Tanzania: a survey of ten hospitals. BMC Health Serv Res. 2013;13:140.
44. Jochberger S, Ismailova F, Lederer W, Mayr VD, Luckner G, Wenzel V, et al. "Helfen Berührt" Study Team. Anesthesia and its allied disciplines in the developing world: a nationwide survey of the Republic of Zambia. Anesth Analg. 2008;106(3):942–8, table of contents.
45. The World Bank. https://data.worldbank.org/indicator/SH.MED.NUMW.P3?view=chart. Accessed 15 July 2017.
46. Munyiginya P, Brysiewicz P, Mill J. Critical care nursing practice and education in Rwanda. Southern African J Crit Care. 2016;32(2):55.
47. Marshall JC, Bosco L, Adhikari NK, Connolly B, Diaz JV, Dorman T, et al. What is an intensive care unit? A report of the task force of the World Federation of Societies of Intensive and Critical Care Medicine. J Crit Care. 2017;37:270–6.
48. Klopotowska JE, Kuiper R, van Kan HJ, de Pont AC, Dijkgraaf MG, Lie-A-Huen L, et al. On-ward participation of a hospital pharmacist in a Dutch intensive care unit reduces prescribing errors and related patient harm: an intervention study. Crit Care. 2010;14(5):R174. https://doi.org/10.1186/cc9278.
49. Riviello ED, Letchford S, Achieng L, Newton MW. Critical care in resource-poor settings: lessons learned and future directions. Crit Care Med. 2011;39(4):860–7.
50. Levine AR, Robertson TE, Papali A, Verceles AC, McCurdy MT. Tele-medicine and point-of-care ultrasound: a new paradigm for resource-constrained settings. Chest. 2016;149(6):1580–1.
51. Papali A, McCurdy MT, Calvello EJ. A "three delays" model for severe sepsis in resource-limited countries. J Crit Care. 2015;30(4):861.e9–14.
52. Mock CN, Quansah R, Addae-Mensah L, Donkor P. The development of continuing education for trauma care in an African nation. Injury. 2005;36(6):725–32.
53. Stephens T, De Silva AP, Beane A, Welch J, Sigera C, De Alwis S, et al. Capacity building for critical care training delivery: development and evaluation of the Network for Improving Critical care Skills Training (NICST) programme in Sri Lanka. Intensive Crit Care Nurs. 2017;39:28–36.
54. De Silva AP, Stephens T, Welch J, Sigera C, De Alwis S, Athapattu P, et al. Nursing intensive care skills training: a nurse led, short, structured, and practical training program, developed and tested in a resource–limited setting. J Crit Care. 2015;30(2):438.e7–11.
55. Thunpattu S, Newey V, Sigera C, De Silva P, Goonarathna A, Aluthge I, et al. The effect of a practical ICU workshop on the knowledge, attitudes and skills of physiotherapists in Sri Lanka. https://www.nicslk.com/posters/150330170324physio%20workshop%20paper.pdf. Accessed 5 Jan 2017.
56. MacLeod JB, Okech M, Labib M, Aphivantrakul P, Lupasha E, Nthele M. Evaluation of trauma and critical care training courses on the knowledge and confidence of participants in Kenya and Zambia. World J Surg. 2011;35:9–16.
57. Macleod JB, Jones T, Aphivantrakul P, Chupp M, Poenaru D. Evaluation of fundamental critical care course in Kenya: knowledge, attitude, and practice. J Surg Res. 2011;167:223–30.
58. Robertson TE, Levine AR, Verceles AC, Buchner JA, Lantry JH 3rd, Papali A, et al. Remote tele-mentored ultrasound for non-physician learners using FaceTime: a feasibility study in a low-income country. J Crit Care. 2017;40:145–8.
59. Albert TJ, Fassier T, Chhuoy M, Bounchan Y, Tan S, Ku N, et al. Bolstering medical education to enhance critical care capacity in Cambodia. Ann Am Thorac Soc. 2015;12(4):491–7.
60. Haglund MM, Kiryabwire J, Parker S, Zomorodi A, MacLeod D, Schroeder R, et al. Surgical capacity building in Uganda through twinning, technology, and training camps. World J Surg. 2011;35(6):1175–82.

61. Ulisubisya M, Jörnvall H, Irestedt L, Baker T. Establishing an Anaesthesia and Intensive Care partnership and aiming for national impact in Tanzania. Glob Health. 2016;12:7. https://doi.org/10.1186/s12992–016–0144–1.
62. W/Tsadik A, Azazh A, Teklu S, Seyum N, Geremew H, Rankin P, et al. Development of emergency medicine and critical care masters program for nurses at Addis Ababa University, School of Medicine. Ethiop Med J. 2014;Suppl 2:21–6.
63. BASIC for Developing Healthcare Systems. https://www.aic.cuhk.edu.hk/web8/BASIC%20DHS.htm. Accessed 24 July 2017.
64. Joynt GM, Zimmerman J, Li TS, Gomersall CD. A systematic review of short courses for nonspecialist education in intensive care. J Crit Care. 2011;26(5):533.e1–10. https://doi.org/10.1016/j.jcrc.2011.01.007.
65. Belle J, Cohen H, Shindo N, Lim M, Velazquez-Berumen A, Ndihokubwayo JB, et al. Influenza preparedness in low-resource settings: a look at oxygen delivery in 12 African countries. J Infect Dev Ctries. 2010;4(7):419–24.
66. Morrissey B, Conroy N, Estelle A. Effect of solar panels on inpatient paediatric mortality in a district hospital in Sierra Leone (abstract). Arch Dis Child. 2015;100(Suppl 3):A114.
67. Turnbull H, Conroy A, Opoka RO, Namasopo S, Kain KC, Hawkes M. Solar-powered oxygen delivery: proof of concept. Int J Tuberc Lung Dis. 2016;20(5):696–703.
68. WHO model list of essential medicines: 17th list, March 2011. Geneva: World Health Organization; 2011. http://apps.who.int/iris/handle/10665/70640. Accessed 1 Mar 2017.
69. Meara JG, Leather AJ, Hagander L, Alkire BC, Alonso N, Ameh EA, et al. Global Surgery 2030: evidence and solutions for achieving health, welfare, and economic development. Lancet. 2015;386:569–624.
70. Papali A, Verceles AC, Augustin ME, Colas LN, Jean-Francois CH, Patel DM, et al. Sepsis in Haiti: prevalence, treatment, and outcomes in a Port-au-Prince referral hospital. J Crit Care. 2017;38:35–40.
71. Wandi F, Peel D, Duke T. Hypoxaemia among children in rural hospitals in Papua New Guinea: epidemiology and resource availability—a study to support a national oxygen programme. Ann Trop Paediatr. 2006;26(4):277–84.
72. Sutherland T, Musafiri S, Twagirumugabe T, Talmor D, Riviello ED. Oxygen as an essential medicine: under- and over-treatment of hypoxemia in low- and high-income nations. Crit Care Med. 2016;44(10):e1015–6.
73. Foran M, Ahn R, Novik J, Tyer-Viola L, Chilufya K, Katamba K, et al. Prevalence of undiagnosed hypoxemia in adults and children in an under-resourced district hospital in Zambia. Int J Emerg Med. 2010;3(4):351–6.
74. Duke T, Peel D, Wandi F, Subhi R, Sa'avu Martin, Matai S. Oxygen supplies for hospitals in Papua New Guinea: a comparison of the feasibility and cost-effectiveness of methods for different settings. P N G Med J 2010;53(3–4):126–138.
75. Bradley BD, Light JD, Ebonyi AO, N'Jai PC, Ideh RC, Ebruke BE, et al. Implementation and 8-year follow-up of an uninterrupted oxygen supply system in a hospital in The Gambia. Int J Tuberc Lung Dis. 2016;20(8):1130–4.
76. Peel D, Howie SRC. Oxygen concentrators for use in tropical countries: a survey. J Clin Eng. 2009;34(4):205–9.
77. Howie SR, Hill S, Ebonyi A, Krishnan G, Njie O, Sanneh M, et al. Meeting oxygen needs in Africa: an options analysis from the Gambia. Bull World Health Organ. 2009;87(10):763–71.
78. http://freewestmedia.com/2016/12/29/south-africas-copper-thieves-putting-lives-at-risk/. Accessed 17 Aug 2017.
79. Duke T, Wandi F, Jonathan M, Matai S, Kaupa M, Saavu M, et al. Improved oxygen systems for childhood pneumonia: a multihospital effectiveness study in Papua New Guinea. Lancet. 2008;372(9646):1328–33.
80. Pittet D, Donaldson L. Clean care is safer care: the first global challenge of the WHO world alliance for patient safety. Infect Control Hosp Epidemiol. 2005;26(11):891–4.

81. Allegranzi B, Nejad SB, Combescure C, Graafmans W, Attar H, Donaldson L, et al. Burden of endemic health-care-associated infection in developing countries: systematic review and meta-analysis. Lancet. 2011;377:228–41.
82. Wasswa P, Nalwadda CK, Buregyeya E, Gitta SN, Anguzu P, Nuwaha F. Implementation of infection control in health facilities in Arua district, Uganda: a cross-sectional study. BMC Infect Dis. 2015;15:268.
83. Horng LM, Unicomb L, Alam MU, Halder AK, Shoab AK, Ghosh PK, et al. Healthcare worker and family caregiver hand hygiene in Bangladeshi healthcare facilities: results from the Bangladesh National Hygiene Baseline Survey. J Hosp Infect. 2016;94(3):286–94.
84. World Health Organization. 2009: WHO guidelines on hand hygiene in health care: a summary first global patient safety challenge clean care is safer care. 2009. http://www.who.int/gpsc/5may/tools/9789241597906/en/. Accessed 3 May 2017.
85. Rosenthal VD, Pawar M, Leblebicioglu H, Navoa-Ng JA, Villamil-Gómez W, Armas-Ruiz A, et al. Impact of the International Nosocomial Infection Control Consortium (INICC) multidimensional hand hygiene approach over 13 years in 51 cities of 19 limited–resource countries from Latin America, Asia, the Middle East, and Europe. Infect Control Hosp Epidemiol. 2013;34(4):415–23.
86. Chakravarthy M, Myatra SN, Rosenthal VD, Udwadia FE, Gokul BN, Divatia JV, et al. The impact of the International Nosocomial Infection Control Consortium (INICC) multicenter, multidimensional hand hygiene approach in two cities of India. J Infect Public Health. 2015;8(2):177–86.
87. Su D, Hu B, Rosenthal VD, Li R, Hao C, Pan W, et al. Impact of the International Nosocomial Infection Control Consortium (INICC) Multidimensional Hand Hygiene Approach in five intensive care units in three cities of China. Public Health. 2015;129(7):979–88.
88. Miranda-Novales MG, Sobreyra-Oropeza M, Rosenthal VD, Higuera F, Armas-Ruiz A, Pérez-Serrato I, et al. Impact of the International Nosocomial Infection Control Consortium (INICC) multidimensional hand hygiene approach during 3 years in 6 hospitals in 3 Mexican cities. J Patient Saf. 2015.
89. Barrera L, Zingg W, Mendez F, Pittet D. Effectiveness of a hand hygiene promotion strategy using alcohol-based handrub in 6 intensive care units in Colombia. Am J Infect Control. 2011;39:633–9.
90. Abaza AF, Amine AE, Hazzah WA. Comparative study on efficacy of different alcohol hand rubs and routine hand wash in a health-care setting, Alexandria, Egypt. J Egypt Public Health Assoc. 2010;85(5–6):273–83.
91. Girou E, Loyeau S, Legrand P, Oppein F, Brun-Buisson C. Efficacy of handrubbing with alcohol based solution versus standard handwashing with antiseptic soap: randomised clinical trial. BMJ. 2002;325(7360):362.
92. Poliquin PG, Vogt F, Kasztura M, Leung A, Deschambault Y, Van den Bergh R, et al. Environmental contamination and persistence of Ebola virus RNA in an Ebola treatment center. J Infect Dis. 2016;214(suppl 3):S145–52.
93. Wolfe MK, Wells E, Mitro B, Desmarais AM, Scheinman P, Lantagne D. Seeking clearer recommendations for hand hygiene in communities facing Ebola: a randomized trial investigating the impact of six hand washing methods on skin irritation and dermatitis. PLoS One. 2016;11(12):e0167378. https://doi.org/10.1371/journal.pone.0167378.
94. Rossoff LJ, Lam S, Hilton E, Borenstein M, Isenberg HD. Is the use of boxed gloves in an intensive care unit safe? Am J Med. 1993;94(6):602–7.
95. Luckey JB, Barfield RD, Eleazer PD. Bacterial count comparisons on examination gloves from freshly opened boxes versus nearly empty boxes and from examination gloves before treatment versus after dental dam isolation. J Endod. 2006;32(7):646–8.
96. Rock C, Harris AD, Reich NG, Johnson JK, Thom KA. Is hand hygiene before putting on nonsterile gloves in the intensive care unit a waste of healthcare worker time?—a randomized controlled trial. Am J Infect Control. 2013;41(11):994–6.
97. Diaz MH, Silkaitis C, Malczynski M, Noskin GA, Warren JR, Zembower T. Contamination of examination gloves in patient rooms and implications for transmission of antimicrobial-resistant microorganisms. Infect Control Hosp Epidemiol. 2008;29(1):63–5.

98. Popp W, Rasslan O, Unahalekhaka A, Brenner P, Fischnaller E, Fathy M, et al. What is the use? An international look at reuse of single-use medical devices. Int J Hyg Environ Health. 2010;213(4):302–7. https://doi.org/10.1016/j.ijheh.2010.04.003. Epub 2010 May 13.
99. Hagos B, Kibwage IO, Mwongera M, Muthotho JN, Githiga IM, Mukindia GG. The microbial and physical quality of recycled gloves. East Afr Med J. 1997;74(4):224–6.
100. Ali Z, Qadeer A, Akhtar A. To determine the effect of wearing shoe covers by medical staff and visitors on infection rates, mortality and length of stay in Intensive Care Unit. Pak J Med Sci. 2014;30(2):272–5.
101. Daschner F, Frank U, Just HM. Proven and unproven methods in hospital infection control in intensive care units. Chemioterapia. 1987;6(3):184–9.
102. Croft LD, Harris AD, Pineles L, Langenberg P, Shardell M, Fink JC, et al. Benefits of Universal Glove and Gown Primary Investigators. The effect of universal glove and gown use on adverse events in intensive care unit patients. Clin Infect Dis. 2015;61(4):545–53. https://doi.org/10.1093/cid/civ315.
103. Harris AD, Pineles L, Belton B, Johnson JK, Shardell M, Loeb M, Newhouse R, et al. Universal glove and gown use and acquisition of antibiotic-resistant bacteria in the ICU: a randomized trial. JAMA. 2013;310(15):1571–80.
104. Huskins WC, Huckabee CM, O'Grady NP, Murray P, Kopetskie H, Zimmer L, et al. Intervention to reduce transmission of resistant bacteria in intensive care. N Engl J Med. 2011;364(15):1407–18.
105. Webster J and Pritchard MA. Gowning by attendants and visitors in newborn nurseries for prevention of neonatal morbidity and mortality. Cochrane Database Syst Rev 2003;(3):CD003670.
106. Mehta Y, Gupta A, Todi S, Myatra SN, Samaddar DP, Vijaya P, et al. Guidelines for prevention of hospital acquired infections. Indian J Crit Care Med. 2014;18(3):149–63.
107. World Health Organization. Guidelines on core components of infection prevention and control programmes at the national and acute health care facility level. http://www.who.int/gpsc/ipc-components-guidelines/en/. Accessed 22 Aug 2017.
108. Smith JD, MacDougall CC, Johnstone J, Copes RA, Schwartz B, Garber GE. Effectiveness of N95 respirators versus surgical masks in protecting health care workers from acute respiratory infection: a systematic review and meta-analysis. CMAJ. 2016;188(8):567–74.
109. Jefferson T, Del Mar CB, Dooley L, Ferroni E, Al-Ansary LA, Bawazeer GA, et al. Physical interventions to interrupt or reduce the spread of respiratory viruses. Cochrane Database Syst Rev. 2011;(7):CD006207.
110. Loeb M, Dafoe N, Mahony J, John M, Sarabia A, Glavin V, et al. Surgical mask vs N95 respirator for preventing influenza among health care workers: a randomized trial. JAMA. 2009;302(17):1865–71.
111. Centers for Disease Control and Prevention. Guideline for isolation precautions: preventing transmission of infectious agents in healthcare settings. 2007. https://www.cdc.gov/infection-control/guidelines/isolation/index.html. Accessed 21 May 2017.
112. World Health Organization. Personal protective equipment for use in a filovirus disease outbreak: rapid advice guideline. 2016. https://www.ncbi.nlm.nih.gov/books/NBK401170/. Accessed 21 May 2017.
113. Pronovost P, Needham D, Berenholtz S, Sinopoli D, Chu H, Cosgrove S, et al. An intervention to decrease catheter-related bloodstream infections in the ICU. N Engl J Med. 2006;355(26):2725–32.
114. Latif A, Kelly B, Edrees H, Kent PS, Weaver SJ, Jovanovic B, et al. Implementing a multifaceted intervention to decrease central line-associated bloodstream infections in SEHA (Abu Dhabi Health Services Company) intensive care units: the Abu Dhabi experience. Infect Control Hosp Epidemiol. 2015;36(7):816–22.
115. Marsteller JA, Sexton JB, Hsu YJ, Hsiao CJ, Holzmueller CG, Pronovost PJ, et al. A multicenter, phased, cluster-randomized controlled trial to reduce central line-associated bloodstream infections in intensive care units*. Crit Care Med. 2012;40(11):2933–9.

116. Lin DM, Weeks K, Bauer L, Combes JR, George CT, Goeschel CA, et al. Eradicating central line-associated bloodstream infections statewide: the Hawaii experience. Am J Med Qual. 2012;27(2):124–9.
117. Hong AL, Sawyer MD, Shore A, Winters BD, Masuga M, Lee H, et al. Decreasing central-line-associated bloodstream infections in Connecticut intensive care units. J Healthc Qual. 2013;35(5):78–87.
118. Sagana R, Hyzy RC. Achieving zero central line-associated bloodstream infection rates in your intensive care unit. Crit Care Clin. 2013;29(1):1–9.
119. Dettenkofer M, Seegers S, Antes G, Motschall E, Schumacher M, Daschner FD. Does the architecture of hospital facilities influence nosocomial infection rates? A systematic review. Infect Control Hosp Epidemiol. 2004;25(1):21–5.
120. Cepeda JA, Whitehouse T, Cooper B, Hails J, Jones K, Kwaku F, et al. Isolation of patients in single rooms or cohorts to reduce spread of MRSA in intensive-care units: prospective two-centre study. Lancet. 2005;365(9456):295–304.
121. Leaf DE, Homel P, Factor PH. Relationship between ICU design and mortality. Chest. 2010;137(5):1022–7.
122. Arabi YM, Phua J, Koh Y, Du B, Faruq MO, Nishimura M, et al; Asian Critical Care Clinical Trials Group. Structure, organization, and delivery of critical care in Asian ICUs. Crit Care Med 2016;44(10):e940–8.
123. Escombe AR, Moore DA, Gilman RH, Navincopa M, Ticona E, Mitchell B, et al. Upper room ultraviolet light and negative air ionization to prevent tuberculosis transmission. PLoS Med. 2009;6(3):e43.
124. Mphaphlele M, Dharmadhikari AS, Jensen PA, Rudnick SN, van Reenen TH, Pagano MA, et al. Institutional Tuberculosis Transmission. Controlled trial of upper room ultraviolet air disinfection: a basis for new dosing guidelines. Am J Respir Crit Care Med. 2015;192(4):477–84.
125. Mehta Y, Gupta A, Todi S, Myatra S, Samaddar DP, Patil V, et al. Guidelines for prevention of hospital acquired infections. Indian J Crit Care Med. 2014;18(3):149–63.
126. World Health Organization. Guide to local production: WHO-recommended handrub formulations. http://www.who.int/gpsc/5may/Guide_to_Local_Production.pdf. Accessed 16 Aug 2017.
127. Iqbal Q, Lubeck-Schricker M, Wells E, Wolfe MK, Lantagne D. Shelf-life of chlorine solutions recommended in Ebola virus disease response. PLoS One. 2016;11(5):e0156136. https://doi.org/10.1371/journal.pone.0156136.
128. Thi Anh Thu L, Thi Hong Thoa V, Thi Van Trang D, Phuc Tien N, Thuy Van D, Thi Kim Anh L, et al. Cost-effectiveness of a hand hygiene program on health care-associated infections in intensive care patients at a tertiary care hospital in Vietnam. Am J Infect Control. 2015;43(12):e93–9.
129. Nthumba PM, Stepita-Poenaru E, Poenaru D, Bird P, Allegranzi B, Pittet D, et al. Cluster-randomized, crossover trial of the efficacy of plain soap and water versus alcohol-based rub for surgical hand preparation in a rural hospital in Kenya. Br J Surg. 2010;97(11):1621–8.
130. Ahmed QA, Memish ZA, Allegranzi B, Pittet D. Muslim health-care workers and alcohol-based handrubs. Lancet. 2006;367(9515):1025–7.
131. Chughtai AA, Seale H, Chi Dung T, Maher L, Nga PT, MacIntyre CR. Current practices and barriers to the use of facemasks and respirators among hospital-based health care workers in Vietnam. Am J Infect Control. 2015;43(1):72–7. https://doi.org/10.1016/j.ajic.2014.10.009.
132. MacIntyre CR, Seale H, Dung TC, Hien NT, Nga PT, Chughtai AA, et al. A cluster randomised trial of cloth masks compared with medical masks in healthcare workers. BMJ Open. 2015;5(4):e006577.
133. World Health Organization. Infection prevention and control (IPC) guidance summary: Ebola guidance package. http://www.who.int//csr/disease/ebola/evid-guidance-summary/en/. Accessed 17 Aug 2017.

134. Lilford RJ, Burn SL, Diaconu KD, Lilford P, Chilton PJ, Bion V, et al. An approach to prioritization of medical devices in low-income countries: an example based on the Republic of South Sudan. Cost Eff Resour Alloc. 2015;13(1):2.
135. Bauserman M, Hailey C, Gado J, Lokangaka A, Williams J, Richards-Kortum R, et al. Determining the utility and durability of medical equipment donated to a rural clinic in a low-income country. Int Health. 2015;7(4):262–5.
136. Clarke DL, Chipps JA, Sartorius B, Bruce J, Laing GL, Brysiewicz P. Mortality rates increase dramatically below a systolic blood pressure of 105-mm Hg in septic surgical patients. Am J Surg. 2016;212(5):941–5.
137. Dünser MW, Ruokonen E, Pettilä V, Ulmer H, Torgersen C, Schmittinger CA, et al. Association of arterial blood pressure and vasopressor load with septic shock mortality: a post hoc analysis of a multicenter trial. Crit Care. 2009;13(6):R181.
138. Vellinga NA, Boerma EC, Koopmans M, Donati A, Dubin A, Shapiro N, et al. International study on microcirculatory shock occurrence in acutely ill patients. Crit Care Med. 2015;43(1):48–56.
139. Seymour CW, Liu VX, Iwashyna TJ, Brunkhorst FM, Rea TD, Scherag A, et al. Assessment of clinical criteria for sepsis: for the third international consensus definitions for sepsis and septic shock (Sepsis-3). JAMA. 2016;315(8):762–74.
140. Riviello ED, Buregeya E, Twagirumugabe T. Diagnosing acute respiratory distress syndrome in resource limited settings: the Kigali modification of the Berlin definition. Curr Opin Crit Care. 2017;23(1):18–23.
141. Lazzerini M, Sonego M, Pellegrin MC. Hypoxaemia as a mortality risk factor in acute lower respiratory infections in children in low and middle-income countries: systematic review and meta-analysis. PLoS One. 2015;10(9):e0136166.
142. Orimadegun AE, Ogunbosi BO, Carson SS. Prevalence and predictors of hypoxaemia in respiratory and non-respiratory primary diagnoses among emergently ill children at a tertiary hospital in south western Nigeria. Trans R Soc Trop Med Hyg. 2013;107(11):699–705.
143. Baker T, Blixt J, Lugazia E, Schell CO, Mulungu M, Milton A, et al. Single deranged physiologic parameters are associated with mortality in a low-income country. Crit Care Med. 2015;43(10):2171–9.
144. Schell CO, Castegren M, Lugazia E, Blixt J, Mulungu M, Konrad D, et al. Severely deranged vital signs as triggers for acute treatment modifications on an intensive care unit in a low-income country. BMC Res Notes. 2015;8:313.
145. Waitt PI, Mukaka M, Goodson P, SimuKonda FD, Waitt CJ, Feasey N, et al. Sepsis carries a high mortality among hospitalised adults in Malawi in the era of antiretroviral therapy scale-up: a longitudinal cohort study. J Infect. 2015;70(1):11–9.
146. Thanachartwet V, Wattanathum A, Sahassananda D, Wacharasint P, Chamnanchanunt S, Khine Kyaw E, et al. Dynamic measurement of hemodynamic parameters and cardiac preload in adults with dengue: a prospective observational study. PLoS One. 2016;11(5):e0156135.
147. Baker T, Schell CO, Lugazia E, Blixt J, Mulungu M, Castegren M, et al. Vital signs directed therapy: improving care in an intensive care unit in a low-income country. PLoS One. 2015;10(12):e0144801.
148. Bur A, Hirschl MM, Herkner H, Oschatz E, Kofler J, Woisetschläger C, et al. Accuracy of oscillometric blood pressure measurement according to the relation between cuff size and upper-arm circumference in critically ill patients. Crit Care Med. 2000;28(2):371–6.
149. Lakhal K, Ehrmann S, Runge I, Legras A, Dequin PF, Mercier E, et al. Tracking hypotension and dynamic changes in arterial blood pressure with brachial cuff measurements. Anesth Analg. 2009;109(2):494–501.
150. Chatterjee A, DePriest K, Blair R, Bowton D, Chin R. Results of a survey of blood pressure monitoring by intensivists in critically ill patients: a preliminary study. Crit Care Med. 2010;38(12):2335–8.
151. Pedersen T, Nicholson A, Hovhannisyan K, Møller AM, Smith AF, Lewis SR. Pulse oximetry for perioperative monitoring. Cochrane Database Syst Rev. 2014;(3):CD002013.

152. Serpa Neto A, Cardoso SO, Ong DS, Espósito DC, Pereira VG, Manetta JA, et al. The use of the pulse oximetric saturation/fraction of inspired oxygen ratio for risk stratification of patients with severe sepsis and septic shock. J Crit Care. 2013;28(5):681–6.
153. Serpa Neto A, Schultz MJ, Festic E. Ventilatory support of patients with sepsis or septic shock in resource-limited settings. Intensive Care Med. 2016;42(1):100–3.
154. Becker DM, Tafoya CA, Becker SL, Kruger GH, Tafoya MJ, Becker TK. The use of portable ultrasound devices in low- and middle-income countries: a systematic review of the literature. Tropical Med Int Health. 2016;21(3):294–311.
155. Thwaites CL, Yen LM, Nga NT, Parry J, Binh NT, Loan HT, et al. Impact of improved vaccination programme and intensive care facilities on incidence and outcome of tetanus in southern Vietnam, 1993–2002. Trans R Soc Trop Med Hyg. 2004;98(11):671–7.
156. Trieu HT, Lubis IN, Qui PT, Yen LM, Wills B, Thwaites CL, Sabanathan S. Neonatal tetanus in Vietnam: comprehensive intensive care support improves mortality. J Pediatric Infect Dis Soc. 2016;5(2):227–30. https://doi.org/10.1093/jpids/piv059.
157. Haniffa R, Lubell Y, Cooper BS, Mohanty S, Alam S, Karki A, et al. Impact of a structured ICU training programme in resource-limited settings in Asia. PLoS One. 2017;12(3):e0173483.
158. Balfour-Lynn RE, Marsh G, Gorayi D, Elahi E, LaRovere J. Non-invasive ventilation for children with acute respiratory failure in the developing world: literature review and an implementation example. Paediatr Respir Rev. 2014;15(2):181–7.
159. Verma AK, Mishra M, Kant S, Kumar A, Verma SK, Chaudhri S, et al. Noninvasive mechanical ventilation: an 18-month experience of two tertiary care hospitals in north India. Lung India. 2013;30(4):307–11.
160. Wilson PT, Morris MC, Biagas KV, Otupiri E, Moresky RT. A randomized clinical trial evaluating nasal continuous positive airway pressure for acute respiratory distress in a developing country. J Pediatr. 2013;162(5):988–92.
161. Chisti MJ, Salam MA, Smith JH, Ahmed T, Pietroni MA, Shahunja KM, et al. Bubble continuous positive airway pressure for children with severe pneumonia and hypoxaemia in Bangladesh: an open, randomised controlled trial. Lancet. 2015;386(9998):1057–65.
162. Jayashree M, KiranBabu HB, Singhi S, Nallasamy K. Use of nasal bubble CPAP in children with hypoxemic clinical pneumonia–report from a resource limited set-up. J Trop Pediatr. 2016;62(1):69–74.
163. Kawaza K, Machen HE, Brown J, Mwanza Z, Iniguez S, Gest A, et al. Efficacy of a low-cost bubble CPAP system in treatment of respiratory distress in a neonatal ward in Malawi. Malawi Med J. 2016;28(3):131–7.
164. Langhan M. Continuous end-tidal carbon dioxide monitoring in pediatric intensive care units. J Crit Care. 2009;24(2):227–30.
165. Erasmus PD. The use of end-tidal carbon dioxide monitoring to confirm endotracheal tube placement in adult and paediatric intensive care units in Australia and New Zealand. Anaesth Intensive Care. 2004;32(5):672–5.
166. Ginosar Y, Shapira SC. The role of an anaesthetist in a field hospital during the cholera epidemic among Rwandan refugees in Goma. Br J Anaesth. 1995;75(6):810–6.
167. Husaini J, Choy YC. End-tidal to arterial carbon dioxide partial pressure difference during craniotomy in anaesthetised patients. Med J Malaysia. 2008;63(5):384–7.
168. Prause G, Hetz H, Lauda P, Pojer H, Smolle-Juettner F, Smolle J. A comparison of the end-tidal-CO_2 documented by capnometry and the arterial pCO_2 in emergency patients. Resuscitation. 1997;35(2):145–8.
169. Totapally BR. Utility of end-tidal carbon dioxide monitoring in critically ill children. Indian J Crit Care Med. 2014;18(6):341–2.
170. Thrush DN, Mentis SW, Downs JB. Weaning with end-tidal CO_2 and pulse oximetry. J Clin Anesth. 1991;3(6):456–60.
171. Healey CJ, Fedullo AJ, Swinburne AJ, Wahl GW. Comparison of noninvasive measurements of carbon dioxide tension during withdrawal from mechanical ventilation. Crit Care Med. 1987;15(8):764–8.

172. Bluemile LW Jr, Webster GD Jr, Elkinton JR. Acute tubular necrosis; analysis of one hundred cases with respect to mortality, complications, and treatment with and without dialysis. AMA Arch Intern Med. 1959;104(2):180–97.
173. Arogundade FA, Sanusi AA, Okunola OO, Soyinka FO, Ojo OE, Akinsola A. Acute renal failure (ARF) in developing countries: which factors actually influence survival. Cent Afr J Med. 2007;53(5–8):34–9.
174. Mer M, Schultz MJ, Adhikari NK (2017) European Society of Intensive Care Medicine (ESICM) Global Intensive Care Working Group and the Mahidol-Oxford Research Unit (MORU), Bangkok, Thailand Core elements of general supportive care for patients with sepsis and septic shock in resource-limited settings Intensive Care Med. https://doi.org/10.1007/s00134-017-4831-z.
175. Park S, Kim DG, Suh GY, Kang JG, Ju YS, Lee YJ, et al. Mild hypoglycemia is independently associated with increased risk of mortality in patients with sepsis: a 3-year retrospective observational study. Crit Care. 2012;16(5):R189.
176. Bagshaw SM, Bellomo R, Jacka MJ, Egi M, Hart GK, George C. The impact of early hypoglycemia and blood glucose variability on outcome in critical illness. Crit Care. 2009;13(3):R91.
177. Casserly B, Phillips GS, Schorr C, Dellinger RP, Townsend SR, Osborn TM, et al. Lactate measurements in sepsis-induced tissue hypoperfusion: results from the Surviving Sepsis Campaign database. Crit Care Med. 43(3):567–73.
178. Mikkelsen ME, Miltiades AN, Gaieski DF, Goyal M, Fuchs BD, Shah CV, et al. Serum lactate is associated with mortality in severe sepsis independent of organ failure and shock. Crit Care Med. 2009;37(5):1670–7.
179. Nguyen HB, Rivers EP, Knoblich BP, Jacobsen G, Muzzin A, Ressler JA, et al. Early lactate clearance is associated with improved outcome in severe sepsis and septic shock. Crit Care Med. 2004;32(8):1637–42.
180. Moore CC, Jacob ST, Pinkerton R, Meya DB, Mayanja-Kizza H, Reynolds SJ, et al. Point-of-care lactate testing predicts mortality of severe sepsis in a predominantly HIV type 1-infected patient population in Uganda. Clin Infect Dis. 2008;46(2):215–22.
181. Mtove G, Nadjm B, Hendriksen IC, Amos B, Muro F, Todd J, et al. Point-of-care measurement of blood lactate in children admitted with febrile illness to an African District Hospital. Clin Infect Dis. 2011;53(6):548–54.
182. Krishna S, Waller DW, ter Kuile F, Kwiatkowski D, Crawley J, Craddock CF, Nosten F, et al. Lactic acidosis and hypoglycaemia in children with severe malaria: pathophysiological and prognostic significance. Trans R Soc Trop Med Hyg. 1994;88:67–73.
183. Molyneux ME, Taylor TE, Wirima JJ, Borgstein A. Clinical features and prognostic indicators in paediatric cerebral malaria: a study of 131 comatose Malawian children. Q J Med. 1989;71:441–59.
184. Subbarao S, Wilkinson KA, van Halsema CL, Rao SS, Boyles T, Utay NS, et al. Raised venous lactate and markers of intestinal translocation are associated with mortality among in-patients with HIV-associated TB in Rural South Africa. J Acquir Immune Defic Syndr. 2015;70(4):406–13.
185. Krishna U, Joshi SP, Modh M. An evaluation of serial blood lactate measurement as an early predictor of shock and its outcome in patients of trauma or sepsis. Indian J Crit Care Med. 2009;13(2):66–73.
186. Ssekitoleko R, Jacob ST, Banura P, Pinkerton R, Meya DB, Reynolds SJ, et al. Hypoglycemia at admission is associated with in hospital mortality in Ugandan patients with severe sepsis. Crit Care Med. 2011;39(10):2271–6.
187. Jallow M, Casals-Pascual C, Ackerman H, Walther B, Walther M, Pinder M, et al. Clinical features of severe malaria associated with death: a 13-year observational study in the Gambia. PLoS One. 2012;7(9):e45645.
188. Jones KL, Donegan S, Lalloo DG. Artesunate versus quinine for treating severe malaria. Cochrane Database Syst Rev. 2007;(4):CD005967.

189. Ramachandran B, Sethuraman R, Ravikumar KG, Kissoon N. Comparison of bedside and laboratory blood glucose estimations in critically ill children with shock. Pediatr Crit Care Med. 2011;12(6):e297–301.
190. Hawkes M, Conroy AL, Opoka RO, Namasopo S, Liles WC, John CC, et al. Performance of point-of-care diagnostics for glucose, lactate, and hemoglobin in the management of severe malaria in a resource-constrained hospital in Uganda. Am J Trop Med Hyg. 2014;90(4):605–8.
191. Meynaar IA, van Spreuwel M, Tangkau PL, Dawson L, Sleeswijk Visser S, Rijks L, et al. Accuracy of AccuChek glucose measurement in intensive care patients. Crit Care Med. 2009;37(10):2691–6.
192. DuBois JA, Slingerland RJ, Fokkert M, Roman A, Tran NK, Clarke W, et al. Bedside glucose monitoring-is it safe? A new, regulatory-compliant risk assessment evaluation protocol in critically ill patient care settings. Crit Care Med. 2017;45(4):567–74.
193. Gu WJ, Zhang Z, Bakker J. Early lactate clearance-guided therapy in patients with sepsis: a meta-analysis with trial sequential analysis of randomized controlled trials. Intensive Care Med. 2015;41(10):1862–3.
194. Burri E, Potocki M, Drexler B, Schuetz P, Mebazaa A, Ahlfeld U, et al. Value of arterial blood gas analysis in patients with acute dyspnea: an observational study. Crit Care. 2011;15(3):R145. https://doi.org/10.1186/cc10268.
195. ARDS Definition Task Force, Ranieri VM, Rubenfeld GD, Thompson BT, Ferguson ND, Caldwell E, Fan E, et al. Acute respiratory distress syndrome: the Berlin Definition. JAMA. 2012;307(23):2526–33. https://doi.org/10.1001/jama.2012.5669.
196. Chawla R, Mansuriya J, Modi N, Pandey A, Juneja D, Chawla A, et al. Acute respiratory distress syndrome: Predictors of noninvasive ventilation failure and intensive care unit mortality in clinical practice. J Crit Care. 2016;31(1):26–30. https://doi.org/10.1016/j.jcrc.2015.10.018.
197. Chittawatanarat K, Morakul S, Thawitsri T. Non-cardiopulmonary monitoring in Thai-ICU (ICU–Resource I study). J Med Assoc Thail. 2014;97(Suppl 1):S31–7.
198. Chittawatanarat K, Wattanathum A, Chaiwat O. Cardiopulmonary monitoring in Thai ICUs (ICU–resource I study). J Med Assoc Thail. 2014;97(Suppl 1):S15–21.
199. Chittawatanarat K, Bunburaphong T, Champunot R. Mechanical ventilators availability survey in Thai ICUs (ICU–resource I study). J Med Assoc Thail. 2014;97 Suppl 1:S1–7.
200. LeBrun DG, Chackungal S, Chao TE, Knowlton LM, Linden AF, Notrica MR, et al. Prioritizing essential surgery and safe anesthesia for the Post 2015 Development Agenda: operative capacities of 78 district hospitals in 7 low- and middle-income countries. Surgery. 2014;155(3):365–73.
201. Bataar O, Lundeg G, Tsenddorj G, Jochberger S, Grander W, Baelani I, et al. Nationwide survey on resource availability for implementing current sepsis guidelines in Mongolia. Bull World Health Organ. 2010;88(11):839–46.
202. Baelani I, Jochberger S, Laimer T, Otieno D, Kabutu J, Wilson I, et al. Availability of critical care resources to treat patients with severe sepsis or septic shock in Africa: a self-reported, continent-wide survey of anaesthesia providers. Crit Care. 2011;15(1):R10.
203. Baelani I, Jochberger S, Laimer T, Rex C, Baker T, Wilson IH, et al. Identifying resource needs for sepsis care and guideline implementation in the Democratic Republic of the Congo: a cluster survey of 66 hospitals in four eastern provinces. Middle East J Anaesthesiol. 2012;21(4):559–75.
204. Mendsaikhan N, Gombo D, Lundeg G, Schmittinger C, Dünser MW. Management of potentially life-threatening emergencies at 74 primary level hospitals in Mongolia: results of a prospective, observational multicenter study. BMC Emerg Med. 2017;17(1):15.
205. Mendsaikhan N, Begzjav T, Lundeg G, Brunauer A, Dünser MW. A Nationwide Census of ICU Capacity and Admissions in Mongolia. PLoS One. 2016;11(8):e0160921.
206. Liyanage T, Ninomiya T, Jha V, Neal B, Patrice HM, Okpechi I, et al. Worldwide access to treatment for end-stage kidney disease: a systematic review. Lancet. 2015;385(9981):1975–82.

207. Gatrad AR, Gatrad S, Gatrad A. Equipment donation to developing countries. Anaesthesia. 2007;62 Suppl 1:90–95.
208. Burn SL, Chilton PJ, Gawande AA, Lilford RJ. Peri-operative pulse oximetry in low-income countries: a cost-effectiveness analysis. Bull World Health Organ. 2014;92(12):858–67.
209. Chen A, Deshmukh AA, Richards-Kortum R, Molyneux E, Kawaza K, Cantor SB. Cost-effectiveness analysis of a low-cost bubble CPAP device in providing ventilatory support for neonates in Malawi—a preliminary report. BMC Pediatr. 2014;14:288.
210. Patel SP, Pena ME, Babcock CI. Cost-effectiveness of noninvasive ventilation for chronic obstructive pulmonary disease-related respiratory failure in Indian hospitals without ICU facilities. Lung India. 2015;32(6):549–56.
211. Poesen K, De Prins M, Van den Berghe G, Van Eldere J, Vanstapel F. Performance of cassette-based blood gas analyzers to monitor blood glucose and lactate levels in a surgical intensive care setting. Clin Chem Lab Med. 2013;51(7):1417–27.
212. Singh S, Bhardawaj A, Shukla R, Jhadav T, Sharma A, Basannar D. The handheld blood lactate analyser versus the blood gas based analyser for measurement of serum lactate and its prognostic significance in severe sepsis. Med J Armed Forces India. 2016;72(4):325–31.
213. Dat VQ, Long NT, Giang KB, Diep PB, Giang TH, Diaz JV. Healthcare infrastructure capacity to respond to severe acute respiratory infection (SARI) and sepsis in Vietnam: a low-middle income country. J Crit Care. 2017;42:109–15. https://doi.org/10.1016/j.jcrc.2017.07.020.
214. Chen W, Janz DR, Shaver CM, Bernard GR, Bastarache JA, Ware LB. Clinical characteristics and outcomes are similar in ARDS diagnosed by oxygen saturation/FiO_2 ratio compared with PaO_2/FiO_2 ratio. Chest. 2015;148(6):1477–83. https://doi.org/10.1378/chest.15-0169.
215. Vukoja M, Riviello E, Gavrilovic S, Adhikari NK, Kashyap R, Bhagwanjee S. A survey on critical care resources and practices in low- and middle-income countries. Glob Heart. 2014;9(3):337-42.e1–5.
216. Schultz MJ, Dunser MW, Dondorp AM, Adhikari NK, Iyer S, Kwizera A, et al. Current challenges in the management of sepsis in ICUs in resource-poor settings and suggestions for the future. Intensive Care Med. 2017;43(5):612–24.
217. Thompson G, O'Horo JC, Pickering BW, Herasevich V. Impact of the electronic medical record on mortality, length of stay, and cost in the hospital and ICU: a systematic review and metaanalysis. Crit Care Med. 2015;43(6):1276–82.
218. Pronovost P, Berenholtz S, Dorman T, Lipsett PA, Simmonds T, Haraden C. Improving communication in the ICU using daily goals. J Crit Care. 2003;18(2):71–5.
219. Narasimhan M, Eisen LA, Mahoney CD, Acerra FL, Rosen MJ. Improving nurse-physician communication and satisfaction in the intensive care unit with a daily goals worksheet. Am J Crit Care. 2006;15(2):217–22.
220. Agarwal S, Frankel L, Tourner S, McMillan A, Sharek PJ. Improving communication in a pediatric intensive care unit using daily patient goal sheets. J Crit Care. 2008;23(2):227–35.
221. Centofanti JE, Duan EH, Hoad NC, Swinton ME, Perri D, Waugh L, et al. Use of a daily goals checklist for morning ICU rounds: a mixed-methods study. Crit Care Med. 2014;42(8):1797–803.
222. Perry V, Christiansen M, Simmons A. A daily goals tool to facilitate indirect nurse-physician communication during morning rounds on a medical-surgical unit. Medsurg Nurs. 2016;25(2):83–7.
223. Cavalcanti AB, Bozza FA, Machado FR, Salluh JI, Campagnucci VP, Vendramim P, et al. Effect of a quality improvement intervention with daily round checklists, goal setting, and clinician prompting on mortality of critically ill patients: a randomized clinical trial. JAMA. 2016;315(14):1480–90.
224. Ferrer R, Artigas A, Levy MM, Blanco J, González-Díaz G, Garnacho-Montero J, et al. Improvement in process of care and outcome after a multicenter severe sepsis educational program in Spain. JAMA. 2008;299(19):2294–303.
225. Barochia AV, Cui X, Vitberg D, Suffredini AF, O'Grady NP, Banks SM, et al. Bundled care for septic shock: an analysis of clinical trials. Crit Care Med. 2010;38(2):668–78.

226. Wang Z, Xiong Y, Schorr C, Dellinger RP. Impact of sepsis bundle strategy on outcomes of patients suffering from severe sepsis and septic shock in china. J Emerg Med. 2013;44(4):735–41.
227. Herrán-Monge R, Muriel-Bombín A, García-García MM, Merino-García PA, Cítores-González R, Fernández-Ratero JA, et al. Mortality reduction and long-term compliance with surviving sepsis campaign: a nationwide multicenter study. Shock. 2016;45(6):598–606.
228. Rhodes A, Phillips G, Beale R, Cecconi M, Chiche JD, De Backer D, et al. The Surviving Sepsis Campaign bundles and outcome: results from the International Multicentre Prevalence Study on Sepsis (the IMPreSS study). Intensive Care Med. 2015;41(9):1620–8.
229. Levy MM, Rhodes A, Phillips GS, Townsend SR, Schorr CA, Beale R, et al. Surviving Sepsis Campaign: association between performance metrics and outcomes in a 7.5-year study. Intensive Care Med. 2014;40(11):1623–33.
230. Jacob ST, Banura P, Baeten JM, Moore CC, Meya D, Nakiyingi L, et al. The impact of early monitored management on survival in hospitalized adult Ugandan patients with severe sepsis: a prospective intervention study*. Crit Care Med. 2012;40(7):2050–8.
231. Papali A, Eoin West T, Verceles AC, Augustin ME, Nathalie Colas L, Jean-Francois CH, et al. Treatment outcomes after implementation of an adapted WHO protocol for severe sepsis and septic shock in Haiti. J Crit Care. 2017;41:222–8.
232. Apisarnthanarak A, Thongphubeth K, Sirinvaravong S, Kitkangvan D, Yuekyen C, Warachan B, et al. Effectiveness of multifaceted hospitalwide qualityimprovement programs featuring an intervention to removeunnecessary urinary catheters at a tertiary care center in Thailand. Infect Control Hosp Epidemiol. 2007;28(7):791–8.
233. Apisarnthanarak A, Thongphubeth K, Yuekyen C, Warren DK, Fraser VJ. Effectiveness of a catheter-associated bloodstream infection bundle in a Thai tertiary care center: a 3-year study. Am J Infect Control. 2010;38(6):449–55.
234. Djogovic D, Green R, Keyes R, Gray S, Stenstrom R, Sweet D, et al. Canadian Association of Emergency Physicians sepsis treatment checklist: optimizing sepsis care in Canadian emergency departments. CJEM. 2012;14(1):36–9.
235. Ballow SL, Kaups KL, Anderson S, Chang M. A standardized rapid sequence intubation protocolfacilitates airway management in critically injured patients. J Trauma Acute Care Surg. 2012;73(6):1401–5.
236. Vukoja M, Kashyap R, Gavrilovic S, Dong Y, Kilickaya O, Gajic O. Checklist for early recognition and treatment of acute illness: International collaboration to improve critical care practice. World J Crit Care Med. 2015;4(1):55–61.
237. Woodhouse D, Berg M, van der Putten J, Houtepen J. Will benchmarking ICUs improve outcome? Curr Opin Crit Care. 2009;15(5):450–5.
238. Rhodes A, Moreno RP, Azoulay E, Capuzzo M, Chiche JD, Eddleston J, et al. Prospectively defined indicators to improve the safety and quality of care for critically ill patients: a report from the Task Force on Safety and Quality of the European Society of Intensive Care Medicine (ESICM). Intensive Care Med. 2012;38(4):598–605.
239. Braun JP, Kumpf O, Deja M, Brinkmann A, Marx G, Bloos F, et al. The German quality indicators in intensive care medicine 2013-second edition. Ger Med Sci. 2013;11:Doc09.
240. Ray B, Samaddar DP, Todi SK, Ramakrishnan N, John G, Ramasubban S. Quality indicators for ICU: ISCCM guidelines for ICUs in India. Indian J Crit Care Med. 2009;13(4):173–206.
241. Swedish Intensive Care Registry. http://www.icuregswe.org/en/About-Intensive-Care/registries/. Accessed 25 May 2017.
242. National Intensive Care Surveillance: a critical care clinical registry and bed availability system for Sri Lanka. http://www.nicslk.com/. Accessed 25 May 2017.
243. Malaysian Registry of Intensive Care. http://mric.org.my/Web/Page/index.aspx. Accessed 25 May 2017.
244. Wong A, Masterson G. Improving quality in intensive care unit practice through clinical audit. J Intensive Care Soc. 2015;16(1):5–8.

245. Colvin JR, Peden C, editors. Raising the Standard: a compendium of audit recipes for continuous quality improvement in anaesthesia. Royal College of Anaesthetists; 2012. http://www.rcoa.ac.uk/system/files/CSQ-ARB-2012_1.pdf.
246. Scales DC, Dainty K, Hales B, Pinto R, Fowler RA, Adhikari NK, et al. A multifaceted intervention for quality improvement in a network of intensive care units: a cluster randomized trial. JAMA. 2011;305(4):363–72.
247. Andrews B, Muchemwa L, Kelly P, Lakhi S, Heimburger DC, Bernard GR. Simplified severe sepsis protocol: a randomized controlled trial of modified early goal-directed therapy in Zambia. Crit Care Med. 2014;42(11):2315–24.
248. Maitland K, Kiguli S, Opoka RO, Engoru C, Olupot-Olupot P, Akech SO, et al. Mortality after fluid bolus in African children with severe infection. N Engl J Med. 2011;364(26):2483–95.

Open Access This chapter is licensed under the terms of the Creative Commons Attribution 4.0 International License (http://creativecommons.org/licenses/by/4.0/), which permits use, sharing, adaptation, distribution and reproduction in any medium or format, as long as you give appropriate credit to the original author(s) and the source, provide a link to the Creative Commons license and indicate if changes were made.

The images or other third party material in this chapter are included in the chapter's Creative Commons license, unless indicated otherwise in a credit line to the material. If material is not included in the chapter's Creative Commons license and your intended use is not permitted by statutory regulation or exceeds the permitted use, you will need to obtain permission directly from the copyright holder.

Recognition of Sepsis in Resource-Limited Settings

4

Arthur Kwizera, Neill K. J. Adhikari, Derek C. Angus, Arjen M. Dondorp, Martin W. Dünser, Emir Festic, Rashan Haniffa, Niranjan Kissoon, Ignacio Martin-Loeches, and Ganbold Lundeg

A. Kwizera
Makerere University College of Health Sciences, Mulago National Referral Hospital, Kampala, Uganda

N. K. J. Adhikari
Sunnybrook Health Sciences Centre, University of Toronto, Toronto, ON, Canada

D. C. Angus
University of Pittsburgh, Pittsburgh, PA, USA

A. M. Dondorp
Faculty of Tropical Medicine, Mahidol University, Bangkok, Thailand

Academic Medical Center, University of Amsterdam, Amsterdam, The Netherlands

Nuffield Department of Clinical Medicine, Oxford Centre for Tropical Medicine and Global Health, University of Oxford, Oxford, UK

M. W. Dünser (✉)
Department of Anesthesiology and Intensive Care Medicine, Kepler University Hospital, Johannes Kepler University Linz, Linz, Austria
e-mail: Martin.Duenser@i-med.ac.at

E. Festic
Mayo Clinic, Jacksonville, FL, USA

R. Haniffa
Faculty of Tropical Medicine, Mahidol University, Bangkok, Thailand

N. Kissoon
British Columbia Children's Hospital, University of British Columbia, Vancouver, CO, Canada

I. Martin-Loeches
St. James's University Hospital, Dublin, Ireland

G. Lundeg
Mongolian National University of Medical Sciences, Ulaanbaatar, Mongolia

© The Author(s) 2019

A. M. Dondorp et al. (eds.), *Sepsis Management in Resource-limited Settings*,
https://doi.org/10.1007/978-3-030-03143-5_4

4.1 Introduction

Sepsis is a life-threatening condition characterized by one or more organ dysfunctions due to a dysregulated host response to infection [1] or, in certain cases, due to direct pathogen effects. Sepsis is not only associated with bacterial or fungal infections but with any other infections such as viral disease, protozoal disease (e.g., malaria), or tropical infections. Although the literature suggests that sepsis is predominantly a healthcare issue in resource-rich countries, the global burden of acute infections is highest in resource-limited areas [2]. Successful sepsis management relies on various components of which early recognition is essential. In this chapter, we summarize recommendations on sepsis recognition, identification of the underlying infection and causative microbiological pathogen, as well as recognition of septic shock in resource-limited settings (Table 4.1).

4.2 Sepsis Recognition

Sepsis is a life-threatening condition due to acute infection that is characterized by one or more organ dysfunctions. From a pathophysiological perspective, organ dysfunction results from a dysregulated response of the host's immune system to the microbiological pathogen [3] and, in certain cases, from direct effects of the pathogen (e.g., sequestration of parasitized red blood cells in malaria, endothelial damage by NS1 [nonstructural protein 1] in dengue, tissue damage by bacterial toxins). Sepsis is not only associated with bacterial or fungal infections but with any other infection such as viral disease, protozoal diseases (e.g., malaria), or other tropical infections. As the benefits of sepsis therapy are delicately time-sensitive with improved mortality and other outcomes observed in patients receiving appropriate therapy early in the course [3, 4], it is critical to recognize sepsis as early as possible upon patient's presentation. Early indicators of severe disease which relate to a fatal outcome select patients needing early and urgent treatment.

The results of a large US health record database including approximately 150,000 patients with suspected acute infection revealed that a quick Sequential (Sepsis-related) Organ Failure Assessment (qSOFA) score could help to identify patients with sepsis outside of an intensive care environment. The qSOFA score indicates the potential presence of sepsis if two of the following three indicators are fulfilled: (1) respiratory rate ≥22 bpm, (2) systolic blood pressure ≤100 mmHg, and (3) any acute change in mental state. Addition of further parameters did not relevantly improve the predictive power of this model [5]. These parameters are also included in different early warning scores [6], whose reasonable power to predict increased mortality of acutely ill patients was confirmed by studies from resource-limited settings [6–9]. A recently published study from Uganda reported that a prognostic index including respiratory rate (≥30 bpm), pulse rate (≥100 bpm), a mean arterial

Table 4.1 Recommendations for the recognition of sepsis in resource-limited settings (with grading)

1	Recognition of sepsis	Define sepsis as the combination of acute infection and two of the following parameters: respiratory rate ≥ 22 bpm, systolic blood pressure ≤ 100 mmHg, and any acute change in mental state (1B); these criteria have not been validated to recognize patients with sepsis from nonbacterial infections such as malaria, dengue, or other tropical infectious diseases (ungraded); diagnose malaria-induced sepsis if malaria and one or more of the following clinical signs occur: impaired consciousness, prostration, respiratory distress, multiple convulsions, hypoglycemia, severe malarial anemia, renal impairment, jaundice, malaria-induced shock, significant bleeding, and hyperparasitemia (1B); diagnose dengue-induced sepsis if dengue infection and any of the following clinical symptoms occur: shock, respiratory distress, severe bleeding, or any organ dysfunction (1B); healthcare workers, irrespective of their proficiency, should be alert to consider sepsis in adults and children with acute infection of any etiology (1C); recognition of sepsis in children is based on different severity indicators (ungraded)
2	Identification of the underlying type of infection	Take a structured patient history and perform a systematic head-to-toe physical examination to identify the underlying type of infection (1A); recognition of local infectious disease epidemiology is crucial (ungraded); depending on their availability, perform additional diagnostic evaluations such as laboratory testing and/or radiographic or ultrasound imaging to identify the source of infection (1B)
3	Identification of the causative microbiological pathogen	If available, obtain microbiological cultures before antimicrobial therapy as long as this does not relevantly delay antimicrobial therapy (1A); take two or more sets of blood cultures and tissue/body secretions from the site of suspected infection (1A); perform microscopy and Gram staining of secretions sampled from the suspected source of infection (1B); if available, test for antibiotic susceptibility of cultured bacteria to guide antibiotic therapy (1B); if resources to test for antibiotic susceptibility are not routinely available, perform intermittent microbiological screening of antimicrobial susceptibility of selected pathogens to inform empirical antimicrobial strategies (2C); use rapid diagnostic tests to diagnose malaria (1A); alternatively, use light microscopy of stained blood smears performed by experienced staff (1A); use direct (early disease phase) or indirect (intermediate or later disease phase) laboratory methods to diagnose specific virus infections such as dengue, influenza, or Ebola virus disease (1A); all patients with an acute infection who are positive for the human immunodeficiency virus, suffer from immunosuppression of other causes (e.g., malnutrition), and had previous tuberculosis infection and/or close contact with person suffering from tuberculosis should be screened for tuberculosis coinfection (1A); use light-emitting diode microscopy of two sputum smears or field PCR for the diagnosis of pulmonary tuberculosis (1A); perform tuberculosis cultures in HIV-positive patients (1A)

(continued)

Table 4.1 (continued)

4	Recognition of septic shock	Define septic shock as the presence of two or more clinical indicators of systemic tissue hypoperfusion independent of the presence of arterial hypotension (1B); if available, measure arterial lactate levels (1A); in patients with dengue sepsis, use a change in arterial blood pressure amplitude of ≤20 mmHg to diagnose shock (1C); do not rely solely on the use of arterial hypotension to diagnose septic shock, as arterial hypotension is typically a preterminal event and associated with an exceedingly high mortality in sepsis patients in resource-limited settings (1C)

Abbreviations: *PCR* polymerase chain reaction, *HIV* human immunodeficiency virus

blood pressure ≥110 or ≤70 mmHg), body temperature (≥38.6 or ≤35.6 °C), and any acute change in mental state could adequately predict hospital mortality in patients with sepsis [10].

It is important to note that the definition of sepsis was established largely based on adult patients suffering from bacterial or fungal infections. The definition has so far not been validated for other infections such as malaria, dengue fever, or tropical infectious diseases, which are highly prevalent in some resource-limited settings. As pathophysiology of malaria and bacterial infections differs [11], it is well conceivable that these criteria have a lower reliability to recognize patients with sepsis due to malaria. A prospective observational study from Uganda reported that out of 216 hospitalized patients with community-acquired infection and the systemic inflammatory response syndrome, only 4% suffered from acute malaria infection [12]. These data indicate that patients with malaria may potentially manifest with alternative signs of infection and might have been unrecognized as such. In 2015, the World Health Organization recommended diagnosing severe malaria in adults with *Plasmodium falciparum* asexual parasitemia and one or more of the following clinical signs: (1) impaired consciousness, (2) prostration (defined as the inability to sit, stand, or walk unassisted), (3) respiratory distress due to acidosis or pulmonary edema, (4) more than two convulsions within 24 h, (4) hypoglycemia, (5) severe malarial anemia, (6) renal impairment, (7) jaundice, (8) malaria-induced shock (for definition see below), (8) significant bleeding, and (9) hyperparasitemia [13]. A malaria prognostic index (including Glasgow Coma Scale <11, admission parasitemia >315,000/μL, pigmented parasites >20%, total bilirubin >58 μmol/L, lactate >5 mmol/L) has shown a high sensitivity (95–100%) and specificity (88–91%) to predict death in Asian adults with falciparum malaria [14]. A post hoc analysis of four studies suggested that normothermia, tachypnea, impaired consciousness, oligo-anuria, shock, and hypo-/hyperglycemia independently predicted death in adults with falciparum malaria [15].

Similarly, in dengue infection, the development of shock, respiratory distress, severe bleeding, or any organ dysfunction has been recommended by the World Health Organization to characterize severe dengue and an increased risk of death [16]. The clinical usefulness and diagnostic reliability of this classification were confirmed in a multicenter study performed in seven countries including 2259 patients from Southeast Asia and Latin America [17].

As the burden of infection-related death in resource-limited areas is highest in children, particularly in those aged <5 years [18], recognition and management of sepsis in this age group is of particular importance. As children differ in several physiologic aspects from adults, the indicators of their life-threatening organ dysfunction may differ as well. These parameters are summarized in a separate part of these expert consensus recommendations dedicated to pediatric sepsis.

One of the key challenges in resource-limited areas is the lack of well-trained healthcare workers, particularly physicians specialized in emergency and critical care medicine [19, 20]. Therefore, it appears unreasonable to limit recognition of sepsis to physicians only. Both physicians and nonphysicians (e.g., medical officers, nurses, and advanced level practitioners) need to be aware of and be able to recognize sepsis. However, they may require specific training and/or experience to do so [21]. Given that the vast majority of children with sepsis in resource-limited areas are presumably managed by non-pediatricians, it is also important that healthcare staff in resource-limited areas is aware of and trained in the specific characteristics of sepsis recognition in children [22]. A shortage in resources should not impede reliable and timely recognition of sepsis as this can generally be achieved using clinical skills only. Similarly, severity of diseases caused by malaria and dengue can be assessed largely by clinical signs. However, to recognize specific symptoms of malaria-induced sepsis or to calculate the malaria prognostic index, it is necessary to determine base deficit, lactate, and total bilirubin and creatinine or urea levels, which may not be routinely available in resource-limited settings.

Sepsis is defined as a life-threatening organ dysfunction due to a dysregulated host response to acute infection or, in certain cases, due to direct effects of the pathogen. Sepsis is not only associated with bacterial or fungal infections but with any other infection such as viral disease, protozoal infections (e.g., malaria), or tropical infections (ungraded). We recommend defining sepsis in adults as the combination of acute infection and the presence of two of the following three parameters: (1) respiratory rate ≥ 22 bpm, (2) systolic blood pressure ≤ 100 mmHg, and (3) any acute change in mental state (1B). These criteria have not been validated to recognize patients with sepsis from nonbacterial infections such as malaria, dengue, or other tropical infectious diseases (ungraded). Until data confirm the predictive value of the new sepsis definition in malaria, we recommend diagnosing malaria-induced sepsis if malaria and one or more of the following clinical signs occur: impaired consciousness, prostration, respiratory distress, multiple convulsions, hypoglycemia, severe malarial anemia, renal impairment, jaundice, malaria-induced shock, significant bleeding, and hyperparasitemia (1B). Until data confirm the predictive value of the new sepsis definition in dengue, we recommend diagnosing dengue-induced sepsis if dengue infection and any of the following clinical symptoms occur: shock, respiratory distress, severe bleeding, or any organ dysfunction (1B). We recommend that healthcare workers, irrespective of their proficiency, should be alert to consider sepsis in adults and children with acute infection of any etiology (1C). Recognition of sepsis in children is based on different severity indicators (ungraded). These are summarized in another chapter of this book.

4.3 Identification of the Underlying Type of Infection

Recognition of acute infection is paramount for both sepsis diagnosis and management. Acute infection can be caused by various microbiological pathogens—bacteria, viruses, parasites, or fungi. The epidemiology of infectious diseases differs globally. While bacterial and fungal infections are observed everywhere in the world, malaria, dengue, and tropical infectious diseases are typically encountered in Central and South America, sub-Saharan Africa, and southern parts of Asia [23]. Although clear data on the epidemiology of sepsis are missing, the global mortality of malaria and thereby the burden of malaria-induced sepsis appear to be exceptionally high in resource-limited countries, particularly in sub-Saharan Africa, India, and Southeast Asia [24]. Tuberculosis is a chronic but sometimes acute bacterial infection caused by *Mycobacterium* spp., highly prevalent in many resource-limited areas [25]. While in high- and upper-middle-income countries, only lower respiratory tract infections are ranked (sixth) among the top ten causes of death; three and four infectious diseases (excluding HIV/AIDS) are among the top ten causes of death in lower-middle- and low-income countries, respectively. In low-income countries, lower respiratory tract infections represent the most common cause of death followed by HIV/AIDS and diarrheal diseases [26]. Viral causes of sepsis, such as dengue, often occur in epidemics.

Clinical skills of structured history taking and systematic physical examination are essential to identify the underlying type of infection. Nonspecific signs of infection include fever, chills, fatigue, malaise, and muscle/joint aches. If associated with a low risk of harm for the patient, sites of suspected infections (e.g., abscess, joints, effusion) can be punctured or incised to verify the infectious focus and sample secretions or tissue for laboratory work-up [2]. Selected laboratory parameters can assist in making the diagnosis of acute infection (e.g., the white blood cell count) but are neither highly sensitive nor specific [27–32]. Diagnostic imaging techniques, where available and preferably portable (e.g., X-ray, ultrasound) [33–35], can be used to answer specific diagnostic questions. Given its increasing portability and availability, the role of ultrasound to diagnose abdominal, joint/soft tissue, and lung infections in resource-limited countries is emphasized [36].

As mainly clinical skills are required, a lack of resources does not relevantly impede identification of the underlying infection. Given that the majority of laboratories in resource-limited settings are capable of routinely determining the white blood cell count [36–38], this parameter may be useful to support the diagnosis of an acute infection. Although ultrasound has been increasingly available in resource-limited settings [36], in many healthcare facilities, ultrasound is not always available, as machines are routinely operated only by selected healthcare workers [39]. In addition, installation of ultrasound services in resource-limited hospitals is usually associated with substantial costs. Maintenance of ultrasound machines is another challenge in these settings. Similarly, X-ray machines are frequently immobile and require supply materials such as X-ray films.

We recommend taking a structured patient history and performing a systematic head-to-toe physical examination to identify the underlying type of infection (1A).

Thereby, recognition of local epidemiology of infectious diseases is crucial (ungraded). Depending on their availability/affordability, we recommend performing additional diagnostic evaluations such as laboratory testing and/or radiographic or ultrasound imaging to identify the source of infection, as guided by the history and physical examination (1B).

4.4 Identification of the Causative Microbiological Pathogen

Definitive (as opposed to empiric) antimicrobial therapy requires identification of the microbiological pathogen of infection [3]. Appropriate antimicrobial therapy is one of the cornerstones of successful sepsis management [3, 4, 40–42]. Knowledge of the causative organism and its susceptibility to antimicrobial agents is a prerequisite for appropriate antimicrobial therapy [3]. Different diagnostic techniques are required for identification of the infectious agents causing bacterial infection, tuberculosis, malaria, and viral diseases.

Microbiological methods are used to specify bacteria and fungi from sampled body fluids and blood as well as to test their susceptibility to antibiotic agents. Microscopy and Gram staining are simple and rapid techniques to identify bacteria and fungi in the sputum, urine, cerebrospinal fluid, ascites, and other body secretions [43–49]. The appearance and staining of bacteria can categorize (Gram positive/negative) and identify selected bacterial species (e.g., meningococci, pneumococci, staphylococci), thus allowing for prompt adjustment of empiric antibiotic therapy. Microbiological cultures of body secretions are the gold standard to grow and specify bacteria. Cultivating bacteria from the blood requires special media known as blood cultures. To achieve a reasonable sensitivity, two or more sets of blood cultures from different puncture sites or indwelling catheters need to be sampled in a sterile fashion [50]. As the shorter time period between the sepsis diagnosis and administration of an appropriate antimicrobial agent may reduce mortality [4], sampling of blood or body secretions for microbiological work-up should not relevantly delay initiation of antimicrobial therapy (e.g., <45 min [3]). The knowledge of antimicrobial susceptibility of the causative pathogen is of crucial importance as any potential resistance of microbiological pathogens against antimicrobial agents may result in inadequate antibiotic therapy. While antimicrobial resistance is a global challenge, the incidence of multidrug resistance is particularly high in many resource-limited areas with rates of resistant bacteria approaching as high as 50% [51–55]. This could explain partially why an observational study from Uganda did not observe a difference in mortality between sepsis patients who received and did not receive an empiric antibiotic therapy [56]. Similarly, resistance of *Plasmodium falciparum* to certain antimalarial drugs such as artemisinin has spread throughout mainland Southeast Asia and has also been detected in sub-Saharan Africa [57–59].

Patients with an acute infection who have a risk of being (co-) infected with tuberculosis should be screened for tuberculosis. Common risk factors are HIV infection, malnutrition, previous tuberculosis infection, and close contact to persons suffering from tuberculosis (e.g., household members, prisoners, healthcare personnel) [60–62]. A study from Uganda reported that one in four HIV-infected patients with severe sepsis had *Mycobacterium tuberculosis* bacteremia [63]. The 2007 WHO international policy on tuberculosis detection recommends light-emitting diode microscopy of two sputum smears for the diagnosis of pulmonary tuberculosis infection [64]. In children, gastric aspirates can be examined alternatively to induced sputum samples. A novel field nucleic acid amplification test (Xpert MTB/RIF) yields diagnostic results and information on rifampicin resistance under 2 h [65]. Despite a more rapid and frequent diagnosis of tuberculosis with this technique, concerns remain as relevant patient outcomes have not been affected so far. Although sputum examination using Ziehl-Neelsen microscopy for acid-fast bacteria is insensitive in HIV-positive subjects, it is frequently performed in laboratories of resource-limited areas, as conventional fluorescence or light-emitting diode microscopy is not commonly available. WHO guidelines recommend performance of tuberculosis cultures in HIV-positive patients [64].

Light microscopy and rapid diagnostic tests are the laboratory methods commonly used to diagnose malaria. Light microscopy of Giemsa-stained blood smears is the standard method applied in many endemic areas to identify *Plasmodium* spp. and estimate parasite density [66, 67]. Depending on the examiner's experience, sensitivity varies but was shown to be very high in expert hands [68]. However, this method is labor intensive and requires specific training [69]. Antigen-detecting rapid diagnostic tests, on the other hand, do not depend on laboratory infrastructure and can be performed by non-laboratory medical personnel [70]. The sensitivity and specificity of rapid diagnostic tests are high (93–98%) and superior to that of light microscopy [71]. As rapid diagnostic tests only yield qualitative results, parasite density cannot be assessed with this method [70]. In addition, depending on the regional malaria epidemiology, different rapid diagnostic tests are required to detect and distinguish between plasmodium species [70].

Laboratory diagnosis of viral diseases, such as dengue, influenza, or Ebola, typically depends on the duration of the illness. During the early phases of infection, virus identification is achieved by direct methods (e.g., detection of viral components or cell cultures), whereas during later phases (after 5–7 days) indirect methods (e.g., serologic detection of serum IgM) are used [16, 72]. For certain viruses, rapid antigen detection tests are available yielding results within a few hours [16].Many of these tests have shown a high sensitivity and specificity such as a point-of-care rapid diagnostic test to detect the Ebola virus [73].

Laboratories in resource-limited areas often lack regular supply of materials to perform microbiological cultures and test for antibiotic susceptibility due to irregular availability of these materials on the local and national markets as well as due to the high cost [36–38]. On the other hand, microscopy and Gram staining are available in many of the laboratories [36–38]. Microscopic analysis and Gram staining can specify selected bacteria and fungi but do not give information on antibiotic susceptibility. In cases where routine microbiological cultures and susceptibility testing are not available, determination of the most common pathogens (e.g., pneumococci, staphylococci, *Escherichia coli*, *Mycobacterium tuberculosis*, *Plasmodium falciparum*, etc.) for each infection site as well as their antimicrobial susceptibility may help to optimize empiric antimicrobial therapy. Accordingly, the World Alliance Against Antibiotic Resistance recommends collection of information on antibiotic resistance in each country/region [74].This recommendation is in line with that of the World Health Organization to regularly monitor drug efficacy for the first-line antimalarial drugs at regular intervals [75].

Laboratory methods to identify malaria are commonly available at healthcare facilities in areas where malaria is endemic [36–38]. The costs of rapid diagnostic tests are higher than those of light microscopy, despite that their use in Africa has increased substantially during the recent years [76]. Regarding tuberculosis detection using polymerase chain reaction tests or virus identification, laboratory tests yielding a high sensitivity and specificity typically require complex technologies, infrastructure requirements, and staff expertise and imply high costs. On the other hand, serologic tests are more affordable although they similarly require specific laboratory facilities which may not be available in many resource-limited settings [36–38]. This may change in cases of viral disease epidemics such as the recent Ebola virus disease epidemic in Western Africa [77]. None of the tests are associated with any direct risks for the patient. However, contamination of microbiological cultures and false-positive or false-negative results of laboratory tests bear the risk of over- or undertreatment, both of which may be associated with harm.

If available/affordable, we recommend obtaining microbiological cultures before antimicrobial therapy as long as this does not relevantly delay antimicrobial therapy (1A). We recommend taking two or more sets of blood cultures and/or tissue/body secretions from the site of suspected infection (1A). We recommend performing microscopy and Gram staining of secretions sampled from the suspected source of infection (1B). If available/affordable, we recommend testing for antibiotic susceptibility of cultured bacteria to guide antibiotic therapy (1B). If resources to test for antibiotic susceptibility are not routinely available, we suggest performing intermittent microbiological screening of antimicrobial susceptibility of selected pathogens to inform empirical antimicrobial strategies (1C). We recommend using rapid diagnostic tests to diagnose malaria (1A). Alternatively, we recommend light microscopy of stained blood smears performed by experienced staff (1A). We recommend using direct (early disease phase) or indirect (intermediate or later disease phase) laboratory methods to diagnose specific virus infections such as dengue, influenza, or Ebola virus disease (1A). All patients with an acute infection who are positive for the human immunodeficiency virus, suffer from immunosuppression of other causes (e.g., malnutrition), and had previous tuberculosis infection and/or close contact with person suffering from tuberculosis should be screened for tuberculosis coinfection (1A). We recommend light-emitting diode microscopy of two sputum smears for the diagnosis of pulmonary tuberculosis (1A). Whenever available/affordable, we recommend using polymerase chain reaction tests (e.g., Gene Xpert) to diagnose tuberculosis or perform tuberculosis cultures in HIV-positive patients (1A).

4.5 Recognition of Septic Shock

Shock is defined as inadequate systemic tissue perfusion with cellular dysoxia/hypoxia [78]. Septic shock has recently been defined as arterial hypotension requiring vasopressor therapy to maintain mean arterial blood pressure at 65 mmHg or greater together with a serum lactate level greater than 2 mmol/L after adequate fluid resuscitation [79]. Systemic tissue hypoperfusion is a critical cofactor in the development of organ dysfunction and death in patients with sepsis [3, 79]. Recognition of septic shock is therefore essential to recognize sepsis patients with a particularly high risk of death.

Critically ill patients with abnormal peripheral perfusion (e.g., cold and clammy skin) following initial resuscitation have more severe metabolic derangements and organ dysfunction than subjects with normal peripheral perfusion [80]. In early septic shock due to bacterial infection, prolonged capillary refill time is strongly associated with organ dysfunction and mortality [81]. Similarly, prolonged capillary refill time is an indicator of disease severity and a high risk of death in malaria [82] and dengue infection [83]. The extent of skin mottling in the lower extremities is associated with organ dysfunction and mortality in sepsis [84]. Given that of all internal organs the kidneys exhibit the highest autoregulatory threshold, renal blood flow is the first to decline in case of decreased cardiac output or peripheral vasodilation [85]. Thus, any episode of oliguria (<0.5 ml/kg/h) potentially indicates renal hypoperfusion. Observational studies found that the longer time during which urine output remains <0.5 mL/kg/h is associated with higher morbidity and mortality in critically ill patients [86]. Elevated lactate levels also predict increased morbidity and mortality in patients with sepsis [87, 88]. Moreover, the duration of hyperlactatemia and the rate of lactate clearance are associated with organ dysfunction and mortality in sepsis. Studies from resource-limited settings confirmed that hyperlactatemia is associated with a high degree of illness severity and an increased mortality from sepsis independent of the underlying pathogen [14, 89]. If patients with sepsis and signs of systemic tissue hypoperfusion develop arterial hypotension [defined as a systolic arterial blood pressure < 90 mmHg or a mean arterial blood pressure < 65 mmHg], the risk of death was shown to be excessively high in resource-limited settings [89–91]. Per the authors' experience, occurrence of arterial hypotension in septic patients with systemic tissue hypoperfusion is typically a preterminal sign, as the therapeutic requirements in these patients often exceed the capabilities of resource-limited healthcare facilities. In patients with severe malaria, arterial hypotension is rare and when present is often associated with bacterial coinfection [11, 13, 92]. The World Health Organization defined dengue shock by the presence of an arterial blood pressure amplitude (systolic minus diastolic arterial blood pressure) ≤20 mmHg [16]. In dengue shock, systolic arterial blood pressure remains normal or even elevated but can drop rapidly preceding terminal cardiovascular collapse [16]. Studies have suggested that the following clinical symptoms result from early plasma leakage and herald dengue shock: abdominal pain, hepatomegaly, high or increasing hematocrit levels, rapid decrease in platelet count, serosal effusions, mucosal bleeding, and lethargy or restlessness [16].

A shortage of resources does not impede the ability to recognize septic shock as the diagnosis is mainly based on clinical indicators. Specific training of healthcare workers to recognize these clinical signs is, however, essential. Using skin mottling to assess skin perfusion in dark complexed patients may not be feasible. However, assessment of capillary refill time is a meaningful alternative that demonstrated similar predictive value for organ dysfunction and death in sepsis [81]. Costs for lactate measurements may be relevant and, in some settings, may even impede use of arterial lactate in sepsis patients. There are no direct patient risks related to diagnosing shock by using clinical techniques. Despite its strong predictive power, arterial lactate measurements are not routinely available or affordable in many resource-limited healthcare facilities [36–38].

We recommend defining septic shock as the presence of two or more clinical indicators of systemic tissue hypoperfusion independent of the presence of arterial hypotension (1B). If available, we recommend measuring arterial lactate levels in patients with sepsis (1A). In patients with dengue sepsis, we recommend using a reduction in the arterial blood pressure amplitude ≤20 mmHg to diagnose shock (1C). We recommend against relying solely on arterial hypotension as a diagnostic criterion for the diagnosis of septic shock, as arterial hypotension is typically a preterminal event and associated with an exceedingly high mortality in sepsis patients in resource-limited settings (1C).

4.6 Conclusions

Sepsis is not only associated with bacterial or fungal infections but with any other infection such as viral disease, protozoal disease (e.g., malaria), or tropical infections. We provided a set of simple, readily available, and affordable recommendations on how to recognize sepsis, identify the underlying type of infection, identify the causative microbiological pathogen, and recognize septic shock in resource-limited settings. As most evidence originates from resource-rich settings, there is an urgent need for related research in resource-limited settings.

References

1. Singer M, Deutschman CS, Seymour CW, Shankar-Hari M, Annane D, Bauer M, Bellomo R, Bernard GR, Chiche JD, Coopersmith CM, Hotchkiss RS, Levy MM, Marshall JC, Martin GS, Opal SM, Rubenfeld GC, van der Poll T, Vincent JL, Angus DC. The third international consensus definitions for sepsis and septic shock (Sepsis-3). JAMA. 2016;315:801–10.
2. The 10 leading causes of death by country income group. WHO factsheets. 2012. http://www.who.int/mediacentre/factsheets/fs310/en/index1.html.
3. Angus DC, van der Poll T. Severe sepsis and septic shock. N Engl J Med. 2013;369:840–51.
4. Kumar A, Roberts D, Wood KE, Light B, Parrillo JE, Sharma S, Suppes R, Feinstein D, Zanotti S, Taiberg L, Gurka D, Kumar A, Cheang M. Duration of hypotension before initiation of effective antimicrobial therapy is the critical determinant of survival in human septic shock. Crit Care Med. 2006;34:1589–96.

5. Seymour CW, Liu VX, Iwashyna TJ, Brunkhorst FM, Rea TD, Scherag A, Rubenfeld G, Kahn JM, Shankar-Hari M, Singer M, Deutschman CS, Escobar GJ, Angus DC. Assessment of clinical criteria for sepsis: for the third international consensus definitions for sepsis and septic shock (Sepsis-3). JAMA. 2016;315:762–74.
6. Ghanem-Zoubi NO, Vardi M, Laor A, Weber G, Bitterman H. Assessment of disease-severity scoring systems for patients with sepsis in general internal medicine departments. Crit Care. 2011;15:R95.
7. Rylance J, Baker T, Mushi E, Mashaga D. Use of an early warning score and ability to walk predicts mortality in medical patients admitted to hospitals in Tanzania. Trans R Soc Trop Med Hyg. 2009;103:790–4.
8. Bulut M, Cebicci H, Sigirli D, Sak A, Durmus O, Top AA, Kaya S, Uz K. The comparison of modified early warning score with rapid emergency medicine score: a prospective multicentre observational cohort study on medical and surgical patients presenting to emergency department. Emerg Med J. 2014;31:476–81.
9. Opio MO, nansubuga G, Kellett J, Clifford M, Murray A. Performance of TOTAL, in medical patients attending a resource-poor hospital in Sub-Saharan Africa and a small Irish rural hospital. Acute Med. 2013;12:135–40.
10. Asiimwe SB, Abdallah A, Ssekitoleko R. A simple prognostic index based on admission vital signs data among patients with sepsis in a resource-limited setting. Cirt Care. 2015;19:86.
11. White NJ, Pukrittayakamee S, Hien TT, Faiz MA, Mokuolu OA, Dondorp AM. Malaria. Lancet. 2014;383:723–35.
12. Auma MA, Siedner MJ, Nyehangane D, Nalusaji A, Nakaye M, Mwanga-Amumpaire J, Muhindo R, Wilson LA, Boum Y II, Moore CC. Malaria is an uncommon cause of adult sepsis in south-western Uganda. Malar J. 2013;12:146.
13. The World Health Organization. Guidelines for the management of malaria. 3rd ed. Geneva: World Health Organization; 2015. isbn:978-92-4-154912-7.
14. Newton PN, Stepniewska K, Dondorp A, Kamolrat S, Chierakul W, Krishna S, Davis TME, Suputtamongkol Y, Angus B, Pukrittayakamee S, Ruangveerayuth R, Hanson J, Day NPJ, White NJ. Prognostic indicators in adults hospitalized with falciparum malaria in Western Thailand. Malar J. 2013;12:229.
15. Hanson J, Lee SJ, Mohanty S, Faiz MA, Anstey NM, Price RN, Charunwatthana P, Yunus EB, Mishra SK, Tjitra E, Rahman R, Nosten F, Htut Y, Maude RJ, ThiHong Chau T, HoanPhu N, Tinh Hien T, White NJ, Day NPJ, Dondorp AM. PLoS One. 2014;9:e87020.
16. Simmons CP, Farrar JJ, van Vinh Chau N, Wills B. Dengue. N Engl J Med. 2012;366:1423–32.
17. Alexander N, Balmaseda A, Coelho IC, Dimaano E, Hien TT, Hung NT, Jänisch T, Kroeger A, Lum LC, Martinez E, Siqueira JB, Thuy TT, Villalobos I, Villegas E, Wills B. Multicentre prospective study on dengue classification in four Southeast Asian and three Latin American countries. Tropical Med Int Health. 2011;16:936–48.
18. The World Health Organization. The top 10 causes of death. http://www.who.int/mediacentre/factsheets/fs310/en/index2.html. Accessed 8 Sept 2015.
19. Jochberger S, Ismailova F, Lederer W, Mayr VD, Luckner G, Wenzel V, Ulmer H, Hasibeder WR, Dünser MW, "HelfenBerührt" Study Team. Anesthesia and its allied disciplines in the developing world: a nationwide survey of the Republic of Zambia. Anesth Analg. 2008;106:942–8.
20. Dünser MW, Bataar O, Tsenddorj G, Lundeg G, Jochberger S, Jakob S, "HelfenBerührt" Study Team. Intensive care medicine in Mongolia's 3 largest cities: outlining the needs. J Crit Care. 2009;24:469.e1–6.
21. Peltola L, Goddia C, Namboya F, Brunkhorst FM, Pollach G. Sepsis—knowledge of non-physician personnel in Africa. A cross-sectional study in Malawian district hospitals. Med Klin Intensivmed Notfmed. 2015;110:49–54.
22. Kissoon N. Out of Africa—a mother's journey. Pediatr Crit Care Med. 2011;12:73–9.
23. Gething PW, Patil AP, Smith DL, Guerra CA, Elyazar IR, Johnston GL, Tatem AJ, Hay SI. A new world malaria map: Plasmodium falciparum endemicity in 2010. Malar J. 2011;10:378.

24. Snow RW, Guerra CA, Noor AM, Myint HY, Hay SI. The global distribution of clinical episodes of Plasmodium falciparum malaria. Nature. 2005;434:214–7.
25. Zumla A, Raviglione M, Hafner R, von Reyn CF. Tuberculosis. N Engl J Med. 2013;368:745–55.
26. The 10 leading causes of death by country income group. 2012. WHO factsheets. http://www.who.int/mediacentre/factsheets/fs310/en/index1.html. Accessed 23 Aug 2015.
27. Chan YL, Tseng CP, Tsay PK, Chang SS, Chiu TF, Chen JC. Procalcitonin as a marker of bacterial infection in the emergency department: an observational study. Crit Care. 2004;8:R12–20.
28. Chan YL, Liao HC, Tsay PK, Chang SS, Chen JC, Liaw SJ. C-reactive protein as an indicator of bacterial infection of adult patients in the emergency department. Chang Gung Med J. 2002;25:437–45.
29. Cheval C, Timsit JF, Garrouste-Orgeas M, Assicot M, De Jonghe B, Misset B, Bohuon C, Carlet J. Procalcitonin (PCT) is useful in predicting the bacterial origin of an acute circulatory failure in critically ill patients. Intensive Care Med. 2000;26(Suppl 2):S153–8.
30. Lagerström F, Engfeldt P, Holmberg H. C-reactive protein in diagnosis of community-acquired pneumonia in adult patients in primary care. Scand J Infect Dis. 2006;38:964–9.
31. Liu A, Bui T, Van Nguyen H, Ong B, Shen Q, Kamalasena D. Serum C-reactive protein as a biomarker for early detection of bacterial infection in the older patient. Age Ageing. 2010;39:559–65.
32. Póvoa P, Coelho L, Almeida E, Fernandes A, Mealha R, Moreira P, Sabino H. C-reactive protein as a marker of infection in critically ill patients. Clin Microbiol Infect. 2005;11:101–8.
33. Ifergan J, Pommier R, Brion MC, Glas L, Rocher L, Bellin MF. Imaging in upper urinary tract infections. Diagn Interv Imaging. 2012;93:509–19.
34. Cardinal E, Bureau NJ, Aubin B, Chhem RK. Role of ultrasound in musculoskeletal infections. Radiol Clin North Am. 2001;39:191–201.
35. Diefenthal HC, Tashjian J. The role of plain films, CT, tomography, ultrasound, and percutaneous needle aspiration in the diagnosis of inflammatory lung disease. Semin Respir Infect. 1988;3:83–105.
36. Chavez MA, Naithani N, Gilman RH, Tielsch JM, Khatry S, Ellington LE, Miranda JJ, Gurung G, Rodriguez S, Checkley W. Agreement between the World Health Organization and lung consolidation identified using point-of-care ultrasound for the diagnosis of childhood pneumonia by general practitioners. Lung. 2015;193:531–8.
37. Baelani I, Jochberger S, Laimer T, Rex C, Baker T, Wilson IH, Grander W, Dünser MW. Identifying resource needs for sepsis care and guideline implementation in the Democratic Republic of the Congo: a cluster survey of 66 hospitals in four eastern provinces. Middle East J Anaesthesiol. 2012;21:559–75.
38. Bataar O, Lundeg G, Tsenddorj G, Jochberger S, Grander W, Baelani I, Wilson I, Baker T, Dünser MW, HelfenBerührt Study Team. Nationwide survey on resource availability for implementing current sepsis guidelines in Mongolia. Bull World Health Organ. 2010;88:839–46.
39. Harris RD, Cho JY, Deneen DR. Compact ultrasound donations to medical facilities in low-resource countries: a survey-based assessment of the current status and trends. J Ultrasound Med. 2012;31:1255–9.
40. Kollef MH, Sherman G, Ward S, Fraser VJ. Inadequate antimicrobial treatment of infections: a risk factor for hospital mortality among critically ill patients. Chest. 1999;115:462–74.
41. Ibrahim EH, Sherman G, Ward S, Fraser VJ, Kollef MH. The influence of antimicrobial treatment of bloodstream infections on patient outcomes in the ICU setting. Chest. 2000;118:146–55.
42. Paul M, Shani V, Muchtar E, Kariv G, Robenshtok E, Leibovici L. Systematic review and meta-analysis of the efficacy of appropriate empiric antibiotic therapy for sepsis. Antimicrob Agents Chemother. 2010;54:4851–63.
43. Holm S, Wahlin A, Wahlqvist L, Wedrén H, Lundgren B. Urine microscopy as screening method for bacteriuria. Acta Med Scand. 1982;211:209–12.
44. Barbin GK, Thorley JD, Reinarz JA. Simplified microscopy for rapid detection of significant bacteriuria in random urine specimens. J Clin Micorbiol. 1978;7:286–9.

45. Salih MA, el Hag AI, Sid Ahmed H, Bushara M, Yasin I, Omer MI, Hofvander Y, Olcen P. Endemic bacterial meningitis in Sudanese children: aetiology, clinical findings, treatment and short-term outcome. Ann Trop Paediatr. 1990;10:203–10.
46. Leman P. Validity of urinalysis and microscopy for detecting urinary tract infection in the emergency department. Eur J Emerg Med. 2002;9:141–7.
47. Alausa KO, Osoba AO, Montefiore D, Sogbetun OA. Laboratory diagnosis of tuberculosis in a developing country 1968-1975. Afr J Med Med Sci. 1977;6:103–8.
48. Shameem S, Vinod Kumar CS, Neelagund YF. Bacterial meningitis: rapid diagnosis and microbial profile: a multicentered study. J Commun Dis. 2008;40:111–20.
49. Heyman SN, Ginosar Y, Niel L, Amir J, Marx N, Shapiro M, Maayan S. Meningococcal meningitis among Rwandan refugees: diagnosis, management, and outcome in a field hospital. Int J Infect Dis. 1998;2:137–42.
50. Shafazand S, Weinacker AB. Blood cultures in the critical care unit: improving utilization and yield. Chest. 2002;122:1727–36.
51. Bataar O, Khuderchuluun C, Lundeg G, Chimeddorj S, Brunauer A, Gradwohl-Matis I, Duenser MW. Rate and pattern of antibiotic resistance and microbiological cultures of sepsis patients in a low-middle-income country's ICU. Middle East J Anaesthesiol. 2013;22:293–300.
52. Iroezindu MO, El C, Isiguzo GC, Mbata GC, Onyedum CC, Kl O, Okoli LE. Sputum bacteriology and antibiotic sensitivity patterns of community-acquired pneumonia in hospitalized adult patients in Nigeria: a 5-year multicentre retrospective study. Scand J Infect Dis. 2014;46:875–87.
53. Matute AJ, Brouwer WP, Hak E, Delgado E, Alonso E, Hoepelman IM. Aetiology and resistance patterns of community-acquired pneumonia in León, Nicaragua. Int J Antimicrob Agents. 2006;28:423–7.
54. Biadglegne F, Rodloff AC, Sack U. Review of the prevalence and drug resistance of tuberculosis in prisons: a hidden epidemic. Epidemiol Infect. 2015;143:887–900.
55. Chittawatanarat K, Jaipakdee W, Chotirosniramit N, Chandacham K, Jirapongcharoenlap T. Microbiology, resistance patterns, and risk factors of mortality in ventilator-associated bacterial pneumonia in a Northern Thai tertiary-care university based general surgical intensive care unit. Infect Drug Resist. 2014;7:203–10.
56. Jacob ST, Moore CC, Banura P, Pinkerton R, Meya D, Opendi P, Reynolds SJ, Kenya-Mugisha N, Mayanja-Kizza H, Scheld WM, Promoting Resource-Limited Interventions for Sepsis Management in Uganda (PRISM-U) Study Group. Severe sepsis in two Ugandan hospitals: a prospective observational study of management and outcomes in a predominantly HIV-1 infected population. PLoS One. 2009;4:e7782.
57. Dondorp AM, Nosten F, Yi P, et al. Artemisinin resistance in Plasmodium falciparum malaria. N Engl J Med. 2009;361:455–67.
58. Ashley EA, Dhorda M, Fairhurst RM, et al. Spread of artemisinin resistance in Plasmodium falciparum malaria, vol. 371; 2014. p. 411–23.
59. Kamau E, Campino S, Amenga-Etego L, et al. K13-propeller polymorphisms in Plasmodium falciparum parasites from sub-Saharan Africa. J Infect Dis. 2015;211:1352–5.
60. Telisinghe L, Fielding KL, Malden JL, Hanifa Y, Churchyard GJ, Grand AD, Charalambous S. High tuberculosis prevalence in a South African prison: the need for routine tuberculosis screening. PLoS One. 2014;9:e87262.
61. Joshi R, Reingold AL, Menzies D, Pai M. Tuberculosis among health-care workers in low- and middle-income countries: a systematic review. PLoS Med. 2006;3:e494.
62. Lienhardt C, Fielding K, Sillah JS, Bah B, Gustafson P, Warndorff D, Palayew M, Lisse I, Donkor S, Diallo S, Manneh K, Adegbola R, Aaby P, Bah-Sow O, Bennett S, McAdam K. Investigation of the risk factors for tuberculosis: a case-control study in three countries in West Africa. Int J Epidemiol. 2005;34:914–23.
63. Jacob ST, Pavlinac PB, Nakiyingi L, Banura P, Baeten JM, Morgan K, Magaret A, Manabe Y, Reynolds SJ, Liles WC, Wald A, Joloba ML, Mayanja-Kizza H, Scheld WM. Mycobacterium tuberculosis bacteremia in a cohort of HIV-infected patients hospitalized with severe sepsis in

Uganda—high frequency, low clinical suspicion and derivation of a clinical prediction score. PLoS One. 2013;8:e70305.

64. World Health Organization. Reduction of number of smears for the diagnosis of pulmonary TB. Geneva: World Health Organization; 2007. http://www.who.int/tb/dots/laboratory/policy/en/index2.html.
65. McNerney R, Cunningham J, Hepple P, Zumla A. New tuberculosis diagnostics and rollout. Int J Infect Dis. 2015;32:81–6.
66. Dowling MA, Shute GT. A comparative study of thick and thin blood films in the diagnosis of scanty malaria parasitaemia. Bull World Heatlh Organ. 1966;34:249–67.
67. Payne D. Use and limitations of light microscopy for diagnosing malaria at the primary health care level. Bull World Health Organ. 1988;66:621–6.
68. Wongsrichanalai C, Barcus MJ, Muth S, Sutamihardja A, Wernsdorfer WH. A review of malaria diagnostic tools: microscopy and rapid diagnostic test (RDT). Am J Trop Med Hyg. 2007;77(6 Suppl):119–27.
69. Murray CK, Gaser RA Jr, Magill AJ, Miller RS. Update on rapid diagnostic testing for malaria. Clin Microbiol Rev. 2008;21:97–110.
70. Wilson ML. Malaria rapid diagnostic tests. Clin Infect Dis. 2012;54:1637–41.
71. Abba K, Deeks JJ, Olliaro P, Naing CM, Jackson SM, Takwoingi Y, Donegan S, Garner P. Rapid diagnostic tests for diagnosing uncomplicated P. falciparum malaria in endemic countries. Cochrane Database Syst Rev. 2011;7:CD008122.
72. Rathakrishnan A, Sekaran SD. New development in the diagnosis of dengue infections. Expert Opin Med Diagn. 2013;7:99–112.
73. Broadhurst MJ, Kelly JD, Miller A, et al. ReEBOV antigen rapid test kit for point-of-care and laboratory-based testing for Ebola virus disease: a field validation study. Lancet. 2015;386:867–74.
74. Carlet J. Ten tips on how to win the war against resistance to antibiotics. Intensive Care Med. 2015;41:899–901.
75. World Health Organization. Assessment and monitoring of antimalarial drug efficacy for the treatment of uncomplicated falciparum malaria. Geneva: World Health Organization; 2003. http://malaria.who.int/docs/ProtocolWHO.pdf.
76. WHO. World malaria report, 2011. Geneva: World Health Organization; 2012.
77. Walkner NF, Brown CS, Youkee D, et al. Evaluation of a point-of-care blood test for identification of Ebola virus disease at Eboalholidng units, Western Area, Sierra Leone, January to February 2015. Euro Surveill. 2015;20:21073.
78. Cecconi M, De Backer D, Antonelli M, Beale R, Bakker J, Hofer C, Jaeschke R, Mebazaa A, Pinsky MR, Teboul JL, Vincent JL, Rhodes A. Consensus on circulatory shock and hemodynamic monitoring. Task force of the European Society of Intensive Care Medicine. Intensive Care Med. 2014;40:1795–815.
79. Shankar-Hari M, Phillips GS, Levy ML, Seymour CW, Liu VX, Deutschman CS, Angus DC, Rubenfeld GD, Singer M, Sepsis Definitions Task Force. Developing a new definition and assessing new clinical criteria for septic shock: for the third international consensus definition for sepsis and septic shock (Sepsis-3). JAMA. 2016;315:775–87.
80. Lima A, Jansen TC, van Bommel J, Ince C, Bakker J. The prognostic value of the subjective assessment of peripheral perfusion in critically ill patients. Crit Care Med. 2009;37:934–8.
81. Ait-Oufella H, Bige N, Boelle PY, Pichereau C, Alves M, Bertinchamp R, Baudel JL, Galbois A, Maury E, Guidet B. Capillary refill time exploration during septic shock. Intensive Care Med. 2014;40:958–64.
82. Evans JA, May J, Ansong D, Antwi S, Asafo-Adjei E, Nguah SB, Osei-Kwakye K, Akoto AO, Ofori AO, Sambian D, Sylverken J, Busch W, Timmann C, Agbenyega T, Horstmann RD. Capillary refill time as an independent prognostic indicator in severe and complicated malaria. J Pedatir. 2006;149:676–81.
83. Biswas HH, Ortega O, Grodon A, Standish K, Balmaseda A, Kuan G, Harris E. Early clinical features of dengue virus infection in Nicaraguan children: a longitudinal analysis. PLoS Negl Trop Dis. 2012;e1562:6.

84. Ait-Oufella H, Lemoinne S, Boelle PY, Galbois A, Baudel JL, Lemant J, Joffre J, Margetis D, Guidet B, Maury E, Offenstadt G. Mottling score predicts survival in septic shock. Intensive Care Med. 2011;37:801–7.
85. Leithe ME, Margorien RD, Hermiller JB, Unverferth DV, Leier CV. Relationship between central hemodynamics and regional blood flow in normal subjects and in patients with congestive heart failure. Circulation. 1984;69:57–64.
86. Macedo E, Malhotra R, Bouchard J, Wynn SK, Mehta RL. Oliguria is an early predictor of higher mortality in critically ill patients. Kidney Int. 2011;80:760–7.
87. Bakker J, Coffernils M, Leon M, Gris P, Vincent JL. Blood lactate levels are superior to oxygen-derived variables in predicting outcome in human septic shock. Chest. 1991;99:956–62.
88. Nguyen HB, Rivers EP, Knoblich BP, Jacobsen G, Muzzin A, Ressler JA, Tomlanovich MC. Early lactate clearance is associated with improved outcome in severe sepsis and septic shock. Crit Care Med. 2004;32:1637–42.
89. Dünser MW, Bataar O, Tsenddorj G, Lundeg G, Torgersen C, Romand JA, Hasibeder WR, HelfenBerührt Study Team. Differences in critical care practice between an industrialized and a developing country. Wien Klin Wochenschr. 2008;120:600–7.
90. Bahloul M, Samet M, Chaari A, Ben Aljia N, Ben Mbarek MN, Chelly H, Dammak H, Ben Hamida C, Rekik N, Kallel H, Bouaziz M. Use of catecholamines for shock. A continuous debate. Tunis Med. 2012;90:291–9.
91. Frikha N, Mebazaa M, Mnif L, El Euch N, Abassi M, Ben Ammar MS. Septic shock in a Tunisian intensive care unit: mortality and predictive factors. 100 cases. Tunis Med. 2005;83:320–5.
92. Bruneel F, Gachot B, Timsit JF, Wolff M, Bédos JP, Régnier B, Vachon F. Shock complicating severe falciparum malaria in European adults. Intensive Care Med. 1997;23:698–701.

Open Access This chapter is licensed under the terms of the Creative Commons Attribution 4.0 International License (http://creativecommons.org/licenses/by/4.0/), which permits use, sharing, adaptation, distribution and reproduction in any medium or format, as long as you give appropriate credit to the original author(s) and the source, provide a link to the Creative Commons license and indicate if changes were made.

The images or other third party material in this chapter are included in the chapter's Creative Commons license, unless indicated otherwise in a credit line to the material. If material is not included in the chapter's Creative Commons license and your intended use is not permitted by statutory regulation or exceeds the permitted use, you will need to obtain permission directly from the copyright holder.

Core Elements of General Supportive Care for Patients with Sepsis and Septic Shock in Resource-Limited Settings

5

Mervyn Mer, Marcus J. Schultz, Neill K. J. Adhikari, Arthur Kwizera, Sanjib Mohanty, Arjen M. Dondorp, Ary Serpa Neto, and Jacobus Preller

M. Mer
Divisions of Critical Care and Pulmonology, Department of Medicine, Faculty of Health Sciences, Charlotte Maxeke Johannesburg Academic Hospital, University of the Witwatersrand, Johannesburg, South Africa

Wits-UQ Critical Care Infection Collaboration, Faculty of Health Sciences, Charlotte Maxeke Johannesburg Academic Hospital, University of the Witwatersrand, Johannesburg, South Africa

M. J. Schultz (✉)
Department of Intensive Care, Academic Medical Center, University of Amsterdam, Amsterdam, The Netherlands

Laboratory of Experimental Intensive Care and Anesthesiology (L.E.I.C.A.), Academic Medical Center, University of Amsterdam, Amsterdam, The Netherlands

Mahidol-Oxford Tropical Medicine Research Unit (MORU), Faculty of Tropical Medicine, Mahidol University, Bangkok, Thailand

N. K. J. Adhikari
Department of Critical Care Medicine, Sunnybrook Health Sciences Centre, Toronto, ON, Canada

Interdepartmental Division of Critical Care, University of Toronto, Toronto, ON, Canada

A. Kwizera
Intensive Care Unit, Mulago National Referral Hospital, Makerere University College of Health Sciences, Kampala, Uganda

Department of Anesthesia, Mulago National Referral Hospital, Makerere University College of Health Sciences, Kampala, Uganda

S. Mohanty
Intensive Care Unit, Ispat General Hospital, Rourkela, Sundargarh, Odisha, India

A. M. Dondorp
Mahidol-Oxford Tropical Medicine Research Unit (MORU), Faculty of Tropical Medicine, Mahidol University, Bangkok, Thailand

© The Author(s) 2019
A. M. Dondorp et al. (eds.), *Sepsis Management in Resource-limited Settings*,
https://doi.org/10.1007/978-3-030-03143-5_5

A. Serpa Neto
Deptartment of Critical Care Medicine, Hospital Israelita Albert Einstein, São Paulo, Brazil

J. Preller
Intensive Care Unit, Addenbrooke's Hospital, Cambridge University Hospitals NHS Foundation Trust, Cambridge, UK

5.1 Introduction

Evidence informing the management of patients with sepsis and septic shock mainly derives from research in resource-rich settings. Knowledge translation to intensive care units (ICUs) in resource-limited settings is limited by restricted availability of skilled staff, equipment, and laboratory support, compounded by infrastructure and logistical challenges. Consequently, we developed recommendations relating to core elements of general supportive care for patients with sepsis and septic shock in resource-limited settings. Our recommendations are built on guidelines from the Surviving Sepsis Campaign [1] and the Global Intensive Care Working Group of the European Society of Intensive Care Medicine [2], as well as on a search for additional recent evidence from resource-limited ICUs.

Clinicians with direct experience in resource-limited ICUs developed recommendations by adapting the Grading of Recommendations Assessment, Development and Evaluation (GRADE) tools [3]. Similar to our group's previous publications (e.g., see [4]), quality of evidence was assessed as high to very low. Recommendations were stated as strong or weak based additionally on indirectness of evidence, magnitude of effects, and availability, feasibility, and safety in resource-limited ICUs. We consulted the World Health Organization's Essential Medicines List when considering the availability of medications (available at http://www.who.int/medicines/publications/essentialmedicines/en/). When necessary, evidence from resource-rich ICUs was adopted after pragmatic experience-based appraisal (see online supplement). We also made several good practice statements [5]. Recommendations and suggestions are summarized in Table 5.1.

5.2 Corticosteroids for Patients with Refractory Shock in Resource-Limited ICUs

Sepsis and septic shock constitute major global health-care problems, particularly in resource-limited countries, where there is a large burden of infectious diseases, and are associated with significant morbidity and mortality [1, 10, 11]. Early and appropriate antimicrobial therapy, intravenous fluids, vasopressors, and source control were necessary, and appropriate supportive care comprises the fundamental principles of therapy in such cases [1, 10].

Several adjunctive therapies for septic shock have been developed and studied, and various treatment strategies evaluated, without improving outcomes [12–15]. Sepsis is associated with systemic inflammation, which may be a significant contributor to the

Table 5.1 Recommendations for core elements of general support for septic patients in resource-limited ICUs

Topic	Recommendation	Relationship to other guidelines
Corticosteroids	We suggest intravenous hydrocortisone (200 mg per day, or equivalent dose of another corticosteroid) in adult patients with septic shock, who despite both adequate fluid resuscitation and vasopressor support remain hemodynamically unstable (low quality of evidence) Remarks: Hemodynamic instability may be defined by systolic blood pressure less than 90 mmHg for more than 1 h despite adequate fluid and vasopressor therapy. Hydrocortisone can be administered by continuous infusion or boluses for 5–7 days, or up to the weaning of vasopressor therapy, followed by tapering of the dose as guided by the clinical response. Bolus dosing does not require an infusion pump and is therefore more feasible. Dosing and pharmacokinetic properties of various corticosteroids are presented in Table 5.2	Same as SSC [1]
Sedation	The group believes that continuous or intermittent sedation be minimized in mechanically ventilated sepsis patients, targeting specific titration end points from sedation scales (ungraded good practice statement) Remarks: Management of intravenous sedation for mechanically ventilated septic patients requires attentive nursing and medical expertise and sufficient staffing to handle risks of agitated delirium and device removal. Adequate pain control should be attained in all patients where necessary (analgesia-first sedation), and lighter sedation targets aimed for in general	Same as SSC [1]
Use of neuromuscular blocking agents	We suggest neuromuscular blockade for maximum of 2 days in mechanically ventilated septic patients with ARDS and PaO_2/FiO_2 ratio <150 mmHg (SpO_2/FiO_2 ratio <190) (moderate quality of evidence) Remark: Attentive nursing and medical care are essential requirements to care for patients on neuromuscular blockade. We suggest monitoring the depth of blockade through train-of-four stimulation when neuromuscular blocking agents are administered by continuous infusion. The safety of continuous neuromuscular blockade in the absence of capnography or arterial blood gas analysis is not established	Same as SSC [1]
	The group believes that neuromuscular blocking agents should not be administered when sedation and analgesia can prevent patient–ventilator dyssynchrony (ungraded good practice statement)	Not addressed
	The group believes that sedation and analgesia should be used before and during neuromuscular blockade to achieve deep sedation (ungraded good practice statement)	Same as recent guideline [6]

(continued)

Table 5.1 (continued)

Topic	Recommendation	Relationship to other guidelines
Venous thromboembolism prophylaxis	We recommend UFH or LMWH to prevent VTE in patients with no contraindications to these medications (moderate quality of evidence)	Same as SSC [1]
	We recommend LMWH over UFH in patients with no contraindications to LMWH, assuming availability of both medications (moderate quality of evidence)	Same as SSC [1]
	We suggest mechanical VTE prophylaxis when UFH and LMWH are contraindicated or unavailable (low quality of evidence) Remark: Mechanical prophylaxis includes GCS and IPC devices; GCS may be less effective than IPC devices but are far more likely to be available	Same as SSC [1]
	We suggest combination of mechanical and pharmacologic prophylaxis if possible (low quality of evidence) Remark: Same as for the previous recommendation	Same as SSC [1]
	The group believes that VTE prophylaxis should be continued until the patient is fully mobile (ungraded good practice statement)	Similar to recent guideline [7]
Stress ulcer prophylaxis	We recommend that stress ulcer prophylaxis be given to patients with sepsis or septic shock with risk factors for GI bleeding (low quality of evidence) Remark: Risk factors for GI bleeding include mechanical ventilation for ≥48 h, coagulopathy, renal replacement therapy, liver disease, multiple comorbidities, and higher organ failure score	Same as SSC [1]
	We suggest that either PPIs or H2RAs be used for stress ulcer prophylaxis (low quality of evidence)	Same as SSC [1]
Blood glucose management	We recommend a protocolized approach to blood glucose management in ICU patients with sepsis, commencing when blood glucose >180 mg/dL (>10 mmol/L), with a target blood glucose value ≤180 mg/dL (≤10 mmol/L) (high quality of evidence)	Same as SSC [1]
	The group believes that blood glucose levels obtained with finger-stick blood glucose tests be interpreted with caution, as these measurements may not accurately estimate arterial blood or plasma glucose values (ungraded good practice statement)	Same as SSC [1]
	The group believes that a simple protocol for blood glucose management should be implemented for all critically ill patients but only if frequent blood glucose monitoring is feasible, safe, and affordable (ungraded good practice statement)	Same as recent guideline [8]
	The group believes that insulin should be administered intravenously rather than subcutaneously in ICU patients with sepsis (ungraded good practice statement)	Not addressed

Enteral feeding	We suggest early enteral feeding as tolerated in patients with sepsis and septic shock (low quality of evidence). Remarks: Additional considerations include starting oral or enteral intake within 24–48 h in adequately resuscitated and hemodynamically stable patients, taking measures to reduce the risk of aspiration, and being aware of the refeeding syndrome in the first few days following enteral nutrition initiation in severely malnourished or starved patients. The risk of aspiration may be increased in enterally fed non-intubated comatose patients with inadequate nursing supervision	Same as SSC [1]
	We suggest either early trophic/hypocaloric or early full enteral feeding in critically ill patients with sepsis or septic shock; if trophic/hypocaloric feeding is the initial strategy, then feeds should be advanced according to patient tolerance (moderate quality of evidence) Remark: We suggest advancing feeds over the first week of ICU stay and note that many patients in low-resource ICUs would be expected to be at high nutrition risk/malnourished and therefore likely to benefit from full enteral feeding	Same as SSC [1]
	We suggest establishing the energy and protein requirements to determine the goals of nutrition therapy using weight-based equations (low quality of evidence)	Consistent with recent guideline [9]
	We suggest a feeding protocol to optimize delivery of EN (moderate quality of evidence)	Consistent with recent guideline [9]
Renal replacement therapy	We suggest that patients with sepsis-induced AKI requiring renal replacement therapy be supported with PD in centers with no current access to renal replacement therapy (very low quality of evidence; case series only) Remark: In centers with functioning IHD programs, we suggest that this modality continue to be used	Not addressed

(continued)

Table 5.1 (continued)

Topic	Recommendation	Relationship to other guidelines
Fluid administration	We suggest conservative fluid administration in patients with sepsis who are not in shock (low quality of evidence; indirect evidence from trials in other forms of critical illness) Remarks: Conservative fluid administration requires development of a protocol (e.g., incorporating shock, oliguria, jugular venous pressure, capillary refill; see supplement for reference to a sample resuscitation protocol incorporating some clinical signs). The protocol should specify the timing of re-evaluation between fluid interventions determined by patient stability. No de-resuscitation protocol has been tested in low-resource ICUs. The role of pressure monitoring via a central venous catheter to direct resuscitation and de-resuscitation is contentious. Conservative fluid administration may be associated with higher levels of blood urea nitrogen, bicarbonate, hemoglobin, and albumin	Not addressed

Additional general comments: Focused attention and careful evaluation of safety aspects and cost-efficiency should be a consideration in every patient and in all settings.

Abbreviations: *ARDS* acute respiratory distress syndrome, *EN* enteral nutrition, *GCS* graduated compression stockings, *GI* gastrointestinal, *H2RA* histamine-2 receptor antagonist, *ICU* intensive care unit, *IHD* intermittent hemodialysis, *IPC* intermittent pneumatic compression, *LMWH* low-molecular-weight heparin, *PD* peritoneal dialysis, *PPI* proton-pump inhibitor, *SSC* Surviving Sepsis Campaign, *UFH* unfractionated heparin, *VTE* venous thromboembolism progression of organ dysfunction and death if uncontrolled [16–20]. Sepsis may also be complicated by impaired corticosteroid metabolism and hypothalamic-pituitary-adrenal axis (HPA) dysfunction in critically ill patients [21–25]. This HPA axis dysfunction in critically ill patients has been referred to as critical illness-related corticosteroid insufficiency (CIRCI) and relates to inadequate corticosteroid activity for the severity of illness as a consequence of decreased adrenal corticosteroid production, as well as tissue resistance to corticosteroids. The process is a dynamic one and may be reversible.

Proinflammatory cytokines and structural damage to the adrenal glands have been implicated in the etiology [17, 18]. The terms "relative" adrenal insufficiency and "functional" adrenal insufficiency have also been used to allude to the same entity [26]. Based on the recognition of the role of excessive inflammation and impaired corticosteroid metabolism in the pathophysiology of multisystem organ dysfunction, corticosteroids have been extensively studied as adjunctive therapy in patients with septic shock over several decades [10, 20, 27–29]. Corticosteroids have the ability to modulate the inflammatory response. They reduce inflammation by decreasing cytokines, adhesion molecules, and other mediators. Corticosteroids halt the activation of various transcription factors and inhibit nuclear factor kappa beta (NF-κB), which plays a crucial role in cytokine gene transcription, thereby ameliorating inflammation [18, 20, 30–33]. Additionally, corticosteroids are pro-apoptotic, assist in maintaining vascular tone by reversing depressed vasopressor sensitivity to catecholamines, maintain endothelium integrity and myocardial contractility, and have an effect on the coagulation cascade by inhibiting platelet aggregation and attenuating tissue factor-mediated activity [20, 34–36].

More recently, the concept of relative adrenal insufficiency as well as of CIRCI has been challenged. This has been based on altered cortisol metabolism in critically ill patients. An increase in cortisol production by a corticotropin-independent mechanism, probably cytokine mediated, and a decrease in cortisol clearance that together contribute to hypercortisolemia and corticotropin suppression have been described [22, 37]. Patients with high cortisol levels have also been shown to have less favorable outcomes [38, 39], which has raised concern about the safety of exogenous administration. Additionally, currently used methods for cortisol measurement have poor agreement, and it has been suggested that the corticotropin stimulation test may not be a valid marker for adrenal dysfunction [40–42].

The use of corticosteroids in the setting of septic shock has been the subject of controversy and uncertainty [1, 19, 43–48]. Initial studies of adjunctive high-dose corticosteroid therapy in patients with septic shock found no evidence of survival benefit [49, 50]. More recent randomized controlled trials (referred to hereafter as "trials") and systematic reviews have suggested that low-dose corticosteroids of longer duration may benefit patients in terms of shock reversal, length of ICU stay, and mortality, with limited adverse effects [1, 19, 28, 29, 47, 51–53]. Adjunctive corticosteroid therapy has been used in a wide array of life-threatening infectious diseases with reported beneficial effects [54–67].

A search of MEDLINE and of references from relevant reviews did not produce any trials that directly addressed the question posed. The search did identify two papers on recommendations for sepsis management in resource-limited settings where some aspects of corticosteroid therapy in refractory shock in resource-limited settings are addressed [2, 68]. A sepsis guideline for Pakistan was also identified, which addressed aspects of corticosteroid administration in patients with sepsis should hemodynamic targets not be met with fluid resuscitation and vasopressor support [69]. Several studies and guidelines from resource-rich ICUs were identified and are included in the discussion.

Trials conducted in the 1980s with high-dose corticosteroids in patients with septic shock failed to demonstrate a mortality benefit, although decreased time to shock reversal was noted in one trial [49, 50, 70, 71]. With the abandonment of the use of high-dose corticosteroids in septic shock, the focus of attention shifted to the concept of relative adrenal insufficiency in septic shock and the use of lower doses of corticosteroids. Promising data emerged using lower doses of corticosteroids (so-called supra-physiological or stress doses of hydrocortisone, 200–300 mg/day), with reports of shock reversal, trends toward earlier resolution of organ dysfunction, and improved mortality [52, 53]. A multicenter trial ($n = 300$) appeared to demonstrate improved 28-day survival in patients with vasopressor-refractory septic shock and relative adrenal insufficiency who were given low-dose intravenous hydrocortisone (50 mg every 6 h) and low-dose fludrocortisone for 7 days [51]. Study patients were hypotensive despite intravenous fluid and vasopressor administration; the benefit was only seen in nonresponders to an adrenocorticotrophic hormone (ACTH) test (blood cortisol level failed to rise appropriately in response to a dose of synthetic ACTH) (hydrocortisone vs. placebo mortality 53% vs. 63%; $p = 0.02$ using survival analysis but not significant in unadjusted chi-square test). Two subsequent meta-analyses found that longer courses (at least 5 days) of low-dose corticosteroids (hydrocortisone 200–300 mg/day) were associated with a decrease in mortality without any significant increase in complications [72]. Based on the available data, the 2004 Surviving Sepsis Campaign guidelines recommended low-dose hydrocortisone in vasopressor-dependent septic shock following appropriate fluid resuscitation [73].

The subsequent Corticosteroid Therapy of Septic Shock (CORTICUS) trial randomized 499 patients with septic shock to receive low-dose intravenous hydrocortisone (50 mg every 6 h) or placebo [74]. The study showed faster shock reversal but no mortality benefit with corticosteroids (hydrocortisone vs. placebo 34.3% vs. 31.5%; $p = 0.51$). The study enrolled all patients with septic shock, including those who did not respond to vasopressors, and the use of the ACTH test did not predict benefit. Corticosteroid administration was associated with an increased incidence of superinfection and new sepsis but was not associated with an increased incidence of polyneuropathy. Various authors have pointed out differences between CORTICUS and the earlier trial [51]: patients in CORTICUS had a much lower severity of illness, could be enrolled for up to 72 h after the onset of shock (vs. 8 h), and were given hydrocortisone for a lesser duration, which may have reduced the potential benefits. Additionally, in the years between the studies, improved management with sepsis bundles and new guidelines may also have reduced corticosteroid benefits. A post hoc subgroup analysis of CORTICUS patients who met the inclusion criteria used in the earlier trial [51] showed a lower 28-day mortality with hydrocortisone [18, 44, 75, 76]. Finally, fludrocortisone was not used in CORTICUS, but a subsequent trial involving 509 patients with septic shock randomized to receive hydrocortisone plus fludrocortisone or hydrocortisone alone later negated its potential benefit (Corticosteroids and Intensive Insulin Therapy for Septic Shock (COIITSS) trial) [77].

The 2008 Surviving Sepsis Campaign guidelines suggested that low-dose hydrocortisone only be given to patients who respond poorly to intravenous fluids and vasopressors and that an ACTH test was not necessary [78]. A different consensus statement by an international task force recommended that low-dose hydrocortisone should be considered in the management of patients with septic shock, especially those who have responded poorly to fluid resuscitation and vasopressors. Intravenous hydrocortisone in a dose of 200 mg/day in four divided doses, or as a bolus of 100 mg followed by a continuous infusion of 10 mg/h, was recommended. The task force suggested continuation for 5–7 days before tapering (rather than abrupt cessation), assuming no recurrence or sepsis or septic shock. They also suggested that tests of adrenal function were not routinely required [17]. A systematic review of corticosteroids in the treatment of sepsis and septic shock involving 17 randomized trials and 3 quasi-randomized trials with acceptable methodological quality suggested beneficial drug effects on shock reversal and 28-day mortality, without increasing the risk of gastroduodenal bleeding, superinfection, or neuromuscular weakness. Corticosteroids were, however, associated with an increased risk of hyperglycemia and hypernatremia [79]. Another systematic review suggested no increased risk of superinfection in patients treated with corticosteroids for septic shock and that corticosteroids significantly reduced the incidence of vasopressor-dependent septic shock [80]. Various reviews and commentaries on the topic have advocated the use of low doses of corticosteroids in refractory septic shock [18, 19, 44, 47, 81].

The 2012 Surviving Sepsis Campaign guidelines suggested 200 mg/day of hydrocortisone to treat patients with septic shock if adequate fluid resuscitation and vasopressor therapy are unable to restore hemodynamic stability (grade 2B). The guidelines recommend against the use of an ACTH stimulation test to identify patients with septic shock who should receive corticosteroid therapy. The guidelines also recommend against the use of corticosteroids to treat sepsis in the absence of shock (grade 1D). Tapering of the administered hydrocortisone is suggested, as is the use of a continuous infusion hydrocortisone (grade 2D) [1]. The 2016 Surviving Sepsis guidelines restated the first recommendation (weak recommendation, low quality of evidence), but did not issue recommendations on the ACTH test, tapering schedule, or continuous vs. intermittent administration.

The timing of corticosteroid therapy was addressed in a retrospective observational study involving 178 critically ill patients with septic shock. Early initiation of low-dose corticosteroids (within 6 h after the onset of septic shock) was associated with a significant 37% reduction in mortality [28]. Another retrospective, multicenter, propensity-matched cohort study involving patients with septic shock who received intravenous low-dose corticosteroid therapy within 48 h of diagnosis of septic shock revealed a beneficial effect on mortality only in patients with the highest severity of illness [45]. In general, data from observational studies on corticosteroids for septic shock have been conflicting, with many studies finding no benefit [45, 82–84] or harm [85, 86].

Recommendations addressing sepsis management in resource-limited settings have advocated the administration of intravenous hydrocortisone (up to 300 mg/day) or prednisolone (up to 75 mg/day) to adult patients requiring escalating dosages of vasopressor support [2]. Additional recommendations include not exceeding 300 mg hydrocortisone or 75 mg prednisolone (to mitigate the risk of additional infections), not administering corticosteroids to patients not requiring vasopressor support unless they are on chronic corticosteroid therapy, and, when vasopressor support is withdrawn, to slowly taper corticosteroids over several days to avoid rebound hypotension. A similar approach has been suggested in another paper addressing the management of sepsis with limited resources [68]. The Sepsis Guidelines for Pakistan, endorsed by the Global Sepsis Alliance, recommends the administration of intravenous hydrocortisone (50 mg every 6 h) should hemodynamic targets not be met following adequate fluid resuscitation and where dose requirements of vasopressors rapidly escalate [69].

A most recent Cochrane systematic review and meta-analysis has evaluated both the rationale and current evidence from 33 randomized trials involving 4268 patients with respect to corticosteroids in septic shock [29]. Corticosteroids reduced 28-day mortality by 13%, significantly decreased the length of ICU and hospital stay, decreased organ dysfunction and failure, and increased the proportion of shock reversal by day 7 by 31%. Length of stay in the ICU was reduced by more than 2 days. Survival benefits were dependent on lower doses of corticosteroids (less than 400 mg of hydrocortisone or equivalent) given for a longer duration of treatment (3 or more days at the full dose). The review also suggested that the sickest patients with sepsis were more likely to derive benefit from corticosteroids. The administration of low-dose corticosteroids was not found to be associated with gastrointestinal bleeding, superinfection, or neuromuscular weakness. In some studies, corticosteroids were associated with mild increases in blood glucose and sodium levels.

Further information will become available after publication of two large trials [87, 88] (planned $n = 3800$ and 1241, respectively), both of which will investigate hydrocortisone (200 mg/day) versus placebo in patients with septic shock; the second trial will also study fludrocortisone.

Corticosteroids given in low-dose are readily available and inexpensive, and evidence exists to support their use in septic patients with refractory shock; various formulations are on the World Health Organization's Essential Medicines List [89]. Data from recent systematic reviews suggest no increased risk of gastrointestinal bleeding, superinfection, or neuromuscular weakness. Their use may, however, be associated with an increased risk of hyperglycemia and hypernatremia.

After reviewing the evidence (no additional trials from resource-limited ICUs) and considering availability, feasibility, affordability, and safety, our recommendation and grading are consistent with the Surviving Sepsis guidelines. We *suggest*

Table 5.2 Characteristics of corticosteroids

Type	Equivalent anti-inflammatory doses (potency)	Mineralocorticoid potency	Biological half-life (hours)
Hydrocortisone	20 mg (1)	1.0	8–12
Cortisone	25 mg (0.8)	0.8	8–12
Prednisolone/prednisone	5 mg (4)	0.8	12–36
Methylprednisolone	4 mg (5)	0.5	12–36
Dexamethasone	0.75 (25)	0	36–54
Fludrocortisone	–	125	18–36

Adapted from [268–270]

intravenous hydrocortisone (200 mg per day, or equivalent dose of another corticosteroid) in adult patients with septic shock, who despite both adequate fluid resuscitation and vasopressor support remain hemodynamically unstable (low quality of evidence). Of note, hemodynamic instability may be defined by systolic blood pressure <90 mmHg for >1 h. Hydrocortisone can be administered by continuous infusion or boluses for 5–7 days, or up to the weaning of vasopressor therapy, followed by tapering of the dose as guided by the clinical response. Bolus dosing does not require an infusion pump and is therefore more feasible. Dosing and pharmacokinetic properties of various corticosteroids are presented in Table 5.2.

5.3 Sedation for Patients with Sepsis in Resource-Limited ICUs

Sedation has been a feature of intensive care since the inception of mechanical ventilation. The earliest ventilators had only mandatory modes, followed by ventilators with insensitive triggers that made patient–ventilator synchronization a challenge. Deep sedation was the pragmatic solution for this problem. Progress in technology and the development of sensitive ventilator trigger outpaced widespread adaptation in sedation practice, despite emerging evidence for the detrimental effects of sedation and specifically deep sedation.

Sedation, especially when deep, has been associated with risk of increased organ dysfunction [90, 91], delirium, cognitive deficit, increased length of stay (LOS) in ICU and hospital, and increased mortality [92]. Strategies to decrease the risk of oversedation include the use of sedation protocols to lighter sedation targets, daily sedation interruptions, or no sedation. Bolus dosing of sedatives is another strategy to titrate sedation to a specified target and prevent oversedation.

A MEDLINE search found no trials that address this question in resource-limited ICUs. The search and references from relevant reviews did not produce any trials that directly addressed the question posed. The 2016 Surviving Sepsis guidelines made a best practice recommendation that continuous or intermittent sedation be minimized in mechanically ventilated sepsis patients, targeting specific titration end points. Earlier comprehensive guidelines [19] on pain, agitation, and delirium recommend that sedative medications be titrated to maintain a light rather than a deep level of sedation in adult ICU patients, unless clinically contraindicated. Neither guideline makes a recommendation about continuous or bolus dosing.

In a single-center prospective observational study [93] of 142 consecutive mechanically ventilated ICU patients, 38.4% received continuous IV sedation (mostly lorazepam [72%] and fentanyl [71%]) to achieve a Ramsay score of 3. A majority (61.6%) received either bolus sedation ($n = 64$) or no intravenous sedation after intubation ($n = 85$). Patients with continuous IV sedation spent more time on mechanical ventilation (by 130 h) and had longer ICU LOS (by 8.7 days) hospital LOS (by 8.2 days; all adjusted $p \leq 0.007$). There were no statistically significant differences in mortality, time of mechanical ventilation (68.5 vs. 45.9 h, $p = 0.07$), or hospital LOS (14.8 vs. 11.3 days, $p = 0.127$) between patients receiving bolus sedation vs. no sedation but a longer ICU LOS (5.7 vs. 4.1 days, $p = 0.017$).

A single-center randomized controlled trial [94] randomized 321 patients to protocol-directed vs. non-protocol-directed sedation and found lower duration of mechanical ventilation (mean 89.1 vs. 124.0 h, $p = 0.003$), lower LOS in ICU (mean 5.7 vs. 7.5 days, $p = 0.013$) and hospital (mean 14.0 vs. 19.9 days, $p < 0.001$), and lower tracheostomy rate (6.2% vs. 13.2%, $p = 0.038$). In the subgroup of patients who received continuous intravenous sedation ($n = 132$, 41.1% of total), the protocol-directed sedation group had a significantly shorter duration of continuous intravenous sedation (3.5 vs. 5.6 days, $p = 0.003$). A Cochrane systematic review (2 trials, $n = 633$) [95] found no differences between patients managed with protocol-directed sedation vs. usual care in efficacy outcomes or adverse events (unplanned extubation or reintubation), but the results of the two included trials conflicted.

Kress et al. [96] randomized 128 patients in a single-center randomized controlled trial to an intervention group sedation with target Ramsay score of 3–4 and daily interruption of continuous sedative infusions. The control group received standard care with no-sedation target or interruption of sedation. Duration of mechanical ventilation and ICU LOS were reduced by 2.4 days ($p = 0.004$) and 3.5 days ($p = 0.02$) in the intervention group, respectively, with no difference in the risk of self-extubation. Subsequent analysis showed fewer complications in the intervention group (2.8% vs. 6.2% in control group, $p = 0.04$) [97] and no increase in the risk of myocardial ischemia [98]. However, a larger multicenter trial ($n = 430$) showed no effect of daily sedation interruption when both groups were managed with a sedation protocol; patients in the daily interruption group received higher doses of benzodiazepines and opiates. A Cochrane systematic review on daily interruption of sedation [99] did not find strong evidence in favor of this approach, although point estimates for efficacy outcomes favored the intervention and a post hoc subgroup analysis of five trials conducted in North America did show reduced duration of mechanical ventilation. There were no differences in risks of unplanned extubation or catheter removal.

Concerns about patient emotional and physical discomfort were raised in a prospective observational study (31 Chinese academic ICUs, $n = 163$). The majority

(79.1%) of patients remembered seriously uncomfortable experiences; protocolized sedation or non-protocolized continuous sedation but not intermittent sedation reduced the risk of complex-mixed discomfort episodes. Of note, 37.4% of patients did not receive any sedation, and only 14.7% received protocolized sedation. The nurse–patient ratio was not stated [100]. Overall, traditional concerns that light sedation or sedation interruptions are associated with worse psychological outcomes seem to be unfounded. Lightly sedated or non-sedated patients may do better than deeply sedated patients [91, 101–103].

To investigate a more extreme version of light sedation, Strom et al. [91] randomized 140 critically ill adults in one center with expected mechanical ventilation >24 h to receive either continuous sedation with propofol for 48 h and lorazepam thereafter, with daily sedation interruptions ($n = 70$), or no sedation ($n = 70$). Both groups received bolus doses of morphine (2.5 or 5 mg) as needed, and the no-sedation group could receive boluses of haloperidol for delirium. The no-sedation group has improvements in ventilator-free days to day 28 and ICU and hospital LOS, but patients who died or who were extubated within 48 h were excluded, and hence the analysis did not include all randomized patients. The no-sedation group also experienced more agitated delirium, and 10/58 patients crossed over to the sedation group. The nurse–patient ratio was 1:1; the no-sedation group needed an additional member of staff on 11 vs. 3 occasions for the sedation group, corresponding to 2.5 days of extra staff time.

Relevant considerations include the following: (1) morphine, midazolam, and diazepam are generic medications and on the World Health Organization's Essential Medicines List [89], although in practice they may not be uniformly available; (2) care of the mechanically ventilated patient with sepsis requires attentive nursing and medical expertise, including the administration and monitoring of intravenous sedation; and (3) depending on staffing models, medical attendance to a patient who self-extubates and requires reintubation may be delayed, particularly outside of weekday daytime hours. Diazepam may be particularly challenging to use because of its active metabolites and long half-life. Systematic reviews have not documented an increased risk of device removal with "light" sedation approaches [95, 99]. Existing literature from high-income countries derives from ICUs with one nurse per one to two patients. These issues point to the need for caution in managing sedation needs in low-resource ICUs, many of which have less nursing staffing.

After reviewing the evidence (no additional trials from low-resource ICUs) and considering availability, feasibility, affordability, and safety, our recommendation and grading are consistent with the Surviving Sepsis guidelines. The group believes that continuous or intermittent sedation be minimized in mechanically ventilated sepsis patients, targeting specific titration end points (ungraded good practice statement).

Of note, management of intravenous sedation for mechanically ventilated septic patients requires attentive nursing and medical expertise and sufficient staffing to handle risks of agitated delirium and device removal. There are no trials of continuous vs. bolus sedation dosing in resource-limited settings.

5.4 Neuromuscular Blocking Agents for Mechanical Ventilation

The role of neuromuscular blocking agents in the ICU is undefined, and there is no clear evidence that neuromuscular blockade in septic mechanically ventilated patients reduces mortality or morbidity. Nevertheless, neuromuscular blocking agents are often administered to critically ill patients to prevent patient–ventilator dyssynchrony [104], a strategy that anecdotally may be practiced more frequently in resource-limited ICUs than in resource-rich settings. Other indications for neuromuscular blockade are to reduce peak airway pressures and to improve chest wall compliance [104] and to reduce oxygen consumption by decreasing the work of breathing and respiratory muscle blood flow [105].

The MEDLINE search did not result in any study from resource-limited ICUs that directly answered the question of interest. We discuss several studies from resource-rich ICUs. The 2016 Surviving Sepsis guidelines suggest using neuromuscular blockers for ≤48 h in adults with sepsis-induced acute respiratory distress syndrome (ARDS) and a PaO_2/FiO_2 ratio <150 mmHg (weak recommendation, moderate quality of evidence). One recent systematic review [106] of three trials (all from France) in patients with ARDS showed improved survival, more ventilator-free days at day 28, higher PaO_2/FiO_2 ratio, and less barotrauma with continuous infusions of the neuromuscular blocking agent cisatracurium for 2 days compared to standard care [107–109]. Most patients in these three trials met criteria for sepsis. The incidence of ICU-acquired weakness was not affected. Several previous observational studies have found an association of neuromuscular blockade with weakness in patients with severe asthma [110–112], although this signal has not been uniform [113, 114]. Several areas of uncertainly remain. First, peripheral nerve monitoring of the depth of neuromuscular blockade (i.e., train-of-four [TOF] stimulation) was only performed in the two smaller trials [107, 108]. Current guidelines [6] suggest that TOF may be useful for monitoring depth blockade but only if incorporated with clinical assessment and suggest that TOF may not be used alone for this purpose. Second, it is uncertain whether a neuromuscular blocking agent other than cisatracurium would have similar effects. Further information about the effects of neuromuscular blockade in the acute respiratory distress syndrome will be available after completion of a large ongoing trial [115].

Selected neuromuscular blocking agents (albeit not cisatracurium) are on the World Health Organization's Essential Medicines List [89] and should therefore be available in resource-limited settings, although in practice they may not be uniformly available. Even if available, associated costs can be substantial when given in a continuous fashion, as this delivery method increases the amount given and requires a syringe pump. The literature is conflicting regarding the benefits of TOF monitoring over clinical judgment to guide administration of neuromuscular blockers [116–118], with only a weak recommendation in favor [6], but it may reduce the amounts given, leading to faster recovery of neuromuscular function, shorter duration of intubation, and lower costs. On the other hand, costs of TOF meters could minimize any financial benefit of neuromuscular blockade. Attentive nursing and medical care are required to care for patients on neuromuscular blockade, with current guidelines suggesting structured physiotherapy and glucose control (to <180 mg/dL, <10 mmol/L) for these patients [6]. The safety of continuous neuromuscular blockade in the absence of capnography or arterial blood gas analysis is not established.

After reviewing the evidence (no additional trials from low-resource ICUs) and considering availability, feasibility, affordability, and safety, our first recommendation and grading are consistent with the Surviving Sepsis guidelines. We *suggest* neuromuscular blockade for a maximum of 2 days in mechanically ventilated septic patients with ARDS and PaO_2/FiO_2 ratio < 150 mmHg (SpO_2/FiO_2 ratio < 190) (moderate quality of evidence). Of note, attentive nursing and medical care are essential requirements to care for patients on neuromuscular blockade. We suggest monitoring the depth of blockade through TOF stimulation when neuromuscular blocking agents are administered by continuous infusion. The safety of continuous neuromuscular blockade in the absence of capnography or arterial blood gas analysis is not established. The conversion of PaO_2/FiO_2 ratio to SpO_2/FiO_2 ratio is from reference [119].

The group believes that neuromuscular blocking agents should not be administered when sedation and analgesia can prevent patient–ventilator dyssynchrony (ungraded good practice statement). The group believes that sedation and analgesia should be used before and during neuromuscular blockade to achieve suitable sedation (ungraded good practice statement). This statement is consistent with recent guidelines [6].

5.5 Deep Venous Thrombosis Prophylaxis in Resource-Limited ICUs

Venous thromboembolism (VTE) is a common and severe complication of critical illness and includes the entities of deep venous thrombosis and pulmonary embolism [120, 121]. VTE is recognized as being the commonest preventable cause of hospital death in resource-rich settings, and evidence strongly supports the value of VTE prophylaxis [122, 123]. Guidelines of many scientific societies strongly recommend that every hospital should have a policy for VTE prophylaxis [122, 123].

Sepsis has been demonstrated to be an independent risk factor for the development of VTE in critically ill patients [7, 120, 124–127]. Therapeutic modalities involved in the management of septic critically ill patients may further contribute to the risk, including mechanical ventilation, central venous catheters, and vasopressors. The inflammatory milieu of sepsis is felt to play an important role in the pathogenesis of VTE [127–130]. Patients with certain forms of infections, such as HIV/AIDS and tuberculosis (TB), which are commonly seen in resource-limited environments, have been shown to be at particularly high risk for VTE [7, 131–135].

An association between mortality and lack of prophylaxis in ICU patients has been demonstrated in both resource-rich and resource-limited settings [136–138].

Data from developing countries, however, has revealed a significant underutilization of VTE prophylaxis [138, 139].

The MEDLINE search did not produce any trials that directly answered this question in resource-limited settings. Several relevant guidelines, recommendations, commentaries, overviews, and studies of VTE prophylaxis were identified, in addition to one retrospective cohort of patients with VTE [140].

The 2016 Surviving Sepsis guidelines [1] make two strong recommendations (moderate quality of evidence): pharmacologic prophylaxis (unfractionated heparin [UFH] or low-molecular-weight heparin [LMWH]) against venous thromboembolism (VTE) in the absence of contraindications to the use of these agents and LMWH rather than UFH for VTE prophylaxis in the absence of contraindications to the use of LMWH. The guidelines also make two weak recommendations (low quality of evidence): combination pharmacologic VTE prophylaxis and mechanical prophylaxis, whenever possible, and mechanical VTE prophylaxis when pharmacologic VTE is contraindicated.

Sepsis guidelines for Pakistan recommend daily pharmacologic prophylaxis (UFH twice daily or LMWH, depending on hospital policy and environment), with intermittent pneumatic compression (IPC) in the case of coagulopathy or low platelets. Where IPC is not available, graduated compression stockings (GCS) are advocated [69]. The South African Guideline on venous thromboembolism recommends pharmacologic prophylaxis with UFH (three times per day) or LMWH until the patient is fully mobile and states that evidence-based data show LMWH to be superior to UFH. Mechanical prophylaxis (GCS or IPC) is suggested as an alternative for patients at high risk of bleeding [7].

VTE prophylaxis has been shown to be effective in a plethora of trials in various populations of acutely ill patients [141–147]. At least two well-conducted systematic reviews further corroborate the efficacy of VTE prophylaxis [148, 149]. Many of the patients studied in these trials had sepsis. The Surviving Sepsis Campaign guidelines and the American College of Chest Physicians guidelines both strongly recommend VTE prophylaxis in the absence of contraindications [1, 123]. Similarly, VTE prophylaxis is advocated in various guidelines, overviews, and commentaries addressing resource-limited settings [2, 124, 138].

Studies have shown that the practice of VTE prophylaxis is suboptimal globally [150, 151]. VTE underutilization, nonadherence to guidelines, and lack of awareness of risk factors have been documented in resource-limited settings [137–139, 152–154]. For example, in an observational study from India, 100% of ICU patients were assessed as being at highest risk for VTE [138]. Just over 25% deemed to be at the highest risk for VTE had sepsis or bloodstream infection; only 11% of the highest risk patients received VTE prophylaxis. VTE has also been documented to be a common finding at autopsy, with many patients noted to be young [155] and to have had septic shock [156].

Guideline adherence and VTE risk stratification are often lacking in resource-limited settings. In a cross-sectional descriptive study conducted in a tertiary care hospital in Nigeria, almost three-fourth of physicians did not perform VTE risk assessment of patients, and only 18.8% follow guidelines on VTE prophylaxis

[157]. Similar data regarding low level of awareness of VTE risk factors has been reported in a national cross-sectional study from Mexico [158]. In an overview of strategies to reduce mortality from bacterial sepsis in adults in developing countries, the authors point out that VTE prophylaxes are both warranted and available in most resource-limited settings [55].

Recently, a prospective multicenter study ($n = 113$) from a high-resource setting [127] found a three- to tenfold higher incidence of VTE in patients admitted with sepsis and septic shock compared to published reports in primarily non-septic ICU patients. The incidence of VTE was 37.2%, and the majority of emboli (88%) were clinically significant pulmonary emboli or DVT. Patients with VTE had a statistically significant increased length of hospital stay of approximately 5 days. Insertion of a central venous catheter and longer duration of mechanical ventilation were additional risk factors. The higher incidence of VTE in this cohort occurred despite pharmacological prophylaxis, with the authors suggesting that higher doses of pharmacological prophylaxis or combination prophylaxis with both heparinoids and mechanical devices may be more effective in septic patients.

Prophylaxis involves both pharmacological and mechanical modalities; the former most frequently includes UFH or LMWH. A systematic review of seven trials ($n = 7226$) of heparin prophylaxis in critically ill patients found that any heparin prophylaxis decreased VTE, with LMWH being superior to UFH for the outcome of pulmonary embolism. There was no effect of any heparin vs. placebo and no effect of LMWH vs. UFH on major bleeding [159]. A Cochrane systematic review of heparin (UFH or LMWH) in acutely ill medical patients (excluding stroke and myocardial infarction; 16 trials, $n = 34{,}369$) revealed a significant reduction in VTE in patients who received any form of heparin prophylaxis. LMWH was superior to UFH and was associated with less major bleeding [160]. The PROTECT Investigators evaluated LMWH versus UFH in 3764 medical–surgical ICU patients and demonstrated no effect on proximal deep vein thrombosis but fewer pulmonary emboli in patients assigned to LMWH [161]. Pharmacological prophylaxis has been shown to be cost-effective for VTE prevention, with LMWH superior to UFH in an economic analysis of PROTECT [162, 163].

Mechanical measures include elastic GCS, IPC, and venous foot pumps. All these modalities have been shown to be beneficial in reducing VTE, likely by increasing venous blood flow and enhancing endogenous fibrinolysis [164]. A recent systematic review (70 trials, $n = 16{,}164$ [165]) found that IPC reduced VTE compared to no IPC prophylaxis and GCS and had similar effect vs. pharmacological prophylaxis but with a reduced risk of bleeding. Adding pharmacological prophylaxis to IPC further reduced the risk of deep venous thrombosis vs. IPC alone.

Pharmacological prophylaxis is generally available in resource-limited ICUs and can be delivered feasibly and safely. The WHO Essential Medicines List includes both heparin and enoxaparin [89]. Mechanical modalities may not be available in many resource-limited ICUs but have the added potential advantage of being reuseable, which would lower costs.

After reviewing the evidence (no additional trials and one guideline from low-resource ICUs) and considering availability, feasibility, affordability, and safety, our recommendations and grading are consistent with the Surviving Sepsis guidelines, except when noted. We *recommend* UFH or LMWH to prevent VTE in patients with no contraindications to these medications (moderate quality of evidence). We *recommend* LMWH over UFH in patients with no contraindications to LMWH assuming availability of both medications (moderate quality of evidence). We *suggest* mechanical VTE prophylaxis when UFH and LMWH are contraindicated or unavailable (low quality of evidence). Of note, mechanical prophylaxis includes GCS and IPC devices; GCS may be less effective than IPC devices but are far more likely to be available. We *suggest* combination mechanical (IPC devices) and pharmacologic prophylaxis if possible (low quality of evidence). Of note, mechanical prophylaxis includes GCS and IPC devices; GCS may be less effective than IPC devices but are far more likely to be available. The group believes that VTE prophylaxis should be continued until the patient is fully mobile (ungraded good practice statement). This statement is consistent with that made in the South African VTE guideline [7].

5.6 Stress Ulcer Prophylaxis in Patients with Sepsis in Resource-Limited ICUs

Stress ulceration of the gastric mucosa in critically ill patients has been studied for many years, with mechanical ventilation for ≥48 h and presence of coagulopathy identified as risk factors [166]. A recent multicenter observational study conducted in 11 high-income countries found that clinically important gastrointestinal (GI) bleeding occurred in 2.6% (95%CI 1.5–3.6%) of patients [167]. In this study, independent risk factors for GI bleeding included ≥3 comorbidities, liver disease, use of renal replacement therapy, coagulopathy, higher organ failure score, and use of acid suppressants at ICU admission (possibly due to confounding by indication). Systematic reviews of trials from mostly high-income countries have shown that either histamine-2 receptor antagonists (H2RAs) or proton-pump inhibitors (PPIs) reduce GI bleeding [168], with some evidence that PPIs are superior [169].

A MEDLINE search of recent literature (2012–2016) did not identify trials addressing this question. Previous systematic reviews [168, 169] included two trials (India) and five trials (Brazil, China, Iran, India) from middle-income countries, respectively.

The 2016 Surviving Sepsis guidelines [1] recommend, based on low quality of evidence, that stress ulcer prophylaxis be given to patients with sepsis or septic shock with risk factors for GI bleeding (strong recommendation) and suggest that either PPIs or H2RAs be used (weak recommendation). New data on the efficacy of stress ulcer prophylaxis will become available after ongoing trials of PPI vs. placebo are completed [170, 171].

Many H2RAs and PPIs are available as generic preparations and in principle should be widely available. Omeprazole and ranitidine (both in oral and injectable forms) are on the WHO Model List of Essential Medicines [89]. Systematic reviews of trials have not shown statistically significant differences in rates of pneumonia among PPIs, H2RAs, or control [168, 169]; trials have not addressed the comparative risk of *C. difficile* infection. Observational studies on the association between risk of *C. difficile* infection and stress ulcer prophylaxis with PPI have produced inconsistent results [172, 173].

After reviewing the evidence (no additional trials from low-resource ICUs) and considering availability, feasibility, affordability, and safety, our recommendations are consistent with the Surviving Sepsis guidelines. We *recommend* that stress ulcer prophylaxis be given to patients with sepsis or septic shock with risk factors for GI bleeding (low quality of evidence). Risk factors for GI bleeding include mechanical ventilation for ≥48 h, coagulopathy, renal replacement therapy, liver disease, multiple comorbidities, and higher organ failure score. We *suggest* that either PPIs or H2RAs be used for stress ulcer prophylaxis (low quality of evidence).

5.7 Glucose Control in Patients with Sepsis in Resource-Limited ICUs

Dysglycemia frequently occurs in critically ill patients. Hyperglycemia may be associated with critical illness or less frequently due to diabetic ketoacidosis [174]. Certain infectious diseases, e.g., malaria, are associated with an increased risk of hypoglycemia, particularly in children and patients with limited glycogen stores, like malnourished patients or subjects with liver disease [175]. Hypoglycemia may also develop as a side effect of continuous insulin infusion for control of critical illness-associated hyperglycemia [176].

While early trials showed reduced mortality and morbidity with continuous intravenous administration of insulin aiming for normoglycemia (80–110 mg/dL, 4.4–6.1 mmol/L) in critically ill adult and pediatric patients [177, 178], subsequent trials of "intensive insulin therapy" suggested harm [176]. Also, almost without exception, "intensive insulin therapy" results in a much higher incidence of severe hypoglycemia (<40 mg/dL, 2.2 mmol/L) [176]. Consequently the international guidelines, including the Surviving Sepsis Campaign guidelines [1], moved from recommending "intensive insulin therapy" to recommending prevention of hyperglycemia (defined as >180 mg/dL, >10 mmol/L). One of the five systematic reviews of "intensive insulin therapy" [179–183] showed "intensive insulin therapy" to be beneficial only in surgical ICU patients (risk ratio, 0.63 [0.44–0.9]) [180], but another review refuted this finding [181].

Blood glucose control with intravenous insulin is a very complex intervention, independent of the targets used [174, 176]. Many different protocols for the titration of intravenous insulin in ICU patients have been published [184]. It is unknown which of these protocols have been implemented in ICUs beyond the centers where they were designed, let alone whether they are effective and safe in other surroundings. It is generally considered important to guide the titration of intravenous insulin in ICU patients by frequent measurements of the blood glucose level [174], a strategy that is time- and blood-consuming and expensive. Also, it is advised to prefer bedside-based blood gas analyzers over finger-stick blood glucose tests, as accuracy of capillary blood glucose monitoring could be too low to guarantee safe and effective titration of intravenous insulin in ICU patients [176].

While insulin infusion is preferred over oral antihyperglycemic agents for blood glucose control in the ICU [174], a large variety of oral antihyperglycemic agents are available that may simplify and possibly improve blood glucose control in the ICU.

The MEDLINE search did not find trials of "intensive insulin therapy" from resource-limited ICUs. The search, however, identified one recent consensus guideline on blood glucose management in India [8] and three small Iranian trials of the oral antidiabetic agent, metformin [185–187]. Major issues of the Indian guideline are discussed, as are the results from the trials of metformin. We do not discuss the importance of preemptive treatment of hypoglycemia in patients with malaria but refer to another set of guidelines from our group, focusing on management of dengue and malaria [188].

The 2016 Surviving Sepsis guidelines [1] recommend a protocolized approach to blood glucose management in ICU patients with sepsis, commencing insulin dosing when two consecutive blood glucose levels are >180 mg/dL. This approach should target an upper blood glucose level ≤180 mg/dL rather than an upper target blood glucose level ≤110 mg/dL (strong recommendation, high quality of evidence). The guidelines suggest the use of arterial blood rather than capillary blood for point-of-care testing using glucose meters if patients have arterial catheters (weak recommendation, low quality of evidence). The guidelines make two best practice statements: blood glucose values should be monitored every 1–2 h until glucose values and insulin infusion rates are stable and then every 4 h thereafter in patients receiving insulin infusions; glucose levels should be obtained with point-of-care testing of capillary blood be interpreted with caution because such measurements may not accurately estimate arterial blood or plasma glucose values.

Recently, a group of experts in the fields of diabetes and intensive care medicine from India framed recommendations regarding blood glucose control and monitoring for Indian ICUs [8]. One recommendation was to use a *simple* protocol for managing hyperglycemia for all critically ill patients, i.e., with no differences between various types of ICUs. The guideline recommended that the blood glucose target should be 140–180 mg/dL (7.8–10.0 mmol/L) in critically ill patients but lower (110–140 mg/dL, 6.1–7.8 mmol/L) in patients after coronary bypass or uncomplicated surgery; blood glucose target values <110 mg/dL (>6.0 mmol/L) should be avoided; and insulin should be stopped when the blood glucose level drops <70 mg/dL (<3.9 mmol/L; Table 5.3 shows the titration protocol of the Indian guideline [8]). Despite absence of trials, the guideline recommended intravenous over subcutaneous insulin because of the latter's unreliable absorption and unpredictable effects and risk of delayed hypoglycemia. Finally, they recommended monitoring capillary blood glucose every hour or more frequently (e.g., every 20–30 min in case of hypoglycemia, until hypoglycemia resolves).

A few small trials have investigated oral antihyperglycemic agents for blood glucose control in ICU patients. Treatment with twice daily oral metformin was shown to be as effective as continuous intravenous administration of insulin in reducing the

Table 5.3 Example of a *simple* protocol of blood glucose control, as proposed for Indian intensive care units

Start intravenous insulin when blood glucose level >180 mg/dL	
Start insulin infusion (U/L) by dividing the blood glucose value in (mg/dL) by 100 and rounding it off to the nearest decimal (e.g., if blood glucose level is 237 mg/dL, then start insulin infusion at a rate of 2 units/h, and, e.g., if blood glucose value is 387 mg/dL, then start insulin infusion at a rate of 4 units/h)	
Titrate intravenous insulin dosage according to the prevailing blood glucose level:	
<110 mg/dL	No insulin
110–149 mg/dL	1.0 unit/h
150–99 mg/dL	2.0 units/h
200–249 mg/dL	2.5 units/h
250–299 mg/dL	3.0 units/h
300–349 mg/dL	3.5 units/h
350–399 mg/dL	4.0 units/h
400–449 mg/dL	4.5 units/h
450–499 mg/dL	5.0 units/h
500–549 mg/dL	5.5 units/h
550–599 mg/dL	6.0 units/h

Adapted from [8]. To convert mg/dL to mmol/L, divide by 18

blood glucose level in a trial in 51 critically ill trauma patients who presented with hyperglycemia [185]. Of note, it remained unclear what blood glucose targets were used in patients treated with insulin, and blood glucose levels were only marginally reduced over the 3-day observation period. Also, it was not mentioned how frequent blood glucose levels were measured, and incidence of hypoglycemia was not reported. In a trial of 24 critically ill patients after major trauma or non-abdominal surgeries, continuous intravenous administration of insulin caused a greater reduction in blood glucose concentration than metformin alone, but the latter strategy required less attention and trained personnel [186]. Hypoglycemia did not occur in this trial. A third trial in 21 ICU patients with systemic inflammatory response syndrome compared oral metformin plus intravenous insulin to intravenous insulin and found reduced insulin requirement and nursing workload with similar glucose control [187]. All trials were at high risk of bias—they lacked a description of randomization and allocation concealment—one trial was described as double-blinded but with no description of procedures [186], and all trials excluded some patients after randomization.

We did not locate trials of subcutaneous vs. intravenous insulin in critically ill patients, but pharmacologic considerations suggest that titration of insulin dose in response to changing plasma glucose values is much more feasible with intravenous administration.

Critical illness-associated hyperglycemia is common, and short-acting insulin is widely available, cheap, and on the WHO Essential Medicines List [89]. Blood glucose control with continuous intravenous insulin is a complex intervention that requires a continuous infusion pump and close monitoring, with an increased risk for hypoglycemia when blood glucose monitoring is insufficient. Choosing a higher glucose threshold and using a *simple* insulin titration protocol applicable for all ICU patients could reduce complexity and costs. Frequent blood glucose measurements, as suggested in the Indian guideline for blood glucose control [8], may only be feasible and affordable when using finger-stick blood glucose tests, but these remain less accurate than more costly venous or arterial blood samples.

Use of the cheap and widely available metformin may simplify blood glucose control in critically ill patients. However, concerns remain over the risk of lactic acidosis [189], uncertain biological availability of orally administered antihyperglycemic agents, and lack of adequate trial data. The US Food and Drug Administration label for metformin advises that metformin is contraindicated in patients with an estimated glomerular filtration rate (eGFR) <30 mL/min/m^2, not recommended when eGFR is 30–45 mL/min/m^2, and should be withheld "in the presence of any condition associated with hypoxemia, dehydration, or sepsis."

After reviewing the evidence (no additional trials from low-resource ICUs) and considering availability, feasibility, affordability, and safety, our recommendations are consistent with the Surviving Sepsis guidelines and the Indian guidelines [8]. We make no recommendations regarding metformin or other oral antidiabetic agents for blood glucose control in the absence of adequate evidence from trials. We *recommend* a protocolized approach to blood glucose management in ICU patients with sepsis, commencing when blood glucose >180 mg/dL (>10 mmol/L), with a target blood glucose value ≤180 mg/dL (≤10 mmol/L) (high quality of evidence). The group believes that blood glucose levels obtained with finger-stick blood glucose tests be interpreted with caution, as these measurements may not accurately estimate arterial blood or plasma glucose values (ungraded good practice statement). The group believes that a simple protocol for blood glucose management should be implemented for all critically ill patients but only if frequent blood glucose monitoring is feasible, safe, and affordable (ungraded good practice statement). The group believes that insulin should be administered intravenously rather than subcutaneously in ICU patients with sepsis (ungraded good practice statement).

5.8 Enteral Feeding in Patients with Sepsis in Resource-Limited ICUs

Nutrition is an integral component of critical care and evidence relating to its efficacy, timing, composition, and route of administration has evolved substantially over the past two decades. Although nutrition is no longer considered a purely supportive element administered to critically ill patients in order to maintain lean body mass, malnutrition and undernutrition remain a commonly encountered entity in patients worldwide. Malnutrition is often unrecognized and is an independent risk factor for increased morbidity, increased length of hospital stay and hospital costs, delayed recovery, readmission, impaired quality of life, and mortality [190]. This entity is of major relevance in resource-limited settings.

Appropriately administered enteral nutrition (EN) is now believed to be associated with a reduction in complications, duration of stay in the ICU, and improved patient outcomes [191, 192]. The provision of enteral nutrition plays a pivotal role in maintaining gut integrity, thereby limiting the potential translocation of microorganisms into the bloodstream, and is thought to favorably modulate stress and the systemic inflammatory response, with subsequent diminution of cellular injury and attenuation of disease severity [191–194]. Additional benefits of enteral nutrition include its role in stress ulcer prophylaxis [2, 68, 191–193] and facilitation of electrolyte replacement.

A MEDLINE and publication search did not produce any trials that directly answered the question posed. The search identified two papers on recommendations for sepsis management in resource-limited settings [2, 68] and a sepsis guideline from Pakistan [69]. Several additional studies and guidelines from resource-rich ICUs were identified and are discussed below.

Published guidelines are not consistent on recommendations for the timing and amount of enteral feeding. The 2016 Surviving Sepsis guidelines suggest early initiation of enteral feeding rather than a complete fast or only IV glucose in critically ill patients with sepsis or septic shock who can be fed enterally (low quality of evidence) and suggest either trophic/hypocaloric or early full enteral feeding in sepsis and septic shock, with advancement of feeds according to tolerance if the former strategy is used (moderate quality of evidence) [1]. The 2015 Canadian Clinical Practice Guidelines (available at www.criticalcarenutrition.com) recommend consideration of intentional underfeeding of calories (not protein) in patients with low nutrition risk, but not high nutrition risk, and recommend against initial trophic feeding in ARDS. The 2016 SCCM/ASPEN guidelines recommend either trophic or full nutrition by EN in patients with ARDS or an expected duration of ventilation of ≥72 h [192].

No trial has specifically addressed early enteral feeding in septic patients. Data from a heterogeneous group of critically ill patients has revealed evidence of benefit of early enteral (≤48 h) nutrition in reducing infectious complications [191, 193, 195–200], length of mechanical ventilation [198, 201], and length of ICU and hospital stays [198, 201], with a trend toward decreased mortality [192].

Several guidelines, recommendations, and opinion papers warn against the use of early enteral nutrition in hemodynamically unstable patients because of the risk of gastrointestinal ischemia [191, 202]. Suggestions regarding the initiation of enteral nutrition for resource-limited environments advocate administration as early as possible but only after the patient has been adequately resuscitated and is fully awake, or if intubated, after hemodynamic function has stabilized [2, 68]. Additionally, patients receiving EN should be assessed for the risk of aspiration, and steps to reduce this risk should be employed. One small trial in Bangladesh of early nasogastric EN in non-intubated patients with malaria and depressed level of consciousness was terminated early because of an increased aspiration risk in the early feeding group [203].

Risk factors for aspiration are described (Table 5.4) [192]. The potential association of bolus EN with aspiration has been shown [204], and recent guidelines

Table 5.4 Risk factors for aspiration

Inability to protect the airway	Neurologic deficits
Reduced/diminished level of consciousness	Age > 70 years
Supine position	Inadequate nurse/patient ratio
Presence of nasoenteric enteral access device	Gastroesophageal reflux
Mechanical ventilation	Transportation out of ICU
Poor oral care	Use of bolus intermittent EN

Adapted from [192]

suggest continuous EN for high-risk patients or those intolerant of bolus gastric EN [192]. Additional benefits of continuous EN may include fewer interruptions in delivery and delivery of an overall greater volume [205–210]. Additional measures to limit the risk of aspiration include the use of promotility agents, elevation of the head of the bed to 30–45°, chlorhexidine oral care, reduction in the levels of sedation and analgesia, and limiting transportation out of the ICU for diagnostic tests and procedures [211]. Measurement of gastric residual volumes has not been shown to reduce aspiration risk. Most recent guidelines, commentaries, and reviews recommend that gastric residuals not be used to monitor ICU patients on EN [202, 212]. Promotility agents, including metoclopramide (10 mg three to four times daily) and erythromycin (3–7 mg/kg per day), have been advocated in resource-rich environments in patients at high risk of aspiration. Adverse effects include dyskinesia in the elderly with metoclopramide and cardiac toxicity and concerns regarding bacterial resistance with erythromycin [192, 202, 213]. This practice may not always be feasible in resource-limited environments. Elevation of the head of the bed to 30–45° [214, 215] and chlorhexidine oral care [216, 217] have been shown to significantly reduce the incidence of pneumonia.

Energy and protein requirements and methods to calculate them in critically ill patients have been the subject of much debate. Weight-based formulations are regarded as acceptable estimates of nutritional requirements in most critically ill patients (criticalcarenutrition.com), based on lack of evidence for indirect calorimetry [218–221].

Nutrition encompasses the provision of macronutrients (protein, lipid, carbohydrate) and micronutrients (vitamins and minerals/trace elements) (Table 5.5). Energy requirements for the critically ill are generally in the range of 25–30 kcal/kg/day, with protein requirements 1.2–2.0 g/kg/day, with 1.5 g/kg/day generally regarded as being appropriate [192, 199, 202, 220, 222]. This calculation is not necessarily applicable in obese patients where high-protein, hypocaloric feeding has more recently been advocated (2.0–2.5 g protein/kg ideal body weight/day and 65–70% of caloric requirements) to maintain lean body mass, promote loss of fat mass, and improve clinical outcome [192, 202, 223–225]. Vitamins and trace elements are organic compounds and ions that usually act as cofactors for enzymes involved in metabolic pathways or are structurally integral components of enzymes

Table 5.5 Suggested average daily nutritional requirements for most critically ill patients

Energy requirements	25 kcal/kg
Macronutrients	
Protein	1.5 g/kg (1 g protein = 4 kcal)
Carbohydrate	4 g/kg (1 g carbohydrate = 3.75 kcal)
Lipid	1 g/kg (1 g lipid/fat = 9.3 kcal)
Electrolytes	
Sodium	1–2 mmol/kg
Potassium	1 mmol/kg
Chloride	1–2 mmol/kg
Calcium	0.1 mmol/kg
Magnesium	0.1 mmol/kg
Phosphate	0.1–0.4 mmol/kg
Vitamins	
Water-soluble—B complex, folate, vitamin C, vitamin B_{12}	
Fat-soluble—A, D, E, K	
Trace elements	
Iron	10 mg
Zinc	15 mg
Copper	3 mg
Iodine	150 μg
Manganese	5 μg
Chromium	200 μg
Selenium	200 μg

Adapted from [192, 199, 202, 218, 235]

that may be involved in electron transfer. The provision of antioxidant vitamins and trace elements has been associated with improved outcome in several trials [192, 226–229], but the signal has not been uniform, and a recent systematic review found no benefit of selenium [230].

Recommendations for resource-limited environments have suggested that EN be administered as early as possible but only after the patient has been fully resuscitated, demonstrates the ability to swallow, and is awake, in which case small amounts of food and drink may be allowed [2, 69]. The Sepsis Guidelines for Pakistan recommend that in basic hospitals (without intensive care backup and with general physicians), oral feeding as tolerated should be commenced within 48 h instead of only intravenous glucose. They suggest that in intermediate setups (hospitals with level 2 ICUs that are managed by non-intensivists and with access to in-house basic laboratory and diagnostic facilities), enteral feeding be considered within 48 h of sepsis, starting with 500 kcal/day and gradually advanced as tolerated. These guidelines advise against full caloric feed in the first week. In tertiary care setups, initiation of EN is recommended within 48 h, with parenteral nutrition (PN) alone or to supplement enteral feeding not recommended for the first 7 days of a severe infection [69].

Type of enteral feed and the selection of an appropriate enteral formulation have been the subjects of many investigations. In resource-limited environments where commercial feeds may not be available or affordable, hospital-prepared foods may be administered to the patient. Recipes may vary according to countries, regions, and available ingredients. Recommendations include the administration of milk supplemented by cooking oil, salt, sugar, soya, and a multivitamin tablet via a nasogastric tube in intubated hemodynamically stable patients [2] to mixtures involving eggs, milk powder, soya, maize oil, rice, squash, flour, sugar, and fruit. Mixing these foodstuffs in a blender with subsequent administration has been suggested (Towey R, Dunser M, Mer M—personal communications) but may result in unpredictable levels of both macro- and micronutrients. Where commercially available feeds are available, a standard polymeric formula is recommended [192]. These preparations contain intact proteins, fats, and carbohydrates (which require digestion prior to absorption), in addition to electrolytes, trace elements, vitamins, and fibers, and tend to be lactose-free. Commonly used ingredients in these products include the casein (protein from milk), soy protein, maize and soya oils, and the carbohydrate maltodextrin. In general, a ready-to-use standard feed will contain 1 kcal and 0.04 g protein per mL and is usually well tolerated [192].

The utilization and employment of feeding protocols are advocated in several guidelines, studies, commentaries, and recommendations. They are associated with an increase in the overall percentage of nutrition provided and may also positively impact outcome [68, 192, 202, 231–234].

Complications of nutritional support include the refeeding syndrome in patients who are severely malnourished or who have undergone a significant period of starvation. The mechanism relates to in a loss of intracellular electrolytes in starvation or undernutrition, followed by an insulin-mediated influx of electrolytes and thiamine into the cells when carbohydrate is provided, which can result in rapid and marked reductions in serum levels of phosphate, magnesium, potassium, and calcium. Patients may also develop lactic acidosis. Clinical features include edema, diarrhea, neuromuscular abnormalities, seizures, coma, cardiac arrhythmias, and respiratory failure. Risk factors for the refeeding syndrome include a BMI of less than 18.5 kg/m^2; weight loss of greater than 10–15% in the prior 3–6 months; little or no nutritional intake for more than 5 days; history of alcohol abuse or drugs including insulin, chemotherapy, antacids, or diuretics; and very low levels of phosphate, potassium, and magnesium. At-risk patients should be identified, and feeding must be commenced slowly. It has been suggested that feeding commence at 5–10 kcal/kg/day with a gradual escalation over 4–7 days. Electrolytes must be closely monitored and replaced. Thiamine and other B vitamins should be given intravenously prior to commencing feeding and then daily for at least 3 days [235].

Overfeeding should be avoided as it may be associated with fluid overload, worsening renal function, hyperglycemia, hyperlipidemia, fatty liver, and hypercapnia (particularly with excess carbohydrate administration) with delayed weaning from mechanical ventilation more difficult. It has also been associated with a less favorable outcome [202, 235].

Enteral feeding is feasible, readily available, and can be made affordable. Parenteral nutrition is generally not available. Patients should be adequately resuscitated, hemodynamically stable, and caution exercised to limit the possibility of aspiration. Where commercial feeds are not available, hospital-prepared foods may be administered. Non-intubated patients, in whom oral feeding is to be initiated, should be awake and able to swallow. Steps in the care of the patient fed enterally with a gastric tube may be remembered using our coined acronym "COPE" and include continuous infusion, oral care with chlorhexidine, prokinetic agent use (as needed and where feasible), and elevation of the head of the bed (30–45°).

After reviewing the evidence (no additional trials from low-resource ICUs) and considering availability, feasibility, affordability, and safety, our recommendations are consistent with the Surviving Sepsis guidelines, except when noted. We make no recommendations regarding PN due to general lack of availability and therefore relevance to resource-limited ICUs. We *suggest* early enteral feeding as tolerated in patients with sepsis and septic shock (low quality of evidence). Additional considerations include starting oral or enteral intake within 24–48 h in adequately resuscitated and hemodynamically stable patients, taking measures to reduce the risk of aspiration, and being aware of the refeeding syndrome in the first few days following EN initiation in severely malnourished or starved patients. The risk of aspiration may be increased in enterally fed non-intubated comatose patients with inadequate nursing supervision. We *suggest* either early trophic/hypocaloric or early full enteral feeding in critically ill patients with sepsis or septic shock; if trophic/hypocaloric feeding is the initial strategy, then feeds should be advanced according to patient tolerance (moderate quality of evidence). We suggest advancing feeds over the first week of ICU stay and note that many patients in low-resource ICUs would be expected to be at high nutrition risk and therefore to benefit from full enteral feeding. We *suggest* establishing the energy and protein requirements to determine the goals of nutrition therapy using weight-based equations (low quality of evidence). This recommendation is consistent with the 2015 Canadian Clinical Practice Guidelines (available at www.criticalcarenutrition.com), which makes no recommendation on indirect calorimetry vs. predictive equations. We *suggest* a feeding protocol to optimize delivery EN (moderate quality of evidence). This recommendation is consistent with the 2015 Canadian Clinical Practice Guidelines (available at www.criticalcarenutrition.com).

5.9 Dialysis in Patients with Sepsis-Induced Acute Kidney Damage in Resource-Limited ICUs

Although population-based data on the burden of acute kidney injury (AKI) are sparse, acute and chronic renal failure have been estimated to account for approximately 3% of all deaths in India [236], and AKI likely contributes to a much higher proportion of deaths from sepsis. In low-resource rural settings, community-acquired AKI is more common than hospital-acquired AKI in medically complex patients and typically affects young previously healthy patients who develop this complication after obstetrical crisis, trauma, poisoning, or sepsis. Many patients with these conditions present late to hospital with established AKI that does not improve with resuscitation [237], raising the importance of renal replacement therapy for these conditions as a bridge to recovery. Logistical barriers to the deployment of IHD in these settings include lack of reliable electricity and water supply. In contrast, gravity-based PD can be implemented and in theory is more sustainable because of the requirement for consumables only.

No recent trials of IHD vs. PD in sepsis were identified in a search of recent MEDLINE references (2012–2016). One trial compared high-volume peritoneal dialysis to extended daily dialysis in ICUs in two Brazilian hospitals [238]; nearly half the enrolled patients had sepsis. Results of the intention-to-treat analysis were not reported, and treatment groups did not appear well-matched at baseline; overall mortality was 64% and did not differ between groups. The search also revealed several observational studies of adults [239–245] or children [242, 245–248] treated with PD or HD, including one study of CRRT under combat conditions [249]. Among these studies, the median mortality was 30%. Several commentaries have described the Saving Young Lives program of the International Society of Nephrology [250–252], designed to establish sustainable acute PD programs in very low-resource settings. Preliminary data describe 175 patients treated over 33 months in 8 hospitals in Africa and Asia, with one-third of patients surviving to discharge with normal renal function [253].

Surviving Sepsis guidelines make no recommendations about the modality of renal replacement in septic patients [1]. A prominent early trial from a single center in Vietnam showed that continuous hemofiltration vs. peritoneal dialysis reduced mortality in patients with severe acute kidney injury due to infection (malaria or sepsis) [254]. More recently, a systematic review and meta-analysis [255] included seven cohort studies and four trials of IHD vs. PD; the trials were conducted in middle-income countries (Nigeria, India, Brazil, and Vietnam), and the observational studies were conducted in high- or middle-income countries. The risk of bias of the trials was not described in detail, although all scored 3 or below on the 5-point Jadad scale, and therefore could be considered as low quality. The quality of the observational studies was not assessed. Meta-analyses showed no difference in mortality (OR in trials 1.50, 95%CI 0.46–4.86; OR in observational studies 0.96, 95%CI 0.53–1.71).

Recent literature has emphasized the high potential for feasible and cost-effective widespread deployment of PD to very low-resource settings, notwithstanding challenges of patient selection, ongoing training, and program sustainability [253].

Our recommendation is not informed by the Surviving Sepsis guidelines. We *suggest* that patients with sepsis-induced AKI requiring renal replacement therapy be supported with PD in centers with no current access to renal replacement therapy (very low quality of evidence; case series only).

Remark: In centers with functioning IHD programs, we suggest that this modality continue to be used.

5.10 Fluid Strategies in Patients with Sepsis in Resource-Limited ICUs

Sepsis is traditionally treated with large volume fluid resuscitation, which frequently causes accumulation of bodily fluids. However, numerous studies have demonstrated that a positive fluid balance is independently associated with organ dysfunction and decreased survival [256–261]. Achieving a negative fluid balance, or "de-resuscitation," could improve organ function and outcome of critically ill patients [262, 263].

The MEDLINE search did not find trials of "de-resuscitation" from resource-limited ICUs. The search, however, identified one recent systematic review including trials and observational studies that collectively enrolled a broad population of patients and compared "conservative" to "nonconservative" fluid strategies [264]. We also discuss one trial of fluid strategies in patients with ARDS [263].

The 2016 Surviving Sepsis guidelines contain recommendations pertaining to initial resuscitation, but do not address fluid management beyond that phase [1].

The best evidence that "de-resuscitation" may improve outcomes of critically ill patients comes from a randomized controlled trial in 1000 patients with ARDS [263]. In this trial, a "conservative" and a "liberal" strategy of fluid management using complex but *explicit* protocols were compared in patients not in shock. In this factorial trial, patients were also randomized to pulmonary artery vs. central venous catheterization. The mean cumulative fluid balance during the first 7 days was significantly more positive in the "liberal" strategy group (6992 ± 502 mL versus −136 ± 491 mL). While the difference in mortality at 60 days (25.5 vs. 28.4%) was not statistically significant, the "conservative" strategy improved oxygenation and lung function and increased the number of ventilator-free days (14.6 ± 0.5 vs. 12.1 ± 0.5 days) as well as the number of ICU-free days (13.4 ± 0.4 vs. 11.2 ± 0.4 days) during the first 28 days. Notably, while the "conservative" strategy did not increase the incidence of shock during the study or the use of dialysis, it did result in higher levels of blood urea nitrogen, bicarbonate, hemoglobin, and albumin. Also, there were no significant differences in the number of failure-free days for other organs other than the lung. Of note, although most patients in this trial met the criteria for sepsis, it is unclear whether a "restrictive" strategy will have similar beneficial effects when given to septic patients (i.e., in the absence of ARDS).

Trials comparing "conservative" with "liberal" strategy of fluid management in patients with sepsis are lacking. One recently published systematic review [264], including observational studies or trials (often testing interventions other than fluid strategies), showed that the cumulative fluid balance after 1 week of ICU stay was 4.4 L more positive in non-survivors compared to survivors. A "conservative" fluid strategy resulted in a less positive cumulative fluid balance of 5.6 L after 1 week of ICU stay, which was associated with a lower mortality compared to patients treated with a more liberal fluid management strategy (odds ratio, 0.42 [0.32–0.55]). It should be noted, however, that this systematic review included studies of a broad population of patients (including elective surgical patients) and did not report the most unbiased analysis possible, i.e., of outcomes in trials of patients randomized to conservative vs. liberal fluid strategies.

It should be noted that the *explicit* protocols for fluid management in the trial in ARDS patients [263] were quite complex. At least every 4 h, patients were assigned to 1 of as many as 20 protocol cells on the basis of 4 variables: central venous pressure or pulmonary artery occlusion pressure, the presence or absence of shock (a mean systemic arterial pressure <60 mmHg or the need for a vasopressor), the presence or absence of oliguria (less than 0.5 mL/kg/h), and the presence or absence of ineffective circulation (cardiac index of less than 2.5 L/min/m^2 or cold, mottled skin with a capillary refilling time of more than 2 s), with each cell being associated with an intervention and a reassessment interval. Apart from this complex approach, the 4-hourly reassessment and the need for a central venous catheter or pulmonary artery catheter could hamper feasibility and affordability in resource-limited ICUs.

Our recommendations are not informed by the Surviving Sepsis guidelines. We *suggest* conservative fluid administration in patients with sepsis who are not in shock (low quality of evidence; indirect evidence from trials in other forms of critical illness). Conservative fluid administration requires development of a protocol (e.g., incorporating shock, oliguria, jugular venous pressure, capillary refill; see reference [265] for a sample resuscitation protocol incorporating some clinical signs). The protocol should specify the timing of re-evaluation between fluid interventions determined by patient stability. No de-resuscitation protocol has been tested in low-resource ICUs. The role of pressure monitoring via a central venous catheter to direct resuscitation and de-resuscitation is contentious [266, 267]. Conservative fluid administration may be associated with higher levels of blood urea nitrogen, bicarbonate, hemoglobin, and albumin.

References

1. Rhodes A, Evans LE, Alhazzani W, Levy MM, Antonelli M, Ferrer R, Kumar A, Sevransky JE, Sprung CL, Nunnally ME, Rochwerg B, Rubenfeld GD, Angus DC, Annane D, Beale RJ, Bellinghan GJ, Bernard GR, Chiche JD, Coopersmith C, De Backer DP, French CJ, Fujishima S, Gerlach H, Hidalgo JL, Hollenberg SM, Jones AE, Karnad DR, Kleinpell RM, Koh Y, Lisboa TC, Machado FR, Marini JJ, Marshall JC, Mazuski JE, McIntyre LA, McLean AS, Mehta S, Moreno RP, Myburgh J, Navalesi P, Nishida O, Osborn TM, Perner A, Plunkett CM, Ranieri M, Schorr CA, Seckel MA, Seymour CW, Shieh L, Shukri KA, Simpson SQ, Singer M, Thompson BT, Townsend SR, Van der Poll T, Vincent JL, Wiersinga WJ, Zimmerman JL, Dellinger RP (2017) Surviving Sepsis Campaign: international guidelines for management of sepsis and septic shock: 2016. Intensive Care Med 43(3):304–377.
2. Dunser MW, Festic E, Dondorp A, Kissoon N, Ganbat T, Kwizera A, Haniffa R, Baker T, Schultz MJ, Global Intensive Care Working Group of European Society of Intensive Care Medicine. Recommendations for sepsis management in resource-limited settings. Intensive Care Med. 2012;38:557–74.
3. Schünemann H, Brożek J, Guyatt G, Oxman A, editors. GRADE handbook for grading quality of evidence and strength of recommendations. Updated October 2013 [guidelinedevelopment.org/handbook]. The GRADE Working Group. 2013.
4. Serpa Neto A, Schultz MJ, Festic E. Ventilatory support of patients with sepsis or septic shock in resource-limited settings. Intensive Care Med. 2016;42:100–3.

5. Guyatt GH, Alonso-Coello P, Schunemann HJ, Djulbegovic B, Nothacker M, Lange S, Murad MH, Akl EA. Guideline panels should seldom make good practice statements: guidance from the GRADE Working Group. J Clin Epidemiol. 2016;80:3–7.
6. Murray MJ, DeBlock H, Erstad B, Gray A, Jacobi J, Jordan C, McGee W, McManus C, Meade M, Nix S, Patterson A, Sands MK, Pino R, Tescher A, Arbour R, Rochwerg B, Murray CF, Mehta S. Clinical practice guidelines for sustained neuromuscular blockade in the adult critically Ill patient. Crit Care Med. 2016;44:2079–103.
7. Jacobson BF, Louw S, Buller H, Mer M, de Jong PR, Rowji P, Schapkaitz E, Adler D, Beeton A, Hsu HC, Wessels P, Haas S, South African Society of Thrombosis and Haemostasis. Venous thromboembolism: prophylactic and therapeutic practice guideline. S Afr Med J. 2013;103:261–7.
8. Mukherjee JJ, Chatterjee PS, Saikia M, Muruganathan A, Das AK, Diabetes Consensus Group. Consensus recommendations for the management of hyperglycaemia in critically ill patients in the Indian setting. J Assoc Physicians India. 2014;62:16–25.
9. Clinical practice guideline for nutrition support in the mechanically ventilated, critically ill adult patient. http://www.criticalcarenutrition.com/. Clinical Evaluation Research Unit, Kingston General Hospital/Queen's University. 2015.
10. Angus DC, van der Poll T. Severe sepsis and septic shock. N Engl J Med. 2013;369:840–51.
11. Fleischmann C, Scherag A, Adhikari NK, Hartog CS, Tsaganos T, Schlattmann P, Angus DC, Reinhart K. International Forum of Acute Care TrialistsAssessment of global incidence and mortality of hospital-treated sepsis. Current estimates and limitations. Am J Respir Crit Care Med. 2016;193:259–72.
12. Sweeney DA, Danner RL, Eichacker PQ, Natanson C. Once is not enough: clinical trials in sepsis. Intensive Care Med. 2008;34:1955–60.
13. Asfar P, Meziani F, Hamel JF, Grelon F, Megarbane B, Anguel N, Mira JP, Dequin PF, Gergaud S, Weiss N, Legay F, Le Tulzo Y, Conrad M, Robert R, Gonzalez F, Guitton C, Tamion F, Tonnelier JM, Guezennec P, Van Der Linden T, Vieillard-Baron A, Mariotte E, Pradel G, Lesieur O, Ricard JD, Herve F, du Cheyron D, Guerin C, Mercat A, Teboul JL, Radermacher P, SEPSIS-PAM Investigators. High versus low blood-pressure target in patients with septic shock. N Engl J Med. 2014;370:1583–93.
14. Angus DC, Barnato AE, Bell D, Bellomo R, Chong CR, Coats TJ, Davies A, Delaney A, Harrison DA, Holdgate A, Howe B, Huang DT, Iwashyna T, Kellum JA, Peake SL, Pike F, Reade MC, Rowan KM, Singer M, Webb SA, Weissfeld LA, Yealy DM, Young JD. A systematic review and meta-analysis of early goal-directed therapy for septic shock: the ARISE, ProCESS and ProMISe Investigators. Intensive Care Med. 2015;41:1549–60.
15. Caironi P, Tognoni G, Masson S, Fumagalli R, Pesenti A, Romero M, Fanizza C, Caspani L, Faenza S, Grasselli G, Iapichino G, Antonelli M, Parrini V, Fiore G, Latini R, Gattinoni L, ALBIOS Study Investigators. Albumin replacement in patients with severe sepsis or septic shock. N Engl J Med. 2014;370:1412–21.
16. Annane D, Bellissant E, Cavaillon JM. Septic shock. Lancet. 2005;365:63–78.
17. Marik PE, Pastores SM, Annane D, Meduri GU, Sprung CL, Arlt W, Keh D, Briegel J, Beishuizen A, Dimopoulou I, Tsagarakis S, Singer M, Chrousos GP, Zaloga G, Bokhari F, Vogeser M, American College of Critical Care Medicine. Recommendations for the diagnosis and management of corticosteroid insufficiency in critically ill adult patients: consensus statements from an international task force by the American College of Critical Care Medicine. Crit Care Med. 2008;36:1937–49.
18. Marik PE. Critical illness-related corticosteroid insufficiency. Chest. 2009;135:181–93.
19. Annane D. Corticosteroids for severe sepsis: an evidence-based guide for physicians. Ann Intensive Care. 2011;1:7.
20. Cohen R. Use of corticosteroids in septic shock. Minerva Anestesiol. 2011;77:190–5.
21. Marik PE, Annane D. Reduced cortisol metabolism during critical illness. N Engl J Med. 2013;369:480–1.
22. Boonen E, Van den Berghe G. Cortisol metabolism in critical illness: implications for clinical care. Curr Opin Endocrinol Diabetes Obes. 2014;21:185–92.

23. Peeters B, Boonen E, Langouche L, Van den Berghe G. The HPA axis response to critical illness: new study results with diagnostic and therapeutic implications. Mol Cell Endocrinol. 2015;408:235–40.
24. Venkatesh B, Cohen J, Cooper M. Ten false beliefs about cortisol in critically ill patients. Intensive Care Med. 2015;41:1817–9.
25. Kertai MD, Fontes ML. Predicting adrenal insufficiency in severe sepsis: the role of plasma-free cortisol. Crit Care Med. 2015;43:715–6.
26. Cooper MS, Stewart PM. Corticosteroid insufficiency in acutely ill patients. N Engl J Med. 2003;348:727–34.
27. Patel GP, Balk RA. Systemic steroids in severe sepsis and septic shock. Am J Respir Crit Care Med. 2012;185:133–9.
28. Park HY, Suh GY, Song JU, Yoo H, Jo IJ, Shin TG, Lim SY, Woo S, Jeon K. Early initiation of low-dose corticosteroid therapy in the management of septic shock: a retrospective observational study. Crit Care. 2012;16:R3.
29. Annane D, Bellissant E, Bollaert PE, Briegel J, Keh D, Kupfer Y. Corticosteroids for treating sepsis. Cochrane Database Syst Rev. 2015:CD002243.
30. van Leeuwen HJ, van der Bruggen T, van Asbeck BS, Boereboom FT. Effect of corticosteroids on nuclear factor-kappaB activation and hemodynamics in late septic shock. Crit Care Med. 2001;29:1074–7.
31. Prigent H, Maxime V, Annane D. Science review: mechanisms of impaired adrenal function in sepsis and molecular actions of glucocorticoids. Crit Care. 2004;8:243–52.
32. Meduri GU, Muthiah MP, Carratu P, Eltorky M, Chrousos GP. Nuclear factor-kappaB- and glucocorticoid receptor alpha- mediated mechanisms in the regulation of systemic and pulmonary inflammation during sepsis and acute respiratory distress syndrome. Evidence for inflammation-induced target tissue resistance to glucocorticoids. Neuroimmunomodulation. 2005;12:321–38.
33. Mesotten D, Vanhorebeek I, Van den Berghe G. The altered adrenal axis and treatment with glucocorticoids during critical illness. Nat Clin Pract Endocrinol Metab. 2008;4:496–505.
34. Annane D, Bellissant E, Sebille V, Lesieur O, Mathieu B, Raphael JC, Gajdos P. Impaired pressor sensitivity to noradrenaline in septic shock patients with and without impaired adrenal function reserve. Br J Clin Pharmacol. 1998;46:589–97.
35. Galon J, Franchimont D, Hiroi N, Frey G, Boettner A, Ehrhart-Bornstein M, O'Shea JJ, Chrousos GP, Bornstein SR. Gene profiling reveals unknown enhancing and suppressive actions of glucocorticoids on immune cells. FASEB J. 2002;16:61–71.
36. Colin G, Annane D. Corticosteroids and human recombinant activated protein C for septic shock. Clin Chest Med. 2008;29:705–12. x
37. Boonen E, Vervenne H, Meersseman P, Andrew R, Mortier L, Declercq PE, Vanwijngaerden YM, Spriet I, Wouters PJ, Vander Perre S, Langouche L, Vanhorebeek I, Walker BR, Van den Berghe G. Reduced cortisol metabolism during critical illness. N Engl J Med. 2013;368:1477–88.
38. Christ-Crain M, Stolz D, Jutla S, Couppis O, Muller C, Bingisser R, Schuetz P, Tamm M, Edwards R, Muller B, Grossman AB. Free and total cortisol levels as predictors of severity and outcome in community-acquired pneumonia. Am J Respir Crit Care Med. 2007;176:913–20.
39. Salluh JI, Bozza FA, Soares M, Verdeal JC, Castro-Faria-Neto HC, Lapa ESJR, Bozza PT. Adrenal response in severe community-acquired pneumonia: impact on outcomes and disease severity. Chest. 2008;134:947–54.
40. Hamrahian AH, Oseni TS, Arafah BM. Measurements of serum free cortisol in critically ill patients. N Engl J Med. 2004;350:1629–38.
41. Gotoh S, Nishimura N, Takahashi O, Shiratsuka H, Horinouchi H, Ono H, Uchiyama N, Chohnabayashi N. Adrenal function in patients with community-acquired pneumonia. Eur Respir J. 2008;31:1268–73.
42. Briegel J, Sprung CL, Annane D, Singer M, Keh D, Moreno R, Mohnle P, Weiss Y, Avidan A, Brunkhorst FM, Fiedler F, Vogeser M, CORTICUS Study Group. Multicenter comparison of

cortisol as measured by different methods in samples of patients with septic shock. Intensive Care Med. 2009;35:2151–6.
43. Sprung CL, Goodman S, Weiss YG. Steroid therapy of septic shock. Crit Care Nurs Clin North Am. 2011;23:171–80.
44. Marik PE. Glucocorticoids in sepsis: dissecting facts from fiction. Crit Care. 2011;15:158.
45. Funk D, Doucette S, Pisipati A, Dodek P, Marshall JC, Kumar A, Cooperative Antimicrobial Therapy of Septic Shock Database Research Group. Low-dose corticosteroid treatment in septic shock: a propensity-matching study. Crit Care Med. 2014;42:2333–41.
46. Allen KS, Kinasewitz GT. The pendulum of corticosteroids in sepsis swings again? Crit Care Med. 2014;42:2442–3.
47. Annane D. Adjunctive treatment in septic shock: what's next? Presse Med. 2016;45:e105–9.
48. Trubelja AD. Current use of steroids in critical care. SOJ Anesthesiol Pain Manag. 2014;1:1–4.
49. Lefering R, Neugebauer EA. Steroid controversy in sepsis and septic shock: a meta-analysis. Crit Care Med. 1995;23:1294–303.
50. Cronin L, Cook DJ, Carlet J, Heyland DK, King D, Lansang MA, Fisher CJ Jr. Corticosteroid treatment for sepsis: a critical appraisal and meta-analysis of the literature. Crit Care Med. 1995;23:1430–9.
51. Annane D, Sebille V, Charpentier C, Bollaert PE, Francois B, Korach JM, Capellier G, Cohen Y, Azoulay E, Troche G, Chaumet-Riffaud P, Bellissant E. Effect of treatment with low doses of hydrocortisone and fludrocortisone on mortality in patients with septic shock. JAMA. 2002;288:862–71.
52. Bollaert PE, Charpentier C, Levy B, Debouverie M, Audibert G, Larcan A. Reversal of late septic shock with supraphysiologic doses of hydrocortisone. Crit Care Med. 1998;26:645–50.
53. Briegel J, Forst H, Haller M, Schelling G, Kilger E, Kuprat G, Hemmer B, Hummel T, Lenhart A, Heyduck M, Stoll C, Peter K. Stress doses of hydrocortisone reverse hyperdynamic septic shock: a prospective, randomized, double-blind, single-center study. Crit Care Med. 1999;27:723–32.
54. Confalonieri M, Urbino R, Potena A, Piattella M, Parigi P, Puccio G, Della Porta R, Giorgio C, Blasi F, Umberger R, Meduri GU. Hydrocortisone infusion for severe community-acquired pneumonia: a preliminary randomized study. Am J Respir Crit Care Med. 2005;171:242–8.
55. Cheng AC, West TE, Limmathurotsakul D, Peacock SJ. Strategies to reduce mortality from bacterial sepsis in adults in developing countries. PLoS Med. 2008;5:e175.
56. Siemieniuk RA, Meade MO, Alonso-Coello P, Briel M, Evaniew N, Prasad M, Alexander PE, Fei Y, Vandvik PO, Loeb M, Guyatt GH. Corticosteroid therapy for patients hospitalized with community-acquired pneumonia: a systematic review and meta-analysis. Ann Intern Med. 2015;163:519–28.
57. Torres A, Sibila O, Ferrer M, Polverino E, Menendez R, Mensa J, Gabarrus A, Sellares J, Restrepo MI, Anzueto A, Niederman MS, Agusti C. Effect of corticosteroids on treatment failure among hospitalized patients with severe community-acquired pneumonia and high inflammatory response: a randomized clinical trial. JAMA. 2015;313:677–86.
58. Cavalcanti AB, Machado FR, Berwanger O. Quality improvement intervention and mortality of critically ill patients—reply. JAMA. 2016;316:879–80.
59. Thwaites GE, Nguyen DB, Nguyen HD, Hoang TQ, Do TT, Nguyen TC, Nguyen QH, Nguyen TT, Nguyen NH, Nguyen TN, Nguyen NL, Nguyen HD, Vu NT, Cao HH, Tran TH, Pham PM, Nguyen TD, Stepniewska K, White NJ, Tran TH, Farrar JJ. Dexamethasone for the treatment of tuberculous meningitis in adolescents and adults. N Engl J Med. 2004;351:1741–51.
60. Strang JI, Kakaza HH, Gibson DG, Girling DJ, Nunn AJ, Fox W. Controlled trial of prednisolone as adjuvant in treatment of tuberculous constrictive pericarditis in Transkei. Lancet. 1987;2:1418–22.
61. Strang JI, Nunn AJ, Johnson DA, Casbard A, Gibson DG, Girling DJ. Management of tuberculous constrictive pericarditis and tuberculous pericardial effusion in Transkei: results at 10 years follow-up. QJM. 2004;97:525–35.

62. Hoffman SL, Punjabi NH, Kumala S, Moechtar MA, Pulungsih SP, Rivai AR, Rockhill RC, Woodward TE, Loedin AA. Reduction of mortality in chloramphenicol-treated severe typhoid fever by high-dose dexamethasone. N Engl J Med. 1984;310:82–8.
63. Mer M, Richards GA. Corticosteroids in life-threatening varicella pneumonia. Chest. 1998;114:426–31.
64. Bozzette SA, Sattler FR, Chiu J, Wu AW, Gluckstein D, Kemper C, Bartok A, Niosi J, Abramson I, Coffman J, et al. A controlled trial of early adjunctive treatment with corticosteroids for Pneumocystis carinii pneumonia in the acquired immunodeficiency syndrome. California Collaborative Treatment Group. N Engl J Med. 1990;323:1451–7.
65. Ewald H, Raatz H, Boscacci R, Furrer H, Bucher HC, Briel M. Adjunctive corticosteroids for Pneumocystis jiroveci pneumonia in patients with HIV infection. Cochrane Database Syst Rev. 2015:CD006150.
66. Brouwer MC, McIntyre P, Prasad K, van de Beek D. Corticosteroids for acute bacterial meningitis. Cochrane Database Syst Rev. 2015:CD004405.
67. McGee S, Hirschmann J. Use of corticosteroids in treating infectious diseases. Arch Intern Med. 2008;168:1034–46.
68. Stephens K. Management of sepsis with limited resources. Update in Anesthesia. 28:145–55.
69. Hashmi M, Khan FH, bin Sarwar Zubairi A, Sultan ST, Haider S, Aftab S, Husain J, ul Haq A, Rao ZA, Khuwaja A, Sultan SF, Rais Z, Baloch R, Salahuddin N, Khan A, Sultan F, Chima K, Ali A, Ali G. Developing local guidelines for management of sepsis in adults: Sepsis Guidelines for Pakistan (SGP). Anaesth Pain Intensive Care. 2015;19:196–208.
70. Sprung CL, Caralis PV, Marcial EH, Pierce M, Gelbard MA, Long WM, Duncan RC, Tendler MD, Karpf M. The effects of high-dose corticosteroids in patients with septic shock. A prospective, controlled study. N Engl J Med. 1984;311:1137–43.
71. Bone RC, Fisher CJ Jr, Clemmer TP, Slotman GJ, Metz CA. Early methylprednisolone treatment for septic syndrome and the adult respiratory distress syndrome. Chest. 1987;92:1032–6.
72. Annane D, Bellissant E, Bollaert PE, Briegel J, Keh D, Kupfer Y. Corticosteroids for severe sepsis and septic shock: a systematic review and meta-analysis. BMJ. 2004;329:480.
73. Dellinger RP, Carlet JM, Masur H, Gerlach H, Calandra T, Cohen J, Gea-Banacloche J, Keh D, Marshall JC, Parker MM, Ramsay G, Zimmerman JL, Vincent JL, Levy MM, Surviving Sepsis Campaign Management Guidelines Committee. Surviving Sepsis Campaign guidelines for management of severe sepsis and septic shock. Crit Care Med. 2004;32:858–73.
74. Sprung CL, Annane D, Keh D, Moreno R, Singer M, Freivogel K, Weiss YG, Benbenishty J, Kalenka A, Forst H, Laterre PF, Reinhart K, Cuthbertson BH, Payen D, Briegel J, Corticus Study Group. Hydrocortisone therapy for patients with septic shock. N Engl J Med. 2008;358:111–24.
75. Marik PE, Pastores SM, Kavanagh BP. Corticosteroids for septic shock [letter]. N Engl J Med. 2008;358:2069–70. author reply 2070-2061
76. Vincent JL. Steroids in sepsis: another swing of the pendulum in our clinical trials. Crit Care. 2008;12:141.
77. COIITSS Study Investigators, Annane D, Cariou A, Maxime V, Azoulay E, D'Honneur G, Timsit JF, Cohen Y, Wolf M, Fartoukh M, Adrie C, Santre C, Bollaert PE, Mathonet A, Amathieu R, Tabah A, Clec'h C, Mayaux J, Lejeune J, Chevret S. Corticosteroid treatment and intensive insulin therapy for septic shock in adults: a randomized controlled trial. JAMA. 2010;303:341–8.
78. Dellinger RP, Levy MM, Carlet JM, Bion J, Parker MM, Jaeschke R, Reinhart K, Angus DC, Brun-Buisson C, Beale R, Calandra T, Dhainaut JF, Gerlach H, Harvey M, Marini JJ, Marshall J, Ranieri M, Ramsay G, Sevransky J, Thompson BT, Townsend S, Vender JS, Zimmerman JL, Vincent JL, International Surviving Sepsis Campaign Guidelines Committee, American Association of Critical-Care Nurses, American College of Chest Physicians, American College of Emergency Physicians, Canadian Critical Care Society, European Society of Clinical Microbiology and Infectious Diseases, European Society of Intensive Care Medicine, European Respiratory Society, International Sepsis Forum, Japanese Association for Acute Medicine, Japanese Society of Intensive Care Medicine,

Society of Critical Care Medicine, Society of Hospital Medicine, Surgical Infection Society, World Federation of Societies of Intensive and Critical Care Medicine. Surviving Sepsis Campaign: international guidelines for management of severe sepsis and septic shock: 2008. Crit Care Med2008;36:296–327.

79. Annane D, Bellissant E, Bollaert PE, Briegel J, Confalonieri M, De Gaudio R, Keh D, Kupfer Y, Oppert M, Meduri GU. Corticosteroids in the treatment of severe sepsis and septic shock in adults: a systematic review. JAMA. 2009;301:2362–75.
80. Sligl WI, Milner DA Jr, Sundar S, Mphatswe W, Majumdar SR. Safety and efficacy of corticosteroids for the treatment of septic shock: a systematic review and meta-analysis. Clin Infect Dis. 2009;49:93–101.
81. Vincent JL, Serrano EC, Dimoula A. Current management of sepsis in critically ill adult patients. Expert Rev Anti-Infect Ther. 2011;9:847–56.
82. Ferrer R, Artigas A, Suarez D, Palencia E, Levy MM, Arenzana A, Perez XL, Sirvent JM, Edusepsis Study Group. Effectiveness of treatments for severe sepsis: a prospective, multicenter, observational study. Am J Respir Crit Care Med. 2009;180:861–6.
83. Levy MM, Dellinger RP, Townsend SR, Linde-Zwirble WT, Marshall JC, Bion J, Schorr C, Artigas A, Ramsay G, Beale R, Parker MM, Gerlach H, Reinhart K, Silva E, Harvey M, Regan S, Angus DC. The Surviving Sepsis Campaign: results of an international guideline-based performance improvement program targeting severe sepsis. Intensive Care Med. 2010;36:222–31.
84. Povoa P, Salluh JI, Martinez ML, Guillamat-Prats R, Gallup D, HR A-K, Thompson BT, Ranieri VM, Artigas A. Clinical impact of stress dose steroids in patients with septic shock: insights from the PROWESS-Shock trial. Crit Care. 2015;19:193.
85. Beale R, Janes JM, Brunkhorst FM, Dobb G, Levy MM, Martin GS, Ramsay G, Silva E, Sprung CL, Vallet B, Vincent JL, Costigan TM, Leishman AG, Williams MD, Reinhart K. Global utilization of low-dose corticosteroids in severe sepsis and septic shock: a report from the PROGRESS registry. Crit Care. 2010;14:R102.
86. Casserly B, Gerlach H, Phillips GS, Lemeshow S, Marshall JC, Osborn TM, Levy MM. Low-dose steroids in adult septic shock: results of the Surviving Sepsis Campaign. Intensive Care Med. 2012;38:1946–54.
87. Venkatesh B, Myburgh J, Finfer S, Webb SA, Cohen J, Bellomo R, McArthur C, Joyce CJ, Rajbhandari D, Glass P, Harward M, ANZICS CTG Investigators. The ADRENAL study protocol: adjunctive corticosteroid treatment in critically ill patients with septic shock. Crit Care Resusc. 2013;15:83–8.
88. Annane D, Buisson CB, Cariou A, Martin C, Misset B, Renault A, Lehmann B, Millul V, Maxime V, Bellissant E, APPROCHSS Investigators for the TRIGGERSEP Network. Design and conduct of the activated protein C and corticosteroids for human septic shock (APROCCHSS) trial [Erratum in: Ann Intensive Care 2016 Dec; 6(1): 79]. Ann Intensive Care. 2016;6:43.
89. WHO model lists of essential medicines. 2015. World Health Organization. http://www.who.int/medicines/publications/essentialmedicines/en/.
90. Strom T, Johansen RR, Prahl JO, Toft P. Sedation and renal impairment in critically ill patients: a post hoc analysis of a randomized trial. Crit Care. 2011;15:R119.
91. Strom T, Martinussen T, Toft P. A protocol of no sedation for critically ill patients receiving mechanical ventilation: a randomised trial. Lancet. 2010;375:475–80.
92. Pandharipande PP, Pun BT, Herr DL, Maze M, Girard TD, Miller RR, Shintani AK, Thompson JL, Jackson JC, Deppen SA, Stiles RA, Dittus RS, Bernard GR, Ely EW. Effect of sedation with dexmedetomidine vs lorazepam on acute brain dysfunction in mechanically ventilated patients: the MENDS randomized controlled trial. JAMA. 2007;298:2644–53.
93. Kollef MH, Levy NT, Ahrens TS, Schaiff R, Prentice D, Sherman G. The use of continuous i.v. sedation is associated with prolongation of mechanical ventilation. Chest. 1998;114:541–8.
94. Brook AD, Ahrens TS, Schaiff R, Prentice D, Sherman G, Shannon W, Kollef MH. Effect of a nursing-implemented sedation protocol on the duration of mechanical ventilation. Crit Care Med. 1999;27:2609–15.

95. Aitken LM, Bucknall T, Kent B, Mitchell M, Burmeister E, Keogh S. Sedation protocols to reduce duration of mechanical ventilation in the ICU: a Cochrane Systematic Review. J Adv Nurs. 2016;72:261–72.
96. Kress JP, Pohlman AS, O'Connor MF, Hall JB. Daily interruption of sedative infusions in critically ill patients undergoing mechanical ventilation. N Engl J Med. 2000;342:1471–7.
97. Schweickert WD, Gehlbach BK, Pohlman AS, Hall JB, Kress JP. Daily interruption of sedative infusions and complications of critical illness in mechanically ventilated patients. Crit Care Med. 2004;32:1272–6.
98. Kress JP, Vinayak AG, Levitt J, Schweickert WD, Gehlbach BK, Zimmerman F, Pohlman AS, Hall JB. Daily sedative interruption in mechanically ventilated patients at risk for coronary artery disease. Crit Care Med. 2007;35:365–71.
99. Burry L, Rose L, McCullagh IJ, Fergusson DA, Ferguson ND, Mehta S. Daily sedation interruption versus no daily sedation interruption for critically ill adult patients requiring invasive mechanical ventilation. Cochrane Database Syst Rev. 2014:CD009176.
100. Ma P, Liu J, Xi X, Du B, Yuan X, Lin H, Wang Y, Su J, Zeng L. Practice of sedation and the perception of discomfort during mechanical ventilation in Chinese intensive care units. J Crit Care. 2010;25:451–7.
101. Kress JP, Gehlbach B, Lacy M, Pliskin N, Pohlman AS, Hall JB. The long-term psychological effects of daily sedative interruption on critically ill patients. Am J Respir Crit Care Med. 2003;168:1457–61.
102. Treggiari MM, Romand JA, Yanez ND, Deem SA, Goldberg J, Hudson L, Heidegger CP, Weiss NS. Randomized trial of light versus deep sedation on mental health after critical illness. Crit Care Med. 2009;37:2527–34.
103. Jackson JC, Girard TD, Gordon SM, Thompson JL, Shintani AK, Thomason JW, Pun BT, Canonico AE, Dunn JG, Bernard GR, Dittus RS, Ely EW. Long-term cognitive and psychological outcomes in the awakening and breathing controlled trial. Am J Respir Crit Care Med. 2010;182:183–91.
104. Murray MJ, Cowen J, DeBlock H, Erstad B, Gray AW, Jr., Tescher AN, McGee WT, Prielipp RC, Susla G, Jacobi J, Nasraway SA, Jr., Lumb PD, Task Force of the American College of Critical Care Medicine of the Society of Critical Care Medicine, American Society of Health-System Pharmacists, American College of Chest Physicians. Clinical practice guidelines for sustained neuromuscular blockade in the adult critically ill patient. Crit Care Med. 2002;30:142–156.
105. Hansen-Flaschen JH, Brazinsky S, Basile C, Lanken PN. Use of sedating drugs and neuromuscular blocking agents in patients requiring mechanical ventilation for respiratory failure. A national survey. JAMA. 1991;266:2870–5.
106. Neto AS, Pereira VG, Esposito DC, Damasceno MC, Schultz MJ. Neuromuscular blocking agents in patients with acute respiratory distress syndrome: a summary of the current evidence from three randomized controlled trials. Ann Intensive Care. 2012;2:33.
107. Forel JM, Roch A, Marin V, Michelet P, Demory D, Blache JL, Perrin G, Gainnier M, Bongrand P, Papazian L. Neuromuscular blocking agents decrease inflammatory response in patients presenting with acute respiratory distress syndrome. Crit Care Med. 2006;34:2749–57.
108. Gainnier M, Roch A, Forel JM, Thirion X, Arnal JM, Donati S, Papazian L. Effect of neuromuscular blocking agents on gas exchange in patients presenting with acute respiratory distress syndrome. Crit Care Med. 2004;32:113–9.
109. Papazian L, Forel JM, Gacouin A, Penot-Ragon C, Perrin G, Loundou A, Jaber S, Arnal JM, Perez D, Seghboyan JM, Constantin JM, Courant P, Lefrant JY, Guerin C, Prat G, Morange S, Roch A, Investigators AS. Neuromuscular blockers in early acute respiratory distress syndrome. N Engl J Med. 2010;363:1107–16.
110. Leatherman JW, Fluegel WL, David WS, Davies SF, Iber C. Muscle weakness in mechanically ventilated patients with severe asthma. Am J Respir Crit Care Med. 1996;153:1686–90.
111. Behbehani NA, Al-Mane F, D'Yachkova Y, Pare P, FitzGerald JM. Myopathy following mechanical ventilation for acute severe asthma: the role of muscle relaxants and corticosteroids. Chest. 1999;115:1627–31.

112. Adnet F, Dhissi G, Borron SW, Galinski M, Rayeh F, Cupa M, Pourriat JL, Lapostolle F. Complication profiles of adult asthmatics requiring paralysis during mechanical ventilation. Intensive Care Med. 2001;27:1729–36.
113. De Jonghe B, Sharshar T, Lefaucheur JP, Authier FJ, Durand-Zaleski I, Boussarsar M, Cerf C, Renaud E, Mesrati F, Carlet J, Raphael JC, Outin H, Bastuji-Garin S, Groupe de Reflexion et d'Etude des Neuromyopathies en R. Paresis acquired in the intensive care unit: a prospective multicenter study. JAMA. 2002;288:2859–67.
114. Kesler SM, Sprenkle MD, David WS, Leatherman JW. Severe weakness complicating status asthmaticus despite minimal duration of neuromuscular paralysis. Intensive Care Med. 2009;35:157–60.
115. Huang DT, Angus DC, Moss M, Thompson BT, Ferguson ND, Ginde A, Gong MN, Gundel S, Hayden DL, Hite RD, Hou PC, Hough CL, Iwashyna TJ, Liu KD, Talmor DS, Yealy DM, Reevaluation of Systemic Early Neuromuscular Blockade Protocol Committee and the National Institutes of Health National Heart, Lung, and Blood Institute Prevention Early Treatment of Acute Lung Injury Network Investigators. Design and rationale of the reevaluation of systemic early neuromuscular blockade trial for acute respiratory distress syndrome. Ann Am Thorac Soc. 2017;14:124–33.
116. Frankel H, Jeng J, Tilly E, St Andre A, Champion H. The impact of implementation of neuromuscular blockade monitoring standards in a surgical intensive care unit. Am Surg. 1996;62:503–6.
117. Rudis MI, Sikora CA, Angus E, Peterson E, Popovich J Jr, Hyzy R, Zarowitz BJ. A prospective, randomized, controlled evaluation of peripheral nerve stimulation versus standard clinical dosing of neuromuscular blocking agents in critically ill patients. Crit Care Med. 1997;25:575–83.
118. Strange C, Vaughan L, Franklin C, Johnson J. Comparison of train-of-four and best clinical assessment during continuous paralysis. Am J Respir Crit Care Med. 1997;156:1556–61.
119. Rice TW, Wheeler AP, Bernard GR, Hayden DL, Schoenfeld DA, Ware LB, National Institutes of Health, National Heart, Lung, and Blood Institute ARDS Network. Comparison of the SpO2/FIO2 ratio and the PaO2/FIO2 ratio in patients with acute lung injury or ARDS. Chest. 2007;132:410–7.
120. Minet C, Potton L, Bonadona A, Hamidfar-Roy R, Somohano CA, Lugosi M, Cartier JC, Ferretti G, Schwebel C, Timsit JF. Venous thromboembolism in the ICU: main characteristics, diagnosis and thromboprophylaxis. Crit Care. 2015;19:287.
121. Di Nisio M, van Es N, Buller HR. Deep vein thrombosis and pulmonary embolism. Lancet. 2017;388:3060–73.
122. Geerts WH, Bergqvist D, Pineo GF, Heit JA, Samama CM, Lassen MR, Colwell CW, American College of Chest Physicians. Prevention of venous thromboembolism: American College of Chest Physicians evidence-based clinical practice guidelines (8th edition). Chest. 2008;133:381S–453S.
123. Kearon C, Akl EA, Ornelas J, Blaivas A, Jimenez D, Bounameaux H, Huisman M, King CS, Morris TA, Sood N, Stevens SM, Vintch JR, Wells P, Woller SC, Moores L. Antithrombotic therapy for VTE disease: CHEST guideline and expert panel report. Chest. 2016;149:315–52.
124. Jacobson BF. Thrombosis—prevention is better than cure. S Afr Med J. 2013;103:231.
125. Shorr AF, Williams MD. Venous thromboembolism in critically ill patients. Observations from a randomized trial in sepsis. Thromb Haemost. 2009;101:139–44.
126. Levine RL, LeClerc JR, Bailey JE, Monberg MJ, Sarwat S. Venous and arterial thromboembolism in severe sepsis. Thromb Haemost. 2008;99:892–8.
127. Kaplan D, Casper TC, Elliott CG, Men S, Pendleton RC, Kraiss LW, Weyrich AS, Grissom CK, Zimmerman GA, Rondina MT. VTE incidence and risk factors in patients with severe sepsis and septic shock. Chest. 2015;148:1224–30.
128. Rondina MT, Schwertz H, Harris ES, Kraemer BF, Campbell RA, Mackman N, Grissom CK, Weyrich AS, Zimmerman GA. The septic milieu triggers expression of spliced tissue factor mRNA in human platelets. J Thromb Haemost. 2011;9:748–58.

129. Rondina MT, Brewster B, Grissom CK, Zimmerman GA, Kastendieck DH, Harris ES, Weyrich AS. In vivo platelet activation in critically ill patients with primary 2009 influenza A(H1N1). Chest. 2012;141:1490–5.
130. Kaplan D, Rondina MT. Response. Chest. 2016;149:1107–8.
131. Ambrosetti M, Ferrarese M, Codecasa LR, Besozzi G, Sarassi A, Viggiani P, Migliori GB, Group ASTS. Incidence of venous thromboembolism in tuberculosis patients. Respiration. 2006;73:396.
132. Malek J, Rogers R, Kufera J, Hirshon JM. Venous thromboembolic disease in the HIV-infected patient. Am J Emerg Med. 2011;29:278–82.
133. Rasmussen LD, Dybdal M, Gerstoft J, Kronborg G, Larsen CS, Pedersen C, Pedersen G, Jensen J, Pedersen L, Sorensen HT, Obel N. HIV and risk of venous thromboembolism: a Danish nationwide population-based cohort study. HIV Med. 2011;12:202–10.
134. Robson SC, White NW, Aronson I, Woollgar R, Goodman H, Jacobs P. Acute-phase response and the hypercoagulable state in pulmonary tuberculosis. Br J Haematol. 1996;93:943–9.
135. White NW. Venous thrombosis and rifampicin. Lancet. 1989;2:434–5.
136. Ho KM, Chavan S, Pilcher D. Omission of early thromboprophylaxis and mortality in critically ill patients: a multicenter registry study. Chest. 2011;140:1436–46.
137. Kapoor VK. Venous thromboembolism in India. Natl Med J India. 2010;23:193–5.
138. Pandey A, Patni N, Singh M, Guleria R. Assessment of risk and prophylaxis for deep vein thrombosis and pulmonary embolism in medically ill patients during their early days of hospital stay at a tertiary care center in a developing country. Vasc Health Risk Manag. 2009;5:643–8.
139. Deheinzelin D, Braga AL, Martins LC, Martins MA, Hernandez A, Yoshida WB, Maffei F, Monachini M, Calderaro D, Campos W Jr, Sguizzatto GT, Caramelli B, Investigators TR. Incorrect use of thromboprophylaxis for venous thromboembolism in medical and surgical patients: results of a multicentric, observational and cross-sectional study in Brazil. J Thromb Haemost. 2006;4:1266–70.
140. Kamerkar DR, John MJ, Desai SC, Dsilva LC, Joglekar SJ. Arrive: a retrospective registry of Indian patients with venous thromboembolism. Indian J Crit Care Med. 2016;20:150–8.
141. Belch JJ, Lowe GD, Ward AG, Forbes CD, Prentice CR. Prevention of deep vein thrombosis in medical patients by low-dose heparin. Scott Med J. 1981;26:115–7.
142. Dahan R, Houlbert D, Caulin C, Cuzin E, Viltart C, Woler M, Segrestaa JM. Prevention of deep vein thrombosis in elderly medical in-patients by a low molecular weight heparin: a randomized double-blind trial. Haemostasis. 1986;16:159–64.
143. Fraisse F, Holzapfel L, Couland JM, Simonneau G, Bedock B, Feissel M, Herbecq P, Pordes R, Poussel JF, Roux L. Nadroparin in the prevention of deep vein thrombosis in acute decompensated COPD. The Association of Non-University Affiliated Intensive Care Specialist Physicians of France. Am J Respir Crit Care Med. 2000;161:1109–14.
144. Gardlund B. Randomised, controlled trial of low-dose heparin for prevention of fatal pulmonary embolism in patients with infectious diseases. The Heparin Prophylaxis Study Group. Lancet. 1996;347:1357–61.
145. Halkin H, Goldberg J, Modan M, Modan B. Reduction of mortality in general medical in-patients by low-dose heparin prophylaxis. Ann Intern Med. 1982;96:561–5.
146. Hirsch DR, Ingenito EP, Goldhaber SZ. Prevalence of deep venous thrombosis among patients in medical intensive care. JAMA. 1995;274:335–7.
147. Samama MM, Cohen AT, Darmon JY, Desjardins L, Eldor A, Janbon C, Leizorovicz A, Nguyen H, Olsson CG, Turpie AG, Weisslinger N. A comparison of enoxaparin with placebo for the prevention of venous thromboembolism in acutely ill medical patients. Prophylaxis in Medical Patients with Enoxaparin Study Group. N Engl J Med. 1999;341:793–800.
148. Attia J, Ray JG, Cook DJ, Douketis J, Ginsberg JS, Geerts WH. Deep vein thrombosis and its prevention in critically ill adults. Arch Intern Med. 2001;161:1268–79.
149. Geerts W, Cook D, Selby R, Etchells E. Venous thromboembolism and its prevention in critical care. J Crit Care. 2002;17:95–104.

150. Cohen AT, Tapson VF, Bergmann JF, Goldhaber SZ, Kakkar AK, Deslandes B, Huang W, Zayaruzny M, Emery L, Anderson FA Jr, Investigators E. Venous thromboembolism risk and prophylaxis in the acute hospital care setting (ENDORSE study): a multinational cross-sectional study. Lancet. 2008;371:387–94.
151. Kahn SR, Panju A, Geerts W, Pineo GF, Desjardins L, Turpie AG, Glezer S, Thabane L, Sebaldt RJ, CURVE Study Investigators. Multicenter evaluation of the use of venous thromboembolism prophylaxis in acutely ill medical patients in Canada. Thromb Res. 2007;119:145–55.
152. Khoury H, Welner S, Kubin M, Folkerts K, Haas S. Disease burden and unmet needs for prevention of venous thromboembolism in medically ill patients in Europe show underutilisation of preventive therapies. Thromb Haemost. 2011;106:600–8.
153. Parikh KC, Oh D, Sittipunt C, Kalim H, Ullah S, Aggarwal SK, Voice Asia Investigators. Venous thromboembolism prophylaxis in medical ICU patients in Asia (VOICE Asia): a multicenter, observational, cross-sectional study. Thromb Res. 2012;129:e152–8.
154. Todi SK, Sinha S, Chakraborty A, Sarkar A, Gupta S, D T. Utilization of deep venous thrombosis prophylaxis in medical/surgical intensive care units. Indian J Critical Care Med. 2003;7:103–5.
155. Kakkar N, Vasishta RK. Pulmonary embolism in medical patients: an autopsy-based study. Clin Appl Thromb Hemost. 2008;14:159–67.
156. Berlot G, Calderan C, Vergolini A, Bianchi M, Viviani M, Bussani R, Torelli L, Lucangelo U. Pulmonary embolism in critically ill patients receiving antithrombotic prophylaxis: a clinical-pathologic study. J Crit Care. 2011;26:28–33.
157. Ekwere TA, Ino-Ekanem BM, Ekanem A. Venous thromboembolism: awareness and practice of thromboprophylaxis among physicians in a tertiary-care hospital. Int J Med Biomed Res. 2015;4.
158. Majluf-Cruz A, Castro Martinez G, Herrera Cornejo MA, Liceaga-Cravioto G, Espinosa-Larranaga F, Garcia-Chavez J. Awareness regarding venous thromboembolism among internal medicine practitioners in Mexico: a national cross-sectional study. Intern Med J. 2012;42:1335–41.
159. Alhazzani W, Lim W, Jaeschke RZ, Murad MH, Cade J, Cook DJ. Heparin thromboprophylaxis in medical-surgical critically ill patients: a systematic review and meta-analysis of randomized trials. Crit Care Med. 2013;41:2088–98.
160. Alikhan R, Bedenis R, Cohen AT. Heparin for the prevention of venous thromboembolism in acutely ill medical patients (excluding stroke and myocardial infarction). Cochrane Database Syst Rev. 2014:CD003747.
161. PROTECT Investigators for the Canadian Critical Care Trials Group and the Australian and New Zealand Intensive Care Society Clinical Trials Group, Cook D, Meade M, Guyatt G, Walter S, Heels-Ansdell D, Warkentin TE, Zytaruk N, Crowther M, Geerts W, Cooper DJ, Vallance S, Qushmaq I, Rocha M, Berwanger O, Vlahakis NE. Dalteparin versus unfractionated heparin in critically ill patients. N Engl J Med. 2011;364:1305–14.
162. Fowler RA, Mittmann N, Geerts W, Heels-Ansdell D, Gould MK, Guyatt G, Krahn M, Finfer S, Pinto R, Chan B, Ormanidhi O, Arabi Y, Qushmaq I, Rocha MG, Dodek P, McIntyre L, Hall R, Ferguson ND, Mehta S, Marshall JC, Doig CJ, Muscedere J, Jacka MJ, Klinger JR, Vlahakis N, Orford N, Seppelt I, Skrobik YK, Sud S, Cade JF, Cooper J, Cook D, Group CCCT, Group AaNZICSCT. Cost-effectiveness of dalteparin vs unfractionated heparin for the prevention of venous thromboembolism in critically ill patients. JAMA. 2014;312:2135–45.
163. Thirugnanam S, Pinto R, Cook DJ, Geerts WH, Fowler RA. Economic analyses of venous thromboembolism prevention strategies in hospitalized patients: a systematic review. Crit Care. 2012;16:R43.
164. Lippi G, Favaloro EJ, Cervellin G. Prevention of venous thromboembolism: focus on mechanical prophylaxis. Semin Thromb Hemost. 2011;37:237–51.
165. Ho KM, Tan JA. Stratified meta-analysis of intermittent pneumatic compression of the lower limbs to prevent venous thromboembolism in hospitalized patients. Circulation. 2013;128:1003–20.

166. Cook DJ, Fuller HD, Guyatt GH, Marshall JC, Leasa D, Hall R, Winton TL, Rutledge F, Todd TJ, Roy P, Lacroix J, Griffith L, Willan A, for the Canadian Critical Care Trials Group. Risk factors for gastrointestinal bleeding in critically ill patients. Canadian Critical Care Trials Group. N Engl J Med. 1994;330:377–81.
167. Krag M, Perner A, Wetterslev J, Wise MP, Borthwick M, Bendel S, McArthur C, Cook D, Nielsen N, Pelosi P, Keus F, Guttormsen AB, Moller AD, Moller MH, SUP-ICU co-authors. Prevalence and outcome of gastrointestinal bleeding and use of acid suppressants in acutely ill adult intensive care patients. Intensive Care Med. 2015;41:833–45.
168. Krag M, Perner A, Wetterslev J, Wise MP, Hylander Moller M. Stress ulcer prophylaxis versus placebo or no prophylaxis in critically ill patients. A systematic review of randomised clinical trials with meta-analysis and trial sequential analysis. Intensive Care Med. 2014;40:11–22.
169. Alshamsi F, Belley-Cote E, Cook D, Almenawer SA, Alqahtani Z, Perri D, Thabane L, Al-Omari A, Lewis K, Guyatt G, Alhazzani W. Efficacy and safety of proton pump inhibitors for stress ulcer prophylaxis in critically ill patients: a systematic review and meta-analysis of randomized trials. Crit Care. 2016;20:120.
170. Krag M, Perner A, Wetterslev J, Wise MP, Borthwick M, Bendel S, Pelosi P, Keus F, Guttormsen AB, Schefold JC, Moller MH, Investigators S-I. Stress ulcer prophylaxis with a proton pump inhibitor versus placebo in critically ill patients (SUP-ICU trial): study protocol for a randomised controlled trial. Trials. 2016;17:205.
171. Alhazzani W, Guyatt G, Marshall JC, Hall R, Muscedere J, Lauzier F, Thabane L, Alshahrani M, English SW, Arabi YM, Deane AM, Karachi T, Rochwerg B, Finfer S, Daneman N, Zytaruk N, Heel-Ansdell D, Cook D, on behalf of the Canadian Critical Care Trials Group. Re-evaluating the inhibition of stress erosions (REVISE): a protocol for pilot randomized controlled trial. Ann Saudi Med. 2016;36:427–33.
172. MacLaren R, Reynolds PM, Allen RR. Histamine-2 receptor antagonists vs proton pump inhibitors on gastrointestinal tract hemorrhage and infectious complications in the intensive care unit. JAMA Intern Med. 2014;174:564–74.
173. Faleck DM, Salmasian H, Furuya EY, Larson EL, Abrams JA, Freedberg DE. Proton pump inhibitors do not increase risk for Clostridium difficile infection in the intensive care unit. Am J Gastroenterol. 2016;111:1641–8.
174. van Hooijdonk RT, Schultz MJ. Insulin and oral anti-hyperglycemic agents. In: Webb AJ, Angus DC, Finfer S, Gattinoni L, Singer M, editors. The Oxford textbook of critical care. 2015.
175. Ogetii GN, Akech S, Jemutai J, Boga M, Kivaya E, Fegan G, Maitland K. Hypoglycaemia in severe malaria, clinical associations and relationship to quinine dosage. BMC Infect Dis. 2010;10:334.
176. Schultz MJ, Harmsen RE, Spronk PE. Clinical review: strict or loose glycemic control in critically ill patients—implementing best available evidence from randomized controlled trials. Crit Care. 2010;14:223.
177. van den Berghe G, Wouters P, Weekers F, Verwaest C, Bruyninckx F, Schetz M, Vlasselaers D, Ferdinande P, Lauwers P, Bouillon R. Intensive insulin therapy in critically ill patients. N Engl J Med. 2001;345:1359–67.
178. Vlasselaers D, Milants I, Desmet L, Wouters PJ, Vanhorebeek I, van den Heuvel I, Mesotten D, Casaer MP, Meyfroidt G, Ingels C, Muller J, Van Cromphaut S, Schetz M, Van den Berghe G. Intensive insulin therapy for patients in paediatric intensive care: a prospective, randomised controlled study. Lancet. 2009;373:547–56.
179. Wiener RS, Wiener DC, Larson RJ. Benefits and risks of tight glucose control in critically ill adults: a meta-analysis. JAMA. 2008;300:933–44.
180. Griesdale DE, de Souza RJ, van Dam RM, Heyland DK, Cook DJ, Malhotra A, Dhaliwal R, Henderson WR, Chittock DR, Finfer S, Talmor D. Intensive insulin therapy and mortality among critically ill patients: a meta-analysis including NICE-SUGAR study data. CMAJ. 2009;180:821–7.
181. Friedrich JO, Chant C, Adhikari NK. Does intensive insulin therapy really reduce mortality in critically ill surgical patients? A reanalysis of meta-analytic data. Crit Care. 2010;14:324.

182. Marik PE, Preiser JC. Toward understanding tight glycemic control in the ICU: a systematic review and metaanalysis. Chest. 2010;137:544–51.
183. Kansagara D, Fu R, Freeman M, Wolf F, Helfand M. Intensive insulin therapy in hospitalized patients: a systematic review. Ann Intern Med. 2011;154:268–82.
184. Wilson M, Weinreb J, Hoo GW. Intensive insulin therapy in critical care: a review of 12 protocols. Diabetes Care. 2007;30:1005–11.
185. Panahi Y, Mojtahedzadeh M, Zekeri N, Beiraghdar F, Khajavi MR, Ahmadi A. Metformin treatment in hyperglycemic critically ill patients: another challenge on the control of adverse outcomes. Iran J Pharm Res. 2011;10:913–9.
186. Mojtahedzadeh M, Jafarieh A, Najafi A, Khajavi MR, Khalili N. Comparison of metformin and insulin in the control of hyperglycaemia in non-diabetic critically ill patients. Endokrynol Pol. 2012;63:206–11.
187. Ansari G, Mojtahedzadeh M, Kajbaf F, Najafi A, Khajavi MR, Khalili H, Rouini MR, Ahmadi H, Abdollahi M. How does blood glucose control with metformin influence intensive insulin protocols? Evidence for involvement of oxidative stress and inflammatory cytokines. Adv Ther. 2008;25:681–702.
188. Dondorp AM, Hoang MN, Mer M, Sepsis in Resource-Limited Settings-Expert Consensus Recommendations Group of the European Society of Intensive Care Med and the Mahidol-Oxford Research Unit in Bangkok, Thailand. Recommendations for the management of severe malaria and severe dengue in resource-limited settings. Intensive Care Med. 2016.
189. Stang M, Wysowski DK, Butler-Jones D. Incidence of lactic acidosis in metformin users. Diabetes Care. 1999;22:925–7.
190. McWhirter JP, Pennington CR. Incidence and recognition of malnutrition in hospital. BMJ. 1994;308:945–8.
191. Dellinger RP, Levy MM, Rhodes A, Annane D, Gerlach H, Opal SM, Sevransky JE, Sprung CL, Douglas IS, Jaeschke R, Osborn TM, Nunnally ME, Townsend SR, Reinhart K, Kleinpell RM, Angus DC, Deutschman CS, Machado FR, Rubenfeld GD, Webb SA, Beale RJ, Vincent JL, Moreno R, Surviving Sepsis Campaign Guidelines Committee including the Pediatric Subgroup. Surviving sepsis campaign: international guidelines for management of severe sepsis and septic shock. Crit Care Med. 2013;41:580–637.
192. Taylor BE, SA MC, Martindale RG, Warren MM, Johnson DR, Braunschweig C, MS MC, Davanos E, Rice TW, Cresci GA, Gervasio JM, Sacks GS, Roberts PR, Compher C, Society of Critical Care Medicine; American Society for Parenteral and Enteral Nutrition. Guidelines for the provision and assessment of nutrition support therapy in the adult critically ill patient: Society of Critical Care Medicine (SCCM) and American Society for Parenteral and Enteral Nutrition (A.S.P.E.N.). Crit Care Med. 2016;44:390–438.
193. Doig GS, Heighes PT, Simpson F, Sweetman EA, Davies AR. Early enteral nutrition, provided within 24 h of injury or intensive care unit admission, significantly reduces mortality in critically ill patients: a meta-analysis of randomised controlled trials. Intensive Care Med. 2009;35:2018–27.
194. Kang W, Kudsk KA. Is there evidence that the gut contributes to mucosal immunity in humans? JPEN J Parenter Enteral Nutr. 2007;31:246–58.
195. Kompan L, Vidmar G, Spindler-Vesel A, Pecar J. Is early enteral nutrition a risk factor for gastric intolerance and pneumonia? Clin Nutr. 2004;23:527–32.
196. Moore EE, Jones TN. Benefits of immediate jejunostomy feeding after major abdominal trauma—a prospective, randomized study. J Trauma. 1986;26:874–81.
197. Singh G, Ram RP, Khanna SK. Early postoperative enteral feeding in patients with nontraumatic intestinal perforation and peritonitis. J Am Coll Surg. 1998;187:142–6.
198. Nguyen NQ, Fraser RJ, Bryant LK, Burgstad C, Chapman MJ, Bellon M, Wishart J, Holloway RH, Horowitz M. The impact of delaying enteral feeding on gastric emptying, plasma cholecystokinin, and peptide YY concentrations in critically ill patients. Crit Care Med. 2008;36:1469–74.
199. Heyland DK, Dhaliwal R, Drover JW, Gramlich L, Dodek P, Canadian Critical Care Clinical Practice Guidelines Committee. Canadian clinical practice guidelines for nutrition support

in mechanically ventilated, critically ill adult patients. JPEN J Parenter Enteral Nutr. 2003;27:355–73.
200. Marik PE, Zaloga GP. Early enteral nutrition in acutely ill patients: a systematic review. Crit Care Med. 2001;29:2264–70.
201. Chuntrasakul C, Siltharm S, Chinswangwatanakul V, Pongprasobchai T, Chockvivatanavanit S, Bunnak A. Early nutritional support in severe traumatic patients. J Med Assoc Thail. 1996;79:21–6.
202. McClave SA, Martindale RG, Rice TW, Heyland DK. Feeding the critically ill patient. Crit Care Med. 2014;42:2600–10.
203. Maude RJ, Hoque G, Hasan MU, Sayeed A, Akter S, Samad R, Alam B, Yunus EB, Rahman R, Rahman W, Chowdhury R, Seal T, Charunwatthana P, Chang CC, White NJ, Faiz MA, Day NP, Dondorp AM, Hossain A. Timing of enteral feeding in cerebral malaria in resource-poor settings: a randomized trial. PLoS One. 2011;6:e27273.
204. Ibrahim EH, Mehringer L, Prentice D, Sherman G, Schaiff R, Fraser V, Kollef MH. Early versus late enteral feeding of mechanically ventilated patients: results of a clinical trial. JPEN J Parenter Enteral Nutr. 2002;26:174–81.
205. Bonten MJ, Gaillard CA, van der Hulst R, de Leeuw PW, van der Geest S, Stobberingh EE, Soeters PB. Intermittent enteral feeding: the influence on respiratory and digestive tract colonization in mechanically ventilated intensive-care-unit patients. Am J Respir Crit Care Med. 1996;154:394–9.
206. Ciocon JO, Galindo-Ciocon DJ, Tiessen C, Galindo D. Continuous compared with intermittent tube feeding in the elderly. JPEN J Parenter Enteral Nutr. 1992;16:525–8.
207. Hiebert JM, Brown A, Anderson RG, Halfacre S, Rodeheaver GT, Edlich RF. Comparison of continuous vs intermittent tube feedings in adult burn patients. JPEN J Parenter Enteral Nutr. 1981;5:73–5.
208. Kocan MJ, Hickisch SM. A comparison of continuous and intermittent enteral nutrition in NICU patients. J Neurosci Nurs. 1986;18:333–7.
209. Steevens EC, Lipscomb AF, Poole GV, Sacks GS. Comparison of continuous vs intermittent nasogastric enteral feeding in trauma patients: perceptions and practice. Nutr Clin Pract. 2002;17:118–22.
210. MacLeod JB, Lefton J, Houghton D, Roland C, Doherty J, Cohn SM, Barquist ES. Prospective randomized control trial of intermittent versus continuous gastric feeds for critically ill trauma patients. J Trauma. 2007;63:57–61.
211. McClave SA, DeMeo MT, DeLegge MH, DiSario JA, Heyland DK, Maloney JP, Metheny NA, Moore FA, Scolapio JS, Spain DA, Zaloga GP. North American Summit on aspiration in the critically ill patient: consensus statement. JPEN J Parenter Enteral Nutr. 2002;26:S80–5.
212. Desai SV, McClave SA, Rice TW. Nutrition in the ICU: an evidence-based approach. Chest. 2014;145:1148–57.
213. SM A-K, LaPointe NM, Kramer JM, Califf RM. What clinicians should know about the QT interval. JAMA. 2003;289:2120–7.
214. Drakulovic MB, Torres A, Bauer TT, Nicolas JM, Nogue S, Ferrer M. Supine body position as a risk factor for nosocomial pneumonia in mechanically ventilated patients: a randomised trial. Lancet. 1999;354:1851–8.
215. van Nieuwenhoven CA, Vandenbroucke-Grauls C, van Tiel FH, Joore HC, van Schijndel RJ, van der Tweel I, Ramsay G, Bonten MJ. Feasibility and effects of the semirecumbent position to prevent ventilator-associated pneumonia: a randomized study. Crit Care Med. 2006;34:396–402.
216. Simmons-Trau D, Cenek P, Counterman J, Hockenbury D, Litwiller L. Reducing VAP with 6 Sigma. Nurs Manag. 2004;35:41–5.
217. Zack JE, Garrison T, Trovillion E, Clinkscale D, Coopersmith CM, Fraser VJ, Kollef MH. Effect of an education program aimed at reducing the occurrence of ventilator-associated pneumonia. Crit Care Med. 2002;30:2407–12.
218. Dickerson RN, Pitts SL, Maish GO 3rd, Schroeppel TJ, Magnotti LJ, Croce MA, Minard G, Brown RO. A reappraisal of nitrogen requirements for patients with critical illness and trauma. J Trauma Acute Care Surg. 2012;73:549–57.

219. McClave SA, Martindale RG, Kiraly L. The use of indirect calorimetry in the intensive care unit. Curr Opin Clin Nutr Metab Care. 2013;16:202–8.
220. McClave SA, Martindale RG, Vanek VW, McCarthy M, Roberts P, Taylor B, Ochoa JB, Napolitano L, Cresci G, ASPEN Board of Directors, American College of Critical Care Medicine, Society of Critical Care Medicine. Guidelines for the provision and assessment of nutrition support therapy in the adult critically ill patient: Society of Critical Care Medicine (SCCM) and American Society for Parenteral and Enteral Nutrition (A.S.P.E.N.). JPEN J Parenter Enteral Nutr. 2009;33:277–316.
221. Neelemaat F, van Bokhorst de van der Schueren MA, Thijs A, Seidell JC, Weijs PJ. Resting energy expenditure in malnourished older patients at hospital admission and three months after discharge: predictive equations versus measurements. Clin Nutr. 2012;31:958–66.
222. Allingstrup MJ, Esmailzadeh N, Wilkens Knudsen A, Espersen K, Hartvig Jensen T, Wiis J, Perner A, Kondrup J. Provision of protein and energy in relation to measured requirements in intensive care patients. Clin Nutr. 2012;31:462–8.
223. Burge JC, Goon A, Choban PS, Flancbaum L. Efficacy of hypocaloric total parenteral nutrition in hospitalized obese patients: a prospective, double-blind randomized trial. JPEN J Parenter Enteral Nutr. 1994;18:203–7.
224. Choban PS, Burge JC, Scales D, Flancbaum L. Hypoenergetic nutrition support in hospitalized obese patients: a simplified method for clinical application. Am J Clin Nutr. 1997;66:546–50.
225. Choban PS, Dickerson RN. Morbid obesity and nutrition support: is bigger different? Nutr Clin Pract. 2005;20:480–7.
226. Angstwurm MW, Engelmann L, Zimmermann T, Lehmann C, Spes CH, Abel P, Strauss R, Meier-Hellmann A, Insel R, Radke J, Schuttler J, Gartner R. Selenium in Intensive Care (SIC): results of a prospective randomized, placebo-controlled, multiple-center study in patients with severe systemic inflammatory response syndrome, sepsis, and septic shock. Crit Care Med. 2007;35:118–26.
227. Berger MM, Chiolero RL. Antioxidant supplementation in sepsis and systemic inflammatory response syndrome. Crit Care Med. 2007;35:S584–90.
228. Mishra V, Baines M, Perry SE, McLaughlin PJ, Carson J, Wenstone R, Shenkin A. Effect of selenium supplementation on biochemical markers and outcome in critically ill patients. Clin Nutr. 2007;26:41–50.
229. Schneider A, Markowski A, Momma M, Seipt C, Luettig B, Hadem J, Wilhelmi M, Manns MP, Wedemeyer J. Tolerability and efficacy of a low-volume enteral supplement containing key nutrients in the critically ill. Clin Nutr. 2011;30:599–603.
230. Manzanares W, Lemieux M, Elke G, Langlois PL, Bloos F, Heyland DK. High-dose intravenous selenium does not improve clinical outcomes in the critically ill: a systematic review and meta-analysis. Crit Care. 2016;20:356.
231. Barr J, Hecht M, Flavin KE, Khorana A, Gould MK. Outcomes in critically ill patients before and after the implementation of an evidence-based nutritional management protocol. Chest. 2004;125:1446–57.
232. Doig GS, Simpson F, Finfer S, Delaney A, Davies AR, Mitchell I, Dobb G, Nutrition Guidelines Investigators of the ANZICS Clinical Trials Group. Effect of evidence-based feeding guidelines on mortality of critically ill adults: a cluster randomized controlled trial. JAMA. 2008;300:2731–41.
233. Heyland DK, Murch L, Cahill N, McCall M, Muscedere J, Stelfox HT, Bray T, Tanguay T, Jiang X, Day AG. Enhanced protein-energy provision via the enteral route feeding protocol in critically ill patients: results of a cluster randomized trial. Crit Care Med. 2013;41:2743–53.
234. Spain DA, McClave SA, Sexton LK, Adams JL, Blanford BS, Sullins ME, Owens NA, Snider HL. Infusion protocol improves delivery of enteral tube feeding in the critical care unit. JPEN J Parenter Enteral Nutr. 1999;23:288–92.
235. Chan S, McCowen KC, Blackburn GL. Nutrition management in the ICU. Chest. 1999;115:145S–8S.
236. Dare AJ, Fu SH, Patra J, Rodriguez PS, Thakur JS, Jha P, Million Death Study Collaborators. Renal failure deaths and their risk factors in India 2001-13: nationally representative estimates from the Million Death Study. Lancet Glob Health. 2017;5:e89–95.

237. Lameire NH, Bagga A, Cruz D, De Maeseneer J, Endre Z, Kellum JA, Liu KD, Mehta RL, Pannu N, Van Biesen W, Vanholder R. Acute kidney injury: an increasing global concern. Lancet. 2013;382:170–9.
238. Ponce D, Berbel MN, Regina de Goes C, Almeida CT, Balbi AL. High-volume peritoneal dialysis in acute kidney injury: indications and limitations. Clin J Am Soc Nephrol. 2012;7:887–94.
239. Callegari J, Antwi S, Wystrychowski G, Zukowska-Szczechowska E, Levin NW, Carter M. Peritoneal dialysis as a mode of treatment for acute kidney injury in sub-Saharan Africa. Blood Purif. 2013;36:226–30.
240. Chijioke A, Makusidi AM, Rafiu MO. Factors influencing hemodialysis and outcome in severe acute renal failure from Ilorin, Nigeria. Saudi J Kidney Dis Transpl. 2012;23:391–6.
241. Godara SM, Kute VB, Trivedi HL, Vanikar AV, Shah PR, Gumber MR, Patel HV, Gumber VM. Clinical profile and outcome of acute kidney injury related to pregnancy in developing countries: a single-center study from India. Saudi J Kidney Dis Transpl. 2014;25:906–11.
242. Kilonzo KG, Ghosh S, Temu SA, Maro V, Callegari J, Carter M, Handelman G, Finkelstein FO, Levin N, Yeates K. Outcome of acute peritoneal dialysis in northern Tanzania. Perit Dial Int. 2012;32:261–6.
243. Maoujoud O, Zajjari Y, Asseraji M, Aatif T, Ahid S, Oualim Z. Commentary: the practice of dialysis in the intensive care unit in a developing country. Ethn Dis. 2014;24:226–8.
244. Okunola OO, Ayodele OE, Adekanle AD. Acute kidney injury requiring hemodialysis in the tropics. Saudi J Kidney Dis Transpl. 2012;23:1315–9.
245. Shah PR, Gireesh MS, Kute VB, Vanikar AV, Gumber MR, Patel HV, Goplani KR, Trivedi HL. Renal involvement in sepsis: a prospective single-center study of 136 cases. Saudi J Kidney Dis Transpl. 2013;24:620–9.
246. Ademola AD, Asinobi AO, Ogunkunle OO, Yusuf BN, Ojo OE. Peritoneal dialysis in childhood acute kidney injury: experience in southwest Nigeria. Perit Dial Int. 2012;32:267–72.
247. Diarrassouba G, Adonis-Koffy L, Niamien E, Yaokreh JB, Coulibaly PA. Acute peritoneal dialysis in African pediatric area experience of pediatric nephrology unit of Yopougon University Hospital (Abidjan, Cote d'Ivoire). Blood Purif. 2015;39:141–4.
248. Mishra OP, Gupta AK, Pooniya V, Prasad R, Tiwary NK, Schaefer F. Peritoneal dialysis in children with acute kidney injury: a developing country experience. Perit Dial Int. 2012;32:431–6.
249. Rifai AO, Murad LB, Sekkarie MA, Al-Makki AA, Zanabli AR, Kayal AA, Soudan KA. Continuous venovenous hemofiltration using a stand-alone blood pump for acute kidney injury in field hospitals in Syria. Kidney Int. 2015;87:254–61.
250. Smoyer WE, Finkelstein FO, McCulloch M, Carter M, Brusselmans A, Feehally J. Saving young lives: provision of acute dialysis in low-resource settings. Lancet. 2015;386:2056.
251. Burki T. Tanzania's model peritoneal dialysis programme. Lancet. 2015;385:1935–6.
252. Callegari JG, Kilonzo KG, Yeates KE, Handelman GJ, Finkelstein FO, Kotanko P, Levin NW, Carter M. Peritoneal dialysis for acute kidney injury in sub-Saharan Africa: challenges faced and lessons learned at Kilimanjaro Christian Medical Centre. Kidney Int. 2012;81:331–3.
253. Smoyer WE, Finkelstein FO, McCulloch MI, Carter M, Brusselmans A, Feehally J. "Saving Young Lives" with acute kidney injury: the challenge of acute dialysis in low-resource settings. Kidney Int. 2016;89:254–6.
254. Phu NH, Hien TT, Mai NT, Chau TT, Chuong LV, Loc PP, Winearls C, Farrar J, White N, Day N. Hemofiltration and peritoneal dialysis in infection-associated acute renal failure in Vietnam. N Engl J Med. 2002;347:895–902.
255. Chionh CY, Soni SS, Finkelstein FO, Ronco C, Cruz DN. Use of peritoneal dialysis in AKI: a systematic review. Clin J Am Soc Nephrol. 2013;8:1649–60.
256. Bagshaw SM, Brophy PD, Cruz D, Ronco C. Fluid balance as a biomarker: impact of fluid overload on outcome in critically ill patients with acute kidney injury. Crit Care. 2008;12:169.
257. Murphy CV, Schramm GE, Doherty JA, Reichley RM, Gajic O, Afessa B, Micek ST, Kollef MH. The importance of fluid management in acute lung injury secondary to septic shock. Chest. 2009;136:102–9.

258. Payen D, de Pont AC, Sakr Y, Spies C, Reinhart K, Vincent JL, Investigators SOiAIP. A positive fluid balance is associated with a worse outcome in patients with acute renal failure. Crit Care. 2008;12:R74.
259. Rivers EP. Fluid-management strategies in acute lung injury—liberal, conservative, or both? N Engl J Med. 2006;354:2598–600.
260. Sakr Y, Vincent JL, Reinhart K, Groeneveld J, Michalopoulos A, Sprung CL, Artigas A, Ranieri VM, Sepsis Occurence in Acutely Ill Patients Investigators. High tidal volume and positive fluid balance are associated with worse outcome in acute lung injury. Chest. 2005;128:3098–108.
261. Acheampong A, Vincent JL. A positive fluid balance is an independent prognostic factor in patients with sepsis. Crit Care. 2015;19:251.
262. Alsous F, Khamiees M, DeGirolamo A, Amoateng-Adjepong Y, Manthous CA. Negative fluid balance predicts survival in patients with septic shock: a retrospective pilot study. Chest. 2000;117:1749–54.
263. National Heart, Lung, and Blood Institute Acute Respiratory Distress Syndrome (ARDS) Clinical Trials Network, Wiedemann HP, Wheeler AP, Bernard GR, Thompson BT, Hayden D, deBoisblanc B, Connors AF Jr, Hite RD, Harabin AL. Comparison of two fluid-management strategies in acute lung injury. N Engl J Med. 2006;354:2564–2575.
264. Malbrain ML, Marik PE, Witters I, Cordemans C, Kirkpatrick AW, Roberts DJ, Van Regenmortel N. Fluid overload, de-resuscitation, and outcomes in critically ill or injured patients: a systematic review with suggestions for clinical practice. Anaesthesiol Intensive Ther. 2014;46:361–80.
265. Andrews B, Muchemwa L, Kelly P, Lakhi S, Heimburger DC, Bernard GR. Simplified severe sepsis protocol: a randomized controlled trial of modified early goal-directed therapy in Zambia. Crit Care Med. 2014;42:2315–24.
266. Eskesen TG, Wetterslev M, Perner A. Systematic review including re-analyses of 1148 individual data sets of central venous pressure as a predictor of fluid responsiveness. Intensive Care Med. 2016;42:324–32.
267. Magder S. Central venous pressure: a useful but not so simple measurement. Crit Care Med. 2006;34:2224–7.
268. Mager DE, Lin SX, Blum RA, Lates CD, Jusko WJ. Dose equivalency evaluation of major corticosteroids: pharmacokinetics and cell trafficking and cortisol dynamics. J Clin Pharmacol. 2003;43:1216–27.
269. Adrenal cortical steroids drug facts and comparisons. St. Louis: Facts and Comparisons, Inc.; 1997. p. 122–28.
270. Schimmer BP, Funder JW. ACTH, adrenal steroids, and pharmacology of the adrenal cortex. In: Brunton LL, Chabner BA, Knollman BC, editors. Goodman and Gilman's the pharmacological basis of therapeutics. New York: McGraw-Hill; 2011.

Open Access This chapter is licensed under the terms of the Creative Commons Attribution 4.0 International License (http://creativecommons.org/licenses/by/4.0/), which permits use, sharing, adaptation, distribution and reproduction in any medium or format, as long as you give appropriate credit to the original author(s) and the source, provide a link to the Creative Commons license and indicate if changes were made.

The images or other third party material in this chapter are included in the chapter's Creative Commons license, unless indicated otherwise in a credit line to the material. If material is not included in the chapter's Creative Commons license and your intended use is not permitted by statutory regulation or exceeds the permitted use, you will need to obtain permission directly from the copyright holder.

Ventilatory Support of Patients with Sepsis or Septic Shock in Resource-Limited Settings

6

Ary Serpa Neto, Marcus J. Schultz, Emir Festic, Neill K. J. Adhikari, Arjen M. Dondorp, Rajyabardhan Pattnaik, Luigi Pisani, Pedro Povoa, Ignacio Martin-Loeches, and C. Louise Thwaites

A. Serpa Neto
Medical Intensive Care Unit, Hospital Israelita Albert Einstein, São Paulo, Brazil

Program of Post-Graduation, Research and Innovation, Faculdade de Medicina do ABC, São Paulo, Brazil

Department of Intensive Care, Academic Medical Center, University of Amsterdam, Amsterdam, The Netherlands

M. J. Schultz (✉)
Department of Intensive Care, Academic Medical Center, University of Amsterdam, Amsterdam, The Netherlands

Laboratory of Experimental Intensive Care and Anesthesiology (L.E.I.C.A), University of Amsterdam, Amsterdam, The Netherlands

Mahidol-Oxford Research Unit (MORU), Faculty of Tropical Medicine, Mahidol University, Bangkok, Thailand

E. Festic
Pulmonary and Critical Care Medicine, Mayo Clinic, Jacksonville, FL, USA

N. K. J. Adhikari
Department of Intensive Care, Sunnybrook Health Sciences Centre, Toronto, ON, Canada

A. M. Dondorp
Department of Intensive Care, Academic Medical Center, University of Amsterdam, Amsterdam, The Netherlands

Mahidol-Oxford Research Unit (MORU), Faculty of Tropical Medicine, Mahidol University, Bangkok, Thailand

L. Pisani
Department of Intensive Care, Academic Medical Center, University of Amsterdam, Amsterdam, The Netherlands

Mahidol-Oxford Research Unit (MORU), Faculty of Tropical Medicine, Mahidol University, Bangkok, Thailand

© The Author(s) 2019

A. M. Dondorp et al. (eds.), *Sepsis Management in Resource-limited Settings*,
https://doi.org/10.1007/978-3-030-03143-5_6

R. Pattnaik
Department of Intensive Care, Ispat General Hospital, Rourkela, Sundargarh, Odisha, India

P. Povoa
Department of Intensive Care, Centro Hospitalar de Lisboa Ocidental,
Hospital de São Francisco Xavier, Lisbon, Portugal

I. Martin-Loeches
Department of Intensive Care, St. James's University Hospital, Dublin, Ireland

C. L. Thwaites
Nuffield Department of Medicine, Centre for Tropical Medicine and Global Health,
University of Oxford, Oxford, UK

6.1 Introduction

Evidence for recommendations on ventilatory support in patients with sepsis or septic shock has been mainly gathered from investigations in resource-rich settings [1, 2]. Often, it is not practical to directly translate this evidence to resource-limited settings. Indeed, intensive care units (ICUs) in these settings are frequently restricted in availability of equipment, laboratory support, and skilled staff [3]. Recommendations and suggestions are summarized in Table 6.1.

6.2 The Diagnosis of the Acute Respiratory Distress Syndrome (ARDS)

ARDS is a combined clinical and radiographic diagnosis, which per the latest consensus definition [4] requires the presence of acute bilateral chest infiltrates (onset within less than 1 week), not primarily caused by hydrostatic pulmonary edema, associated with hypoxemia based on PaO_2 to FiO_2 ratio (P/F) of less than 300 mm Hg and requiring at least 5 cm H_2O of positive end-expiratory pressure (PEEP). Therefore, in order to diagnose ARDS, performance of a chest radiograph (CXR) and arterial blood gas analysis (ABG) is necessary. However, the availability (or the lack of) of CXR and ABG in resource-limited settings might preclude their timely performance and utility in diagnosing septic patient with ARDS. It is not clear whether the mere diagnosis of ARDS would impact care and/or outcomes of patients with sepsis or septic shock with acute respiratory failure. There is a growing body of evidence suggesting that the diagnostic utility of the ultrasound exam of the lung compares well with that of the CXR [5–9]. When coupled with the performance of point-of-care echocardiogram, the diagnosis of non-cardiogenic pulmonary edema can be achieved in acutely hypoxemic patients, including those with sepsis [10–12].

Low oxygen saturation to FiO_2 ratio (S/F) within 6 h of presentation to emergency room was found to predict early development of ARDS [13]. A secondary analysis of the ARDS Network trial of a lower tidal volume ventilator strategy showed that S/F correlated with P/F in patients with ARDS [14]. Another study suggests that ARDS patients diagnosed by S/F have very similar clinical characteristics and outcomes

Table 6.1 Recommendations and suggestions on ventilatory support in patients with sepsis or septic shock in resource-limited settings (with grading)

1	ARDS diagnosis	Use CXR and ABG in septic patients with acute respiratory failure to diagnose ARDS (2B); where feasible, ultrasound exam of the lungs and heart may be used to narrow down the diagnosis of non-cardiogenic pulmonary edema (2D); oxygen pulse saturation relative to delivered oxygen concentration (S/F) may be an alternative for the arterial oxygen pressure relative to delivered oxygen concentration (P/F) for decision-making and continuous monitoring in settings where blood gas analyzers are absent (2D); patients with acute respiratory failure with or without ARDS diagnosis should be managed employing the principles of lung-protective mechanical ventilation (2B)
2	Semi-recumbent position	For ventilated septic patients, use elevated head-of-bed position ranging from 30° to 45° unless their hemodynamic state precludes this (1B); lower patient's position to less than 30° head-of-bed elevation transiently for the necessary procedures and during the resuscitation of the shock state until hemodynamic status is improved (1B) or longer in cases of sacral decubitus ulcer (1C)
3	NIV	Use invasive mechanical ventilation in cases of severe hemodynamic disturbance (i.e., shock) and/or severe hypoxemia (1A). NIV could be used in selected cases of mild respiratory failure with preserved or relatively stable hemodynamic status (2A); frequent reassessments of therapeutic effect of NIV are required in order to prevent delay in intubation and mechanical ventilation (1B)
4	Spontaneous breathing trials	Use spontaneous breathing trials early and regularly, preferably daily, in all ventilated patients (1A) (notably, to increase the success of this strategy, excessive sedation should be prevented); use the low level of pressure support technique (2D); perform spontaneous breathing trials, and extubate if the trial is passed successfully only at times sufficient staff is available (2D); develop a local guideline for spontaneous breathing trials (2C)
5	Tidal volume size	Use low tidal volume ventilation in patients with ARDS diagnosis (1A) and in all ventilated patients (2B) (i.e., prevent tidal volumes higher than 10 ml/kg PBW, and consider tidal volumes of 5–7 ml/kg PBW in all patients); titrate tidal volume size using PBW and not the actual body weight (2D); timely recognize under-ventilation, where respiratory rates should be adjusted (2D); accept higher respiratory rates (i.e., do not increase sedation if the respiratory rate rises with the use of lower tidal volumes) (2C); end-tidal CO_2 monitoring could be helpful in timely recognition of under- or overventilation (2D)
6	PEEP	Use a minimum level of PEEP (5 cm H_2O) in all patients with sepsis or septic shock with acute respiratory failure (2B); consider using higher levels of PEEP only in patients with moderate or severe ARDS (2A); if lack of CXR and ABG availability hampers making an ARDS diagnosis, we suggest against liberal use of higher levels of PEEP (2D); when the team is trained and experienced in using respiratory dynamic compliance, PEEP could be titrated based on this parameter (2D); so-called PEEP/FiO_2 tables could be used for titrating PEEP, but this approach generally requires frequent ABGs (2B); patients who need higher levels of PEEP are preferably closely monitored, preferably by using an arterial line, as hypotension and circulatory depression may develop (1A)

(continued)

Table 6.1 (continued)

7	FiO_2 vs. PEEP	Low FiO_2 is preferred over high FiO_2 (2B); the target should be PaO_2 > 8 kPa [60 mm Hg] and/or SpO_2 88–95% (2A); PEEP/FiO2 tables can be used to find the best PEEP/FiO2 combination (2B); staff with experience in using PEEP could prefer to use higher levels of PEEP to treat hypoxia; in centers with little experience in using PEEP, the initial response to hypoxia should be higher FiO_2 before using higher levels of PEEP (2D)
8	Recruitment maneuvers	Use recruitment maneuvers in patients with moderate or severe ARDS (2B) and in patients with refractory hypoxemia in whom an ARDS diagnosis cannot be made due to lack of CXR and/or ABG (2D) and only when the staff is trained and experienced in performing these maneuvers (2D); use the simplest maneuver, i.e., "sustained inflation" (2D); when using recruitment maneuvers, the patient should be closely monitored, preferably by using an arterial line, to promptly detect hemodynamic compromise (2B)
9	Modes of ventilation	We recommend using "volume-controlled" modes of ventilation over "pressure-controlled" modes of ventilation (2D); we cannot recommend on whether assisted ventilation ("support" mode) is preferred over assist ventilation ("controlled mode") in all patients; use a short course of muscle paralysis (< 48 h) and thus controlled ventilation, only in patients with moderate or severe ARDS (2B)

Abbreviations: *CO_2* carbon dioxide, *CXR* chest radiograph, *ABG* arterial blood gas, *ARDS* acute respiratory distress syndrome, *PBW* predicted body weight, *PEEP* positive end-expiratory pressure, *NIV* noninvasive ventilation
Grading: see online supplement for explanations

Table 6.2 Proposed S/F values as correlates to existing P/F thresholds

	P/F = 300	P/F = 200	P/F = 100
Pandharipande et al.	370	240	115
Rice et al.	315	235	–
Lobete et al.	296	236	146
Khemani et al.	264	221	–
Bilan et al.	235	181	–

Data from [14, 17–20]

compared with patients diagnosed by P/F [15]. A retrospective study from Brazil showed that a low S/F at ICU admission was associated with increased risk of death in patients with severe sepsis or septic shock [16]. However, diagnosis of ARDS or its severity categorization based on S/F alone can be difficult given a wide variability in S/F relative to P/F observed in the studies on the topic [13–20]. In addition to oxygenation impairment, bilateral infiltrates on CXR at the time of hospital presentation have also been shown to predict development of early ARDS [21].

We *suggest* using CXR and ABG in septic patients with acute respiratory failure, if available (2B). In the absence of CXR availability, frequent physical exams and the overall clinical picture will prove beneficial in monitoring patient's respiratory status and decision-making (2D). Where feasible, ultrasound exam of the lungs and heart may be used to narrow down the diagnosis of non-cardiogenic pulmonary edema (2D). In the absence of ABG availability, the S/F could be an alternative for the P/F in decision-making and continuous monitoring of an individual patient (2B) (Table 6.2).

Patients with sepsis-related acute respiratory failure with or without ARDS diagnosis should be managed employing the principles of lung-protective mechanical ventilation (2B). In the questions to follow, recommendations may vary depending on the availability of CXR and ABG (i.e., the feasibility to make diagnosis of ARDS).

6.3 The Semi-recumbent Position

Position of the septic patient with acute respiratory failure necessitating oxygen and ventilator support may have important implications in the treatment. Currently, it is recommended that ventilated patients be positioned in the bed so the head of bed is elevated at the 30° to 45° (i.e., "semi-recumbent"). This position may be important for at least two reasons: (1) decreased risk of aspiration and (2) decreased work of breathing. Some patients with a profound hemodynamic disturbance despite the resuscitation may need to transiently be placed in a flat or even in a Trendelenburg position. Others, especially obese patients or those with states that increase abdominal pressure may benefit from the higher angle, sitting position to allow better gravity support for the diaphragmatic excursions, which may reduce bibasilar atelectasis and improve ventilation–perfusion matching.

Although it may be expected that the maintenance of the head-of-bed elevation at 30° to 45° may increase the workload of nurses and other bedside providers, a single study from Brazil showed that among other interventions, maintenance of the head of bed at 30° to 45° did not additionally increase the workload of nursing professionals in the ICU [22]. A randomized controlled trial (RCT) from Vietnam, however, suggests that a semi-recumbent position does not prevent the occurrence of healthcare-associated pneumonia in severe tetanus patients [23]. Nevertheless, other RCTs from resource-rich ICUs established the role of semi-recumbent position in the prevention of aspiration and ventilator-associated pneumonia in critically ill patients [24–26]. The actual degree of elevation of head of bed needs to be individualized based on the hemodynamic and respiratory status [27], as well as the risk of pressure sores/decubitus ulcers [28].

The semi-recumbent position should be feasible even in the most resource-limited settings, where despite the lack of special hospital beds, pillows and other soft material items can be used for the upper back and head support. In practice, it could be hard to sustain 30° with pillows alone. Frequent reassessments of the angle of elevation with a target of 30° to 45° should be instituted. Whether this single intervention further increases the workload of bedside providers will depend on the local, site-specific circumstances including the degree of involvement of family members in the nursing care. Of note, the semi-recumbent position may not be suitable for some patients, such as those with acute thoracic spine fracture.

We *recommend* that the vast majority of ventilated septic patients should be placed in the semi-recumbent position with an elevated head of bed ranging from 30° to 45° unless their hemodynamic state precludes this (1B). Patient's position could be lowered to less than 30° head-of-bed elevation transiently for the necessary procedures and during the resuscitation of the shock state until hemodynamic status is improved (1B) or longer in cases of sacral decubitus ulcer (1C).

6.4 Noninvasive Ventilation (NIV)

One of the primary goals in sepsis-induced acute respiratory failure is to ensure and maintain the tissue oxygen delivery. This can be provided by simple oxygen supplementation as well as by NIV or invasive mechanical ventilation, which in addition to oxygen supplementation provides positive-pressure ventilation. Generally, patients with mild oxygen saturation impairments and noncomplicated hemodynamic status (i.e., non-shock states) can be managed with simple oxygen supplementation. NIV has potentially advantageous role in acute respiratory failure over the simple administration of oxygen [29] or invasive mechanical ventilation [30]. However, frequently patients initially started on NIV fail to improve and require intubation and invasive mechanical ventilation. Moreover, the delay in intubation and MV has been associated with adverse outcomes [31].

A prospective cohort study from Brazil showed that more than half of ICU patients initially placed on NIV (54%) required subsequent intubation and mechanical ventilation, and failure of NIV was the strongest predictor of hospital mortality [31]. A 1-year observational study from India showed that almost all patients with moderate to severe acute respiratory failure required invasive mechanical ventilation (40/41) and that almost 2/3 of patients (11/17) initially managed with NIV subsequently required intubation and invasive mechanical ventilation [32]. The remaining evidence stems from resource-rich ICUs and suggests discretionary use of NIV in cases of sepsis-associated acute respiratory failure and concomitant immunosuppressed state [33], hypercapnia due to obstructive lung disease [34, 35], or hydrostatic pulmonary edema, with relatively preserved mental status and absence of shock [30, 34]. NIV could also be attempted in patients with mild hemodynamic and respiratory impairments with frequent reassessments of work of breathing, oxygenation and ventilation and prompt intubation, and invasive mechanical ventilation in cases of failure to improve after 1–2 h of intensive resuscitation and monitoring [36].

In individual ICU settings, where both NIV and invasive mechanical ventilation are available, evidence from resource-rich settings could be translated. However, it is of utmost importance that patients placed on NIV are closely monitored and assessed, so in cases of insufficient improvement, they can be intubated and placed on invasive mechanical ventilation without delays. Therefore, it is important to stress the need for appropriate staffing, which will allow close monitoring and frequent reassessments. Another potential safety concern is when NIV is applied using high tidal volumes because of underlying metabolic acidosis. Given potential for volume-induced lung injury, these patients may need invasive mechanical ventilation with adequate sedation (and maybe even short-term muscle paralysis) if there is no improvement after short-term NIV (i.e., within 1–2 h).

Based on the evidence from resource-rich ICUs, we *recommend* the use of invasive mechanical ventilation in cases of severe hemodynamic disturbance manifested as shock or severe hypoxemia (1A). We *suggest* that NIV could be used in selected cases of mild respiratory failure with preserved or relatively stable hemodynamic status (2A), especially in the above-described specific patient populations. This suggestion does not depend on the availability or lack of CXR or ABG for ARDS diagnosis. Once NIV is started, continuous resuscitation efforts and frequent reassessments of therapeutic effect of NIV are required in order to prevent delay in intubation and MV (1B).

6.5 Spontaneous Breathing Trials

Preventing unnecessary long ventilatory support is essential in preventing harm from intubation and mechanical ventilation. Successful completion of spontaneous breathing trials, which include a low level of pressure support, continuous positive airway pressure, or the use of a T-piece, increases the likelihood of successful discontinuation of ventilation.

Three well-performed trials in resource-rich ICUs [37–39] clearly showed benefit from early spontaneous breathing trials, i.e., shorter duration of ventilation. A recent meta-analysis found no evidence of a difference between spontaneous breathing trials using low levels of pressure support and spontaneous breathing trials using a T-piece [40].

Spontaneous breathing trials are available and affordable, in particular if no additional techniques are used (e.g., when a spontaneous breathing trial uses a low level of pressure support). It could be safer to perform spontaneous breathing trials using low level of pressure support technique than spontaneous breathing trials using a T-piece, as with the first approach a minimum ventilatory support is guaranteed. Spontaneous breathing trials could be time-consuming, in particular for ICUs with restricted staffing, but if successfully implemented, this intervention could save resources including labor because it shortens duration of ventilation. For practical reasons, tracheal extubation of patients in whom a trial of spontaneous breathing is successful should take place when there is sufficient staffing around (i.e., during daytimes), as such reducing the risk of re-intubation with no adequate staffing promptly available. Notably, to increase the success of this strategy, oversedation should be prevented.

We *recommend* using spontaneous breathing trials regularly, preferably daily, in all ventilated patients in low resource-limited ICUs (1A), and we *suggest* using the low level of pressure support technique (2D). We *suggest* performing spontaneous breathing trials and to extubate if the trial is successful only when sufficient staff is available to re-intubate those patients that may still need ventilatory support (2D). Nurses and physicians should develop local protocols for spontaneous breathing trials (2C). Of note, the effectiveness of using spontaneous breathing trials depends on sedation practices.

6.6 Low Tidal Volumes

"Lung-protective" ventilation with low tidal volumes improves survival of patients with ARDS in resource-rich settings [41, 42], and this can be translated to resource-limited ICUs. Delays in diagnosing ARDS may delay timely use of low tidal volumes, a problem that could be encountered in low- and middle-income countries

(LMICs) (see also *question 1*). Restricting low tidal volume ventilation to patients with ARDS diagnosis thus could lead to underuse or delayed use of this intervention, which is not an additional burden to limited resources. Notably, evidence is growing for the benefit of low tidal volume ventilation in patients without ARDS [43–45].

One RCT in ARDS patients from Brazil showed a bundle of a low tidal volume (6 ml/kg PBW) *plus* a level of PEEP above the lower inflection point on the static pressure–volume curve, compared with a bundle of conventional tidal volumes (12 ml/kg PBW) *plus* the lowest level of PEEP to maintain acceptable oxygenation, improved 28-day survival in patients with ARDS [46]. One observational study from Korea in patients with ARDS due to H1N1 [47] compared outcomes in tidal volume size tertiles (≤7 ml/kg PBW, 7–9 ml/kg PBW, and >9 ml/kg PBW) [47]. In this study, use of low tidal volumes was associated with a higher ICU survival and a higher number of ventilation-free days, ICU-free days, and hospital-free days.

The findings are in line with two meta-analyses [41, 42], including several well-performed RCTs [46, 48–51] that confirmed the benefit from low tidal volume ventilation in patients with ARDS. The precise titration of the size of tidal volumes for an individual patient could require adjustment for such factors as the presence of a profound metabolic acidosis and high obligate minute ventilation (tidal volumes may need to be as large as 8 ml/kg PBW) and the plateau pressure achieved and the level of PEEP chosen (tidal volumes may need to be as small as 4 ml/kg PBW). Notably, it is crucial to use predicted body weight for calculating the size of tidal volumes and not to use actual body weight (although actual body weight is usually equal to PBW in the normally nourished or undernourished patient).

Several recent meta-analyses [43–45], including one RCT [52] and several large observational studies in critically ill patients without ARDS in HICs [53–55], suggested a decreased risk of developing ARDS, shorter duration of ventilation, and shorter stay in hospital with low tidal volume volumes.

There are no studies on the use of end-tidal carbon dioxide (CO_2) monitoring as an alternative to ABG monitoring for patients receiving ventilation, including in LMICs, although one guideline suggests capnography to guide ventilator management [56]. Infrequent ABG in low-resource settings may preclude the early detection of harmful hypercapnia. While moderate hypercapnia is acceptable, severe hypercapnia should be prevented by closely monitoring minute ventilation. Also, in patients with brain injury, $PaCO_2$ control may be more important than in other patients. However, metabolic acidosis is frequently seen in patients with sepsis or septic shock, which may limit ventilation strategies that may cause hypercapnia. Low tidal volume ventilation comes with higher respiratory rates, which may create a feeling of discomfort, not necessarily for the patient but for the staff, which may unnecessarily trigger use of (more) sedation.

We *recommend* using low tidal volume ventilation in patients with ARDS diagnosis (1A) and *suggest* using low tidal volumes in all ventilated patients with sepsis or septic shock when lack of CXR or ABG availability hampers a timely ARDS diagnosis (i.e., prevent tidal volumes higher than 10 ml/kg PBW and consider tidal volumes of 5–7 ml/kg PBW in all patients) (2B). Notably, tidal volume size titration must use PBW and not the actual body weight (1A). Staff should be trained in timely recognition of under-ventilation, where respiratory rates should be adjusted (2D). Staff should be trained in accepting higher respiratory rates and not using more sedation (2C). Of note, we found no literature on preferred tidal volume sizes in patients with chronic obstructive pulmonary disease, but these patients may tolerate ventilation with low tidal volumes. End-tidal CO_2 monitoring could be helpful in timely recognition of endotracheal tube dislodgement or under- or overventilation (2D).

6.7 PEEP

PEEP prevents atelectasis, as such preventing ventilation–perfusion mismatch. PEEP, however, could also induce regional overdistension, which could increase dead space and injure lung tissue. Moreover, higher levels of PEEP could cause hemodynamic compromise, especially in patients with sepsis or septic shock. Higher levels of PEEP have only been found beneficial in patients with more severe forms of ARDS [57].

One recent observational study from Brazil showed no association between the level of PEEP applied and outcome in patients without ARDS [16]. In this study the median level of PEEP was 6 cm H_2O. The findings of this study were at least in part in line with results from a RCT in patients without ARDS in the USA that showed no differences in the occurrence of ARDS and other pulmonary complications when ventilating with 8 cm H_2O of PEEP or no PEEP [58]. However, while one recent RCT in the Netherlands comparing a strategy using low tidal volumes (6 ml/kg PBW) with a strategy using conventional tidal volumes (10 ml/kg PBW) in patients without ARDS found an independent association between use of higher levels of PEEP and the development of lung injury [52], one RCT in patients without ARDS in Spain showed a lower incidence of ventilator-associated pneumonia and a lower risk of hypoxemia with 5–8 cm H_2O of PEEP compared to no PEEP [59]. Mortality was not affected in the last RCT, however, and differences in the incidence of ventilator-associated pneumonia could have reflected more a difference in the occurrence of atelectasis than a true difference in pulmonary infection rates.

One RCT in patients with ARDS from Brazil showed that a strategy that uses low tidal volumes (6 ml/kg predicted body weight, PBW) *plus* a level of PEEP above the lower inflection point of the static pressure–volume curve to be superior to a strategy that uses conventional tidal volumes (12 ml/kg PBW) *plus* the lowest level of PEEP to maintain acceptable oxygenation with respect to 28-day survival [46]. It is uncertain whether benefit came from use of lower tidal volumes, higher levels of PEEP, or both. Three large multicenter randomized controlled trials conducted in patients with ARDS in HICs individually showed no benefit from use of higher levels of PEEP, titrated on the pulmonary compliance or based on the P/F, compared to lower levels of PEEP [60–62], but a meta-analysis showed that use of higher levels of PEEP was beneficial in patients with more severe forms of ARDS [57].

A minimum level of PEEP is easily applied and safe as most if not all ventilators allow setting a certain level of PEEP, and the benefit from prevention of atelectasis could outweigh the risk of regional overdistension. Because of the increased risk of hemodynamic instability with higher levels of PEEP, continuous hemodynamic monitoring, preferably by using an arterial line, will be necessary to guarantee safety. It can be a challenge to suspect and detect regional overdistension, and it could be difficult to find the best level of PEEP in an individual patient when physicians are untrained and inexperienced in using respiratory compliance and the P/F.

We *suggest* using at least a minimum level of PEEP (5 cm H_2O) in all patients with sepsis or septic shock with acute respiratory failure in resource-limited ICUs (2B). Based on the available evidence, we *suggest* using higher levels of PEEP only in patients with moderate or severe ARDS (2A). If lack of CXR and ABG availability hampers making an ARDS diagnosis, we *suggest* against liberal use of higher levels of PEEP (2D), but when the team is trained and experienced in using respiratory compliance, PEEP could be titrated based on this parameter (2D). Alternatively, so-called PEEP/FiO_2 tables could be used for titrating PEEP, but this approach generally requires frequent ABGs (2B) or use of SpO_2 to titrate FiO_2. Patients who need higher levels of PEEP should be closely monitored, as hypotension may develop (1A).

6.8 Low Oxygen Fractions with High PEEP or High Oxygen Fractions with Low PEEP

When high levels of PEEP are considered dangerous, or when it is difficult or impossible to find the best level of PEEP in an individual patient (see *question 6*) and when the team is inexperienced in performing recruitment maneuvers (see *question 8*), hypoxemia may trigger use of higher FiO_2. High FiO_2, however, induces the production of large amounts of reactive oxygen species that overwhelm natural antioxidant defenses, which could then injure cellular structures and consequently may induce pulmonary injury. In particular inflamed lungs are more susceptible to oxygen toxicity. Furthermore, ventilation with high FiO_2 could induce reabsorption atelectasis.

While studies suggest that "normoxia" should be targeted in patients with ARDS, there is increasing evidence for harm from strategies that use high FiO_2 aiming for higher blood oxygen levels in general ICU patients [63, 64]. Associations between ventilation strategies that use high FiO_2 and increased mortality have also been found in patients following resuscitation from cardiac arrest [65] and patients with ischemic stroke [66] or traumatic brain injury [67]. Two recent meta-analyses confirm arterial hyperoxia to be associated with worse hospital outcome in various subsets of critically ill patients [68, 69]. As discussed above (*question 6*), higher levels of PEEP have only been found beneficial in patients with more severe forms of ARDS [57].

Table 6.3 Allowable combinations of PEEP and FiO_2

Strategy in which first FiO_2 is raised in response to hypoxemia (originally called the low PEEP group)														
FiO_2	0.21	0.3	0.4	0.4	0.5	0.5	0.6	> 0.6						
PEEP	5	5	5	8	8	10	10	10						
Strategy in which first PEEP is raised in response to hypoxemia (originally called the high PEEP group)														
FiO_2	0.21	0.3	0.4	0.4	0.5	0.5	0.5	0.6	0.7	0.8	0.8	0.9	0.9	1.0
PEEP	5–12	14	14	16	16	18	20	20	20	20	22	22	22	> 22

Adapted from [58]

A certain extent of hypoxemia with a target $PaO_2 > 8$ kPa [60 mmHg] has been suggested to be safe [51]. A SpO_2 of 88–95% could be targeted when ABGs are not or only scarcely available [51].

Using "PEEP/FiO_2 tables" with the aim to ventilate patients with ARDS with the lowest level of PEEP and the lowest level of FiO_2 is feasible and safe in LMICs, but this approach mandates frequent ABGs or use of SpO_2 to titrate FiO_2 [47–49]. Implementation of this strategy could be more complex in LMICs where ABGs typically are less often available. Alternatively, SpO_2 could be used to titrate PEEP and FiO_2. Also, when continuous hemodynamic monitoring is lacking, use of high levels of PEEP could be dangerous. In such settings it could be safer to prefer higher FiO_2 than higher levels of PEEP.

Based on the available evidence, we *suggest* being cautious with liberal use of high FiO_2 (2B). The target should be $PaO_2 > 8$ kPa [60 mmHg] and/or SpO_2 88–95% (2A). PEEP/FiO_2 tables can be used to find the best PEEP/FiO_2 combination in individual patients in LMICs (2B). We *suggest* preferring low FiO_2 with high levels of PEEP, if the team is trained and experienced in (safe) the use of higher levels of PEEP; if not, it is probably safer to use high FiO_2 with lower levels of PEEP (2D). An example of a "PEEP/FiO_2 table" is provided (Table 6.3) [60].

6.9 Recruitment Maneuvers

It is generally considered necessary to combine higher levels of PEEP with recruitment maneuvers, as early use of recruitment maneuvers could open additional lung units that remain closed when only applying higher levels of PEEP. Recruitment maneuvers, however, are complex interventions that could also cause pulmonary and extra-pulmonary harm, especially in inexperienced hands.

In an RCT from Brazil [46], the two arms of the study also differed in respect to using recruitment maneuvers. The same applies for other RCTs comparing higher levels of PEEP with lower levels of PEEP in patients with ARDS in HICs [60–62]. One systematic review of four randomized controlled trials investigating the benefit of recruitment maneuvers remained inconclusive [70]; a more recent meta-analysis suggested that strategies that use recruitment maneuvers are associated with a lower mortality in patients with ARDS [71].

Recruitment maneuvers can cause episodes of severe hemodynamic compromise [61], especially in patients with sepsis or septic shock. Recruitment maneuvers could also induce regional overdistension. In HIC the performance of recruitment maneuvers is seen as a complex intervention, with associated risks if not applied properly [61]. Therefore, it is only applied in patients with refractory and severe hypoxemia and only in patients with a stabilized circulation and preferably with an arterial line in situ.

The recruitment maneuvers are variable, which is a general limitation of the technique because it is not standardized. The earliest recruitment maneuver ever used during mechanical ventilation is probably the "sigh," which consists of increasing tidal volume or level of PEEP [72]. However, there is a potential safety concern given that this maneuver transiently elevates plateau pressure above the recommended threshold of 30 cm H_2O, in patients with ARDS. The most frequently investigated recruitment maneuver, due to its apparent simplicity, is the sustained inflation, which consists of pressurizing the airways at a specific level and maintaining it for a given duration. A common combination is the application of 40 cm H_2O airway pressure for 40 s ("40/40") [73]. Sustained inflation is transient and simple recruitment maneuver, which is likely an overall safe procedure as it can potentially obviate the need for ongoing use of higher intrathoracic pressures. High PEEP and pressure-controlled ventilation with a fixed driving pressure (i.e., the level of inspiratory pressure minus the level of PEEP) are other ways to perform recruitment maneuvers [74].

The use of recruitment maneuvers during ventilation is feasible and safe, but only in experienced hands. The lack of experience and absence of hemodynamic monitoring may hamper the safe and widespread use in LMICs. Moreover, it can be challenging to detect overdistension. Of all recruitment maneuvers, sustained inflation is probably the simplest and the safest maneuver.

We *suggest* using recruitment maneuvers in resource-limited ICUs in patients with moderate or severe ARDS (2B) and suggest using recruitment maneuvers in patients in resource-limited ICUs with refractory hypoxemia in whom a diagnosis of ARDS cannot be made due to lack of CXR and/or ABG (2D), but only when the staff is trained and experienced in performing these maneuvers (2D). We *suggest* using the simplest maneuver, i.e., "sustained inflation" (2D). When using recruitment maneuvers, the patient should be closely monitored to detect hemodynamic compromise (2B).

6.10 Ventilation Modes

Traditionally reserved for use in weaning patients from ventilation, assisted ventilation modes are now used in all phases of ventilation. Controlled ventilation is associated with incapability of reversing alveolar collapse in dependent lung parts and an increased risk of ventilator-induced diaphragmatic dysfunction. Assisted ventilation could be preferred over controlled ventilation, because assisted ventilation can be tolerated with reduced sedation requirements, and may be associated with less hemodynamic deterioration, and lung protection compared to controlled ventilation [75, 76].

"Volume-controlled" ventilation and "pressure-controlled" ventilation are not different ventilatory modes but are different control variables within a mode [77]. "Volume-controlled" ventilation offers the safety of a preset tidal volume and minute ventilation, while "pressure-controlled" ventilation offers a flow that better mimics the flow during inspiration of a spontaneously breathing individual. Investigations comparing the effects of "volume-controlled" ventilation and "pressure-controlled" ventilation are not well controlled and offer no evidence for benefit of the one mode over the other [77].

One small RCT, including patients with and patients without ARDS, demonstrated shorter length of stay in the ICU with use of assisted ventilation compared to controlled ventilation [78]. Another RCT in patients with ARDS showed a higher number of ventilator-free days with assisted ventilation, although the difference was not statistically significant, but in both groups, some sort of support was applied [79]. Beneficial effects of assisted ventilation could include improvement of gas exchange, hemodynamics, and non-pulmonary organ perfusion and function, as well as improved quality of sleep, and are associated with a decreased need for sedation and paralysis [80].

Assisted ventilation is available, feasible, and affordable in all patients in LMICs, where its use is probably also safe. One exception could be patients with severe and early ARDS in whom a short course of muscle paralysis, and thus use of controlled ventilation, has been found to be beneficial [81], though evidence for benefit of a short course of muscle paralysis in these patients in LMICs is lacking. Notably, with assisted ventilation tidal volumes are usually larger than with controlled ventilation. This is probably due to an active diaphragm, which largely prevents dorsal atelectasis. A rise in tidal volumes >6 ml/kg PBW, while using the lowest level of pressure support, may not be a reason to switch back to controlled ventilation. Since minute volume and tidal volume size are guaranteed with "volume-controlled" modes of ventilation and not with "pressure-controlled" modes of ventilation, "volume-controlled" modes could be safer than "pressure-controlled" modes, in particular in settings with restricted physician and nursing staff.

Therefore we *suggest* using "volume-controlled" modes of ventilation rather than "pressure-controlled" modes of ventilation in resource-limited settings. However, teams with experience and expertise in "pressure-controlled" modes of ventilation could continue to use this mode (2D). We *make no recommendations* regarding assisted ventilation over controlled ventilation in all patients in LMICs. We *suggest* a short course of muscle paralysis (<48 h) and thus the use of controlled ventilation, in patients with severe ARDS (2B).

References

1. Rhodes A, Evans LE, Alhazzani W, Levy MM, Antonelli M, Ferrer R, Kumar A, Sevransky JE, Sprung CL, Nunnally ME, Rochwerg B, Rubenfeld GD, Angus DC, Annane D, Beale RJ, Bellinghan GJ, Bernard GR, Chiche JD, Coopersmith C, De Backer DP, French CJ, Fujishima

S, Gerlach H, Hidalgo JL, Hollenberg SM, Jones AE, Karnad DR, Kleinpell RM, Koh Y, Lisboa TC, Machado FR, Marini JJ, Marshall JC, Mazuski JE, McIntyre LA, McLean AS, Mehta S, Moreno RP, Myburgh J, Navalesi P, Nishida O, Osborn TM, Perner A, Plunkett CM, Ranieri M, Schorr CA, Seckel MA, Seymour CW, Shieh L, Shukri KA, Simpson SQ, Singer M, Thompson BT, Townsend SR, Van der Poll T, Vincent JL, Wiersinga WJ, Zimmerman JL, Dellinger RP. Surviving sepsis campaign: international guidelines for management of sepsis and septic shock: 2016. Crit Care Med. 2017;45:486–552.

2. Rhodes A, Evans LE, Alhazzani W, Levy MM, Antonelli M, Ferrer R, Kumar A, Sevransky JE, Sprung CL, Nunnally ME, Rochwerg B, Rubenfeld GD, Angus DC, Annane D, Beale RJ, Bellinghan GJ, Bernard GR, Chiche JD, Coopersmith C, De Backer DP, French CJ, Fujishima S, Gerlach H, Hidalgo JL, Hollenberg SM, Jones AE, Karnad DR, Kleinpell RM, Koh Y, Lisboa TC, Machado FR, Marini JJ, Marshall JC, Mazuski JE, McIntyre LA, McLean AS, Mehta S, Moreno RP, Myburgh J, Navalesi P, Nishida O, Osborn TM, Perner A, Plunkett CM, Ranieri M, Schorr CA, Seckel MA, Seymour CW, Shieh L, Shukri KA, Simpson SQ, Singer M, Thompson BT, Townsend SR, Van der Poll T, Vincent JL, Wiersinga WJ, Zimmerman JL, Dellinger RP. Surviving sepsis campaign: international guidelines for management of sepsis and septic shock: 2016. Intensive Care Med. 2017;43:304–77.
3. Schultz MJ, Dunser MW, Dondorp AM, Adhikari NK, Iyer S, Kwizera A, Lubell Y, Papali A, Pisani L, Riviello BD, Angus DC, Azevedo LC, Baker T, Diaz JV, Festic E, Haniffa R, Jawa R, Jacob ST, Kissoon N, Lodha R, Martin-Loeches I, Lundeg G, Misango D, Mer M, Mohanty S, Murthy S, Musa N, Nakibuuka J, Serpa Neto A, Nguyen Thi Hoang M, Nguyen Thien B, Pattnaik R, Phua J, Preller J, Povoa P, Ranjit S, Talmor D, Thevanayagam J, Thwaites CL, Global Intensive Care Working Group of the European Society of Intensive Care Medicine. Current challenges in the management of sepsis in ICUs in resource-poor settings and suggestions for the future. Intensive Care Med. 2017;43:612–24.
4. Force ADT, Ranieri VM, Rubenfeld GD, Thompson BT, Ferguson ND, Caldwell E, Fan E, Camporota L, Slutsky AS. Acute respiratory distress syndrome: the Berlin Definition. JAMA. 2012;307:2526–33.
5. Lichtenstein D, Goldstein I, Mourgeon E, Cluzel P, Grenier P, Rouby JJ. Comparative diagnostic performances of auscultation, chest radiography, and lung ultrasonography in acute respiratory distress syndrome. Anesthesiology. 2004;100:9–15.
6. Bouhemad B, Zhang M, Lu Q, Rouby JJ. Clinical review: bedside lung ultrasound in critical care practice. Crit Care. 2007;11:205.
7. Volpicelli G, Elbarbary M, Blaivas M, Lichtenstein DA, Mathis G, Kirkpatrick AW, Melniker L, Gargani L, Noble VE, Via G, Dean A, Tsung JW, Soldati G, Copetti R, Bouhemad B, Reissig A, Agricola E, Rouby JJ, Arbelot C, Liteplo A, Sargsyan A, Silva F, Hoppmann R, Breitkreutz R, Seibel A, Neri L, Storti E, Petrovic T, International Liaison Committee on Lung Ultrasound for International Consensus Conference on Lung Ultrasound. International evidence-based recommendations for point-of-care lung ultrasound. Intensive Care Med. 2012;38:577–91.
8. Lichtenstein DA, Meziere GA, Lagoueyte JF, Biderman P, Goldstein I, Gepner A. A-lines and B-lines: lung ultrasound as a bedside tool for predicting pulmonary artery occlusion pressure in the critically ill. Chest. 2009;136:1014–20.
9. Bass CM, Sajed DR, Adedipe AA, West TE. Pulmonary ultrasound and pulse oximetry versus chest radiography and arterial blood gas analysis for the diagnosis of acute respiratory distress syndrome: a pilot study. Crit Care. 2015;19:282.
10. Melamed R, Sprenkle MD, Ulstad VK, Herzog CA, Leatherman JW. Assessment of left ventricular function by intensivists using hand-held echocardiography. Chest. 2009;135:1416–20.
11. Chimot L, Legrand M, Canet E, Lemiale V, Azoulay E. Echocardiography in hemodynamic monitoring. Chest. 2010;137:501–2.
12. Kaplan A, Mayo PH. Echocardiography performed by the pulmonary/critical care medicine physician. Chest. 2009;135:529–35.
13. Festic E, Bansal V, Kor DJ, Gajic O, US Critical Illness and Injury Trials Group: Lung Injury Prevention Study Investigators (USCIITG–LIPS). SpO2/FiO2 ratio on hospital admission is

an indicator of early acute respiratory distress syndrome development among patients at risk. J Intensive Care Med. 2015;30:209–16.

14. Rice TW, Wheeler AP, Bernard GR, Hayden DL, Schoenfeld DA, Ware LB, National Institutes of Health, National Heart, Lung, and Blood Institute ARDS Network. Comparison of the SpO2/FIO2 ratio and the PaO2/FIO2 ratio in patients with acute lung injury or ARDS. Chest. 2007;132:410–7.
15. Chen W, Janz DR, Shaver CM, Bernard GR, Bastarache JA, Ware LB. Clinical characteristics and outcomes are similar in ARDS diagnosed by SpO2/FiO2 ratio compared with PaO2/FiO2 ratio. Chest. 2015;148(6):1477–83.
16. Serpa Neto A, Cardoso SO, Ong DS, Esposito DC, Pereira VG, Manetta JA, Slooter AJ, Cremer OL. The use of the pulse oximetric saturation/fraction of inspired oxygen ratio for risk stratification of patients with severe sepsis and septic shock. J Crit Care. 2013;28:681–6.
17. Bilan N, Dastranji A, Ghalehgolab Behbahani A. Comparison of the spo2/fio2 ratio and the pao2/fio2 ratio in patients with acute lung injury or acute respiratory distress syndrome. J Cardiovasc Thorac Res. 2015;7:28–31.
18. Khemani RG, Thomas NJ, Venkatachalam V, Scimeme JP, Berutti T, Schneider JB, Ross PA, Willson DF, Hall MW, Newth CJ, Pediatric Acute Lung Injury and Sepsis Network Investigators (PALISI). Comparison of SpO2 to PaO2 based markers of lung disease severity for children with acute lung injury. Crit Care Med. 2012;40:1309–16.
19. Lobete C, Medina A, Rey C, Mayordomo-Colunga J, Concha A, Menendez S. Correlation of oxygen saturation as measured by pulse oximetry/fraction of inspired oxygen ratio with Pao2/fraction of inspired oxygen ratio in a heterogeneous sample of critically ill children. J Crit Care. 2013;28(538):e531–7.
20. Pandharipande PP, Shintani AK, Hagerman HE, St Jacques PJ, Rice TW, Sanders NW, Ware LB, Bernard GR, Ely EW. Derivation and validation of Spo2/Fio2 ratio to impute for Pao2/Fio2 ratio in the respiratory component of the Sequential Organ Failure Assessment score. Crit Care Med. 2009;37:1317–21.
21. Rackley CR, Levitt JE, Zhuo H, Matthay MA, Calfee CS. Clinical evidence of early acute lung injury often precedes the diagnosis of ALI. J Intensive Care Med. 2013;28:241–6.
22. Colaco AD, Nascimento ER. Nursing intervention bundle for enteral nutrition in intensive care: a collective construction. Rev Esc Enferm USP. 2014;48:844–50.
23. Loan HT, Parry J, Nga NT, Yen LM, Binh NT, Thuy TT, Duong NM, Campbell JI, Thwaites L, Farrar JJ, Parry CM. Semi-recumbent body position fails to prevent healthcare-associated pneumonia in Vietnamese patients with severe tetanus. Trans R Soc Trop Med Hyg. 2012;106:90–7.
24. Torres A, Serra-Batlles J, Ros E, Piera C, Puig de la Bellacasa J, Cobos A, Lomena F, Rodriguez-Roisin R. Pulmonary aspiration of gastric contents in patients receiving mechanical ventilation: the effect of body position. Ann Intern Med. 1992;116:540–3.
25. Orozco-Levi M, Torres A, Ferrer M, Piera C, el-Ebiary M, de la Bellacasa JP, Rodriguez-Roisin R. Semirecumbent position protects from pulmonary aspiration but not completely from gastroesophageal reflux in mechanically ventilated patients. Am J Respir Crit Care Med. 1995;152:1387–90.
26. Drakulovic MB, Torres A, Bauer TT, Nicolas JM, Nogue S, Ferrer M. Supine body position as a risk factor for nosocomial pneumonia in mechanically ventilated patients: a randomised trial. Lancet. 1999;354:1851–8.
27. Gocze I, Strenge F, Zeman F, Creutzenberg M, Graf BM, Schlitt HJ, Bein T. The effects of the semirecumbent position on hemodynamic status in patients on invasive mechanical ventilation: prospective randomized multivariable analysis. Crit Care. 2013;17:R80.
28. Metheny NA, Frantz RA. Head-of-bed elevation in critically ill patients: a review. Crit Care Nurse. 2013;33:53–66. quiz 67
29. Ferrer M, Esquinas A, Leon M, Gonzalez G, Alarcon A, Torres A. Noninvasive ventilation in severe hypoxemic respiratory failure: a randomized clinical trial. Am J Respir Crit Care Med. 2003;168:1438–44.

30. Antonelli M, Conti G, Rocco M, Bufi M, De Blasi RA, Vivino G, Gasparetto A, Meduri GU. A comparison of noninvasive positive-pressure ventilation and conventional mechanical ventilation in patients with acute respiratory failure. N Engl J Med. 1998;339:429–35.
31. Azevedo LC, Park M, Salluh JI, Rea-Neto A, Souza-Dantas VC, Varaschin P, Oliveira MC, Tierno PF, dal-Pizzol F, Silva UV, Knibel M, Nassar AP Jr, Alves RA, Ferreira JC, Teixeira C, Rezende V, Martinez A, Luciano PM, Schettino G, Soares M, ERICC (Epidemiology of Respiratory Insufficiency in Critical Care) investigators. Clinical outcomes of patients requiring ventilatory support in Brazilian intensive care units: a multicenter, prospective, cohort study. Crit Care. 2013;17:R63.
32. Bhadade RR, de Souza RA, Harde MJ, Khot A. Clinical characteristics and outcomes of patients with acute lung injury and ARDS. J Postgrad Med. 2011;57:286–90.
33. Hilbert G, Gruson D, Vargas F, Valentino R, Gbikpi-Benissan G, Dupon M, Reiffers J, Cardinaud JP. Noninvasive ventilation in immunosuppressed patients with pulmonary infiltrates, fever, and acute respiratory failure. N Engl J Med. 2001;344:481–7.
34. Meduri GU, Turner RE, Abou-Shala N, Wunderink R, Tolley E. Noninvasive positive pressure ventilation via face mask. First-line intervention in patients with acute hypercapnic and hypoxemic respiratory failure. Chest. 1996;109:179–93.
35. Plant PK, Owen JL, Elliott MW. Early use of non-invasive ventilation for acute exacerbations of chronic obstructive pulmonary disease on general respiratory wards: a multicentre randomised controlled trial. Lancet. 2000;355:1931–5.
36. Delclaux C, L'Her E, Alberti C, Mancebo J, Abroug F, Conti G, Guerin C, Schortgen F, Lefort Y, Antonelli M, Lepage E, Lemaire F, Brochard L. Treatment of acute hypoxemic nonhypercapnic respiratory insufficiency with continuous positive airway pressure delivered by a face mask: a randomized controlled trial. JAMA. 2000;284:2352–60.
37. Ely EW, Baker AM, Dunagan DP, Burke HL, Smith AC, Kelly PT, Johnson MM, Browder RW, Bowton DL, Haponik EF. Effect on the duration of mechanical ventilation of identifying patients capable of breathing spontaneously. N Engl J Med. 1996;335:1864–9.
38. Girard TD, Kress JP, Fuchs BD, Thomason JW, Schweickert WD, Pun BT, Taichman DB, Dunn JG, Pohlman AS, Kinniry PA, Jackson JC, Canonico AE, Light RW, Shintani AK, Thompson JL, Gordon SM, Hall JB, Dittus RS, Bernard GR, Ely EW. Efficacy and safety of a paired sedation and ventilator weaning protocol for mechanically ventilated patients in intensive care (Awakening and Breathing Controlled trial): a randomised controlled trial. Lancet. 2008;371:126–34.
39. Kress JP, Pohlman AS, O'Connor MF, Hall JB. Daily interruption of sedative infusions in critically ill patients undergoing mechanical ventilation. N Engl J Med. 2000;342:1471–7.
40. Ladeira MT, Vital FM, Andriolo RB, Andriolo BN, Atallah AN, Peccin MS. Pressure support versus T-tube for weaning from mechanical ventilation in adults. Cochrane Database Syst Rev. 2014;5:CD006056.
41. Burns KE, Adhikari NK, Slutsky AS, Guyatt GH, Villar J, Zhang H, Zhou Q, Cook DJ, Stewart TE, Meade MO. Pressure and volume limited ventilation for the ventilatory management of patients with acute lung injury: a systematic review and meta-analysis. PLoS One. 2011;6:e14623.
42. Putensen C, Theuerkauf N, Zinserling J, Wrigge H, Pelosi P. Meta-analysis: ventilation strategies and outcomes of the acute respiratory distress syndrome and acute lung injury. Ann Intern Med. 2009;151:566–76.
43. Serpa Neto A, Cardoso SO, Manetta JA, Pereira VG, Esposito DC, Pasqualucci Mde O, Damasceno MC, Schultz MJ. Association between use of lung-protective ventilation with lower tidal volumes and clinical outcomes among patients without acute respiratory distress syndrome: a meta-analysis. JAMA. 2012;308:1651–9.
44. Serpa Neto A, Simonis FD, Barbas CS, Biehl M, Determann RM, Elmer J, Friedman G, Gajic O, Goldstein JN, Horn J, Juffermans NP, Linko R, de Oliveira RP, Sundar S, Talmor D, Wolthuis EK, de Abreu MG, Pelosi P, Schultz MJ. Association between tidal volume size, duration of ventilation, and sedation needs in patients without acute respiratory distress syndrome: an individual patient data meta-analysis. Intensive Care Med. 2014;40:950–7.

45. Serpa Neto A, Simonis FD, Barbas CS, Biehl M, Determann RM, Elmer J, Friedman G, Gajic O, Goldstein JN, Linko R, Pinheiro de Oliveira R, Sundar S, Talmor D, Wolthuis EK, Gama de Abreu M, Pelosi P, Schultz MJ. Lung protective ventilation with low tidal volumes and the occurrence of pulmonary complications in patients without ARDS: a systematic review and individual patient data metaanalysis. Crit Care Med. 2015;43(10):2155–63.
46. Amato MB, Barbas CS, Medeiros DM, Magaldi RB, Schettino GP, Lorenzi-Filho G, Kairalla RA, Deheinzelin D, Munoz C, Oliveira R, Takagaki TY, Carvalho CR. Effect of a protective-ventilation strategy on mortality in the acute respiratory distress syndrome. N Engl J Med. 1998;338:347–54.
47. Oh DK, Lee MG, Choi EY, Lim J, Lee HK, Kim SC, Lim CM, Koh Y, Hong SB, Korean Society of Critical Care Medicine HNc. Low-tidal volume mechanical ventilation in patients with acute respiratory distress syndrome caused by pandemic influenza A/H1N1 infection. J Crit Care. 2013;28:358–64.
48. Brochard L, Roudot-Thoraval F, Roupie E, Delclaux C, Chastre J, Fernandez-Mondejar E, Clementi E, Mancebo J, Factor P, Matamis D, Ranieri M, Blanch L, Rodi G, Mentec H, Dreyfuss D, Ferrer M, Brun-Buisson C, Tobin M, Lemaire F. Tidal volume reduction for prevention of ventilator-induced lung injury in acute respiratory distress syndrome. The Multicenter Trail Group on Tidal Volume reduction in ARDS. Am J Respir Crit Care Med. 1998;158:1831–8.
49. Stewart TE, Meade MO, Cook DJ, Granton JT, Hodder RV, Lapinsky SE, Mazer CD, McLean RF, Rogovein TS, Schouten BD, Todd TR, Slutsky AS. Evaluation of a ventilation strategy to prevent barotrauma in patients at high risk for acute respiratory distress syndrome. Pressure- and Volume-Limited Ventilation Strategy Group. N Engl J Med. 1998;338:355–61.
50. Brower RG, Shanholtz CB, Fessler HE, Shade DM, White P Jr, Wiener CM, Teeter JG, Dodd-o JM, Almog Y, Piantadosi S. Prospective, randomized, controlled clinical trial comparing traditional versus reduced tidal volume ventilation in acute respiratory distress syndrome patients. Crit Care Med. 1999;27:1492–8.
51. Acute Respiratory Distress Syndrome Network, Brower RG, Matthay MA, Morris A, Schoenfeld D, Thompson BT, Wheeler A. Ventilation with lower tidal volumes as compared with traditional tidal volumes for acute lung injury and the acute respiratory distress syndrome. N Engl J Med. 2000;342:1301–8.
52. Determann RM, Royakkers A, Wolthuis EK, Vlaar AP, Choi G, Paulus F, Hofstra JJ, de Graaff MJ, Korevaar JC, Schultz MJ. Ventilation with lower tidal volumes as compared with conventional tidal volumes for patients without acute lung injury: a preventive randomized controlled trial. Crit Care. 2010;14:R1.
53. Elmer J, Hou P, Wilcox SR, Chang Y, Schreiber H, Okechukwu I, Pontes-Neto O, Bajwa E, Hess DR, Avery L, Duran-Mendicuti MA, Camargo CA Jr, Greenberg SM, Rosand J, Pallin DJ, Goldstein JN. Acute respiratory distress syndrome after spontaneous intracerebral hemorrhage*. Crit Care Med. 2013;41:1992–2001.
54. Linko R, Okkonen M, Pettila V, Perttila J, Parviainen I, Ruokonen E, Tenhunen J, Ala-Kokko T, Varpula T, FINNALI-study group. Acute respiratory failure in intensive care units. FINNALI: a prospective cohort study. Intensive Care Med. 2009;35:1352–61.
55. Yilmaz M, Keegan MT, Iscimen R, Afessa B, Buck CF, Hubmayr RD, Gajic O. Toward the prevention of acute lung injury: protocol-guided limitation of large tidal volume ventilation and inappropriate transfusion. Crit Care Med. 2007;35:1660–6. quiz 1667
56. Walsh BK, Crotwell DN, Restrepo RD. Capnography/Capnometry during mechanical ventilation: 2011. Respir Care. 2011;56:503–9.
57. Briel M, Meade M, Mercat A, Brower RG, Talmor D, Walter SD, Slutsky AS, Pullenayegum E, Zhou Q, Cook D, Brochard L, Richard JC, Lamontagne F, Bhatnagar N, Stewart TE, Guyatt G. Higher vs lower positive end-expiratory pressure in patients with acute lung injury and acute respiratory distress syndrome: systematic review and meta-analysis. JAMA. 2010;303:865–73.
58. Pepe PE, Hudson LD, Carrico CJ. Early application of positive end-expiratory pressure in patients at risk for the adult respiratory-distress syndrome. N Engl J Med. 1984;311:281–6.

59. Manzano F, Fernandez-Mondejar E, Colmenero M, Poyatos ME, Rivera R, Machado J, Catalan I, Artigas A. Positive-end expiratory pressure reduces incidence of ventilator-associated pneumonia in nonhypoxemic patients. Crit Care Med. 2008;36:2225–31.
60. Brower RG, Lanken PN, MacIntyre N, Matthay MA, Morris A, Ancukiewicz M, Schoenfeld D, Thompson BT, National Heart L, Blood Institute ACTN. Higher versus lower positive end-expiratory pressures in patients with the acute respiratory distress syndrome. N Engl J Med. 2004;351:327–36.
61. Meade MO, Cook DJ, Guyatt GH, Slutsky AS, Arabi YM, Cooper DJ, Davies AR, Hand LE, Zhou Q, Thabane L, Austin P, Lapinsky S, Baxter A, Russell J, Skrobik Y, Ronco JJ, Stewart TE, Lung Open Ventilation Study Investigators. Ventilation strategy using low tidal volumes, recruitment maneuvers, and high positive end-expiratory pressure for acute lung injury and acute respiratory distress syndrome: a randomized controlled trial. JAMA. 2008;299:637–45.
62. Mercat A, Richard JC, Vielle B, Jaber S, Osman D, Diehl JL, Lefrant JY, Prat G, Richecoeur J, Nieszkowska A, Gervais C, Baudot J, Bouadma L, Brochard L, Expiratory Pressure (Express) Study Group. Positive end-expiratory pressure setting in adults with acute lung injury and acute respiratory distress syndrome: a randomized controlled trial. JAMA. 2008;299:646–55.
63. Altemeier WA, Sinclair SE. Hyperoxia in the intensive care unit: why more is not always better. Curr Opin Crit Care. 2007;13:73–8.
64. de Jonge E, Peelen L, Keijzers PJ, Joore H, de Lange D, van der Voort PH, Bosman RJ, de Waal RA, Wesselink R, de Keizer NF. Association between administered oxygen, arterial partial oxygen pressure and mortality in mechanically ventilated intensive care unit patients. Crit Care. 2008;12:R156.
65. Kilgannon JH, Jones AE, Shapiro NI, Angelos MG, Milcarek B, Hunter K, Parrillo JE, Trzeciak S, Emergency Medicine Shock Research Network (EMShockNet) Investigators. Association between arterial hyperoxia following resuscitation from cardiac arrest and in-hospital mortality. JAMA. 2010;303:2165–71.
66. Cornet AD, Kooter AJ, Peters MJ, Smulders YM. Supplemental oxygen therapy in medical emergencies: more harm than benefit? Arch Intern Med. 2012;172:289–90.
67. Davis DP, Meade W, Sise MJ, Kennedy F, Simon F, Tominaga G, Steele J, Coimbra R. Both hypoxemia and extreme hyperoxemia may be detrimental in patients with severe traumatic brain injury. J Neurotrauma. 2009;26:2217–23.
68. Damiani E, Adrario E, Girardis M, Romano R, Pelaia P, Singer M, Donati A. Arterial hyperoxia and mortality in critically ill patients: a systematic review and meta-analysis. Crit Care. 2014;18:711.
69. Helmerhorst HJ, Roos-Blom MJ, van Westerloo DJ, de Jonge E. Association between arterial hyperoxia and outcome in subsets of critical illness: a systematic review, metaanalysis, and meta-regression of cohort studies. Crit Care Med. 2015;43(7):1508–19.
70. Fan E, Wilcox ME, Brower RG, Stewart TE, Mehta S, Lapinsky SE, Meade MO, Ferguson ND. Recruitment maneuvers for acute lung injury: a systematic review. Am J Respir Crit Care Med. 2008;178:1156–63.
71. Suzumura EA, Figueiro M, Normilio-Silva K, Laranjeira L, Oliveira C, Buehler AM, Bugano D, Passos Amato MB, Ribeiro Carvalho CR, Berwanger O, Cavalcanti AB. Effects of alveolar recruitment maneuvers on clinical outcomes in patients with acute respiratory distress syndrome: a systematic review and meta-analysis. Intensive Care Med. 2014;40:1227–40.
72. Levine M, Gilbert R, Auchincloss JH Jr. A comparison of the effects of sighs, large tidal volumes, and positive end expiratory pressure in assisted ventilation. Scand J Respir Dis. 1972;53:101–8.
73. Grasso S, Mascia L, Del Turco M, Malacarne P, Giunta F, Brochard L, Slutsky AS, Marco Ranieri V. Effects of recruiting maneuvers in patients with acute respiratory distress syndrome ventilated with protective ventilatory strategy. Anesthesiology. 2002;96:795–802.
74. Borges CR, Lake DF. Oxidative protein folding: nature's knotty challenge. Antioxid Redox Signal. 2014;21:392–5.
75. Saddy F, Sutherasan Y, Rocco PR, Pelosi P. Ventilator-associated lung injury during assisted mechanical ventilation. Semin Respir Crit Care Med. 2014;35:409–17.

76. Guldner A, Pelosi P, Gama de Abreu M. Spontaneous breathing in mild and moderate versus severe acute respiratory distress syndrome. Curr Opin Crit Care. 2014;20:69–76.
77. Campbell RS, Davis BR. Pressure-controlled versus volume-controlled ventilation: does it matter? Respir Care. 2002;47:416–24. discussion 424-416
78. Putensen C, Zech S, Wrigge H, Zinserling J, Stuber F, Von Spiegel T, Mutz N. Long-term effects of spontaneous breathing during ventilatory support in patients with acute lung injury. Am J Respir Crit Care Med. 2001;164:43–9.
79. Varpula T, Valta P, Niemi R, Takkunen O, Hynynen M, Pettila VV. Airway pressure release ventilation as a primary ventilatory mode in acute respiratory distress syndrome. Acta Anaesthesiol Scand. 2004;48:722–31.
80. McMullen SM, Meade M, Rose L, Burns K, Mehta S, Doyle R, Henzler D, Canadian Critical Care Trials Group (CCCTG). Partial ventilatory support modalities in acute lung injury and acute respiratory distress syndrome-a systematic review. PLoS One. 2012;7:e40190.
81. Neto AS, Pereira VG, Esposito DC, Damasceno MC, Schultz MJ. Neuromuscular blocking agents in patients with acute respiratory distress syndrome: a summary of the current evidence from three randomized controlled trials. Ann Intensive Care. 2012;2:33.

Open Access This chapter is licensed under the terms of the Creative Commons Attribution 4.0 International License (http://creativecommons.org/licenses/by/4.0/), which permits use, sharing, adaptation, distribution and reproduction in any medium or format, as long as you give appropriate credit to the original author(s) and the source, provide a link to the Creative Commons license and indicate if changes were made.

The images or other third party material in this chapter are included in the chapter's Creative Commons license, unless indicated otherwise in a credit line to the material. If material is not included in the chapter's Creative Commons license and your intended use is not permitted by statutory regulation or exceeds the permitted use, you will need to obtain permission directly from the copyright holder.

7 Hemodynamic Assessment and Support in Sepsis and Septic Shock in Resource-Limited Settings

David Misango, Rajyabardhan Pattnaik, Tim Baker, Martin W. Dünser, Arjen M. Dondorp, and Marcus J. Schultz

7.1 Introduction

Recommendations for care in patients with sepsis or septic shock are largely based on evidence originating from resource-rich settings [1]. It is increasingly appreciated that these recommendations cannot be directly generalized to resource-limited

D. Misango
Department of Anaesthesiology and Critical Care Medicine, Aga Khan University Hospital, Nairobi, Kenya

R. Pattnaik
Department of Intensive Care Medicine, Ispat General Hospital, Rourkela, Sundargarh, Odisha, India

T. Baker
Department of Anesthesia, Intensive Care and Surgical Services, Karolinska University Hospital, Stockholm, Sweden

Department of Public Health Sciences, Karolinska Institutet, Stockholm, Sweden

M. W. Dünser (✉)
Department of Anesthesia and Intensive Care, Kepler University Hospital, Johannes Kepler University Linz, Linz, Austria

A. M. Dondorp
Mahidol–Oxford Tropical Medicine Research Unit (MORU), Faculty of Tropical Medicine, Mahidol University, Bangkok, Thailand

Nuffield Department of Clinical Medicine, Oxford Centre for Tropical Medicine and Global Health, University of Oxford, Oxford, UK

Department of Intensive Care, Academic Medical Center, Amsterdam, The Netherlands

M. J. Schultz
Mahidol–Oxford Tropical Medicine Research Unit (MORU), Faculty of Tropical Medicine, Mahidol University, Bangkok, Thailand

Department of Intensive Care, Academic Medical Center, Amsterdam, The Netherlands

© The Author(s) 2019

A. M. Dondorp et al. (eds.), *Sepsis Management in Resource-limited Settings*,
https://doi.org/10.1007/978-3-030-03143-5_7

settings for several reasons, including restrictions in human and material resources but also concerns regarding costs and safety [2, 3]. It is even possible that the efficacy and effectiveness of certain strategies differ between resource-rich and resource-limited settings. Indeed, efficacy and effectiveness could depend on the type of sepsis, and it is well known that non-bacterial sepsis is much more common in resource-limited than in resource-rich settings [3].

In this chapter, we aim to answer five practical questions regarding hemodynamic assessment and support in sepsis and septic shock in resource-limited settings. As recognition of hypoperfusion and return to normal perfusion, and detection of fluid responsiveness, could avoid under- and over-resuscitation as well as under- and overuse of vasoactive agents, (1) there is need for affordable bedside tools for tissue perfusion monitoring and (2) a better understanding of practicalities of passive leg raise tests in these settings; as costs and availability of, but also indications for, intravenous fluids could be different in resource-limited settings, (3) advises regarding the preferable type of intravenous fluid to be used during fluid resuscitation, as well as (4) amounts and timing of intravenous fluids for sepsis shock in resource-limited ICUs, are essential. Finally, seen the limited availability of vasopressors and inotropes, and the risks associated with their use, (5) recommendations on their indications, titrations, and ways of administration in settings with limited resources are highly necessary. Recommendations and suggestions are summarized in Table 7.1.

7.2 Simple Bedside Tools to Assess Tissue Perfusion

Timely detection of tissue hypoperfusion is one crucial aspect of hemodynamic assessment in patients with sepsis or septic shock. Several studies showed that capillary refill times >5 s following initial hemodynamic optimization are associated with worsening organ failures [4–6]. Normalization of capillary refill time was prognostic of survival in septic shock patients [7]. During early septic shock, capillary refill time was found to be a good predictor of short-term mortality [8] and related to perfusion of the liver, spleen, kidneys, and intestines in adults [9]. There was noticeable variation, though, in how capillary refill times were checked, at least in investigations involving children (Table 7.2), and several factors may affect the accuracy capillary refill time, like the ambient temperature and light, the site of measurement, and the amount of pressure applied to the capillary bed [10]. There was debate on whether capillary refill time is subject to interobserver variability [10, 11]. One study in India suggests capillary refill time to be insensitive to detect tissue hypoperfusion in patients with malaria [12].

Mottling, patchy skin discolorations due to heterogenic small-vessel vasoconstriction that usually start around the knees and elbows in patients with shock could also reflect abnormal skin perfusion. A simply to apply at the bedside score, using a scale from 0 (“no mottling”) to 5 (“grave mottling”) (Table 7.3 and Fig. 7.1) related

Table 7.1 Recommendations for fluid management and hemodynamic support in patients with sepsis or septic shock in resource-limited settings (with grading)

1	Simple bedside tools to assess tissue perfusion	We suggest using capillary refill time, skin mottling scores, and, if affordable, skin temperature gradients to assess adequacy of tissue perfusion in pediatric and adult sepsis and septic shock, either alone or in combination (UG). It remains uncertain whether these tools are effective in severe malaria. These tools are noninvasive and safe and come at no additional or low costs, though costs of temperature probes could still be too high for certain resource-limited settings. This recommendation remains weak, mainly because of the absence of evidence that these bedside tools can adequately guide important decisions in hemodynamic support
2	The passive leg raise test and other simple tools to replace direct measurements of cardiac output	We suggest using the passive leg raise test to guide fluid resuscitation in sepsis or septic shock in resource-limited settings (2A). It is uncertain whether the passive leg raise test has predictive values in all types of sepsis and septic shock, like in severe malaria or severe dengue. We suggest using the passive leg raise test in children but only in those above the age of 5 (2C). We recommend direct measurement of changes in cardiac output when performing a passive leg raise test (1C) and suggest using changes in pulse pressure if the former is not possible (2C)
3	Fluid strategies	We recommend crystalloid solutions as the initial fluid of choice in patients with bacterial severe sepsis or septic shock (1B) and recommend against the use of synthetic colloid solutions (1B). We recommend the same for patients with severe falciparum malaria (1B). We also recommend using crystalloids and not colloids in severe dengue with compensated shock for initial fluid resuscitation (1B), but there is insufficient evidence to recommend fluid choices in severe dengue with hypotensive shock. In order to avoid delays in initial resuscitation, it is advisable that wards carrying for patients with sepsis or septic shock stockpile crystalloid solutions for their immediate availability, to avoid delaying initial fluid resuscitation (UG)
4	Amounts and timing of IV fluids	We recommend that fluid resuscitation is initiated in patients with sepsis and suspected hypovolemia as early as possible, ideally within the first 30 min after recognition, and to start with 30 mL/kg over the first 3 h (1A). Larger amounts of fluid may be needed in patient that remains fluid responsive (e.g., according to the results of a passive leg raise test) and still shows signs of tissue hypoperfusion (e.g., according to the capillary refill time, the skin mottling score, or skin temperature gradients) (1C). We recommend being extremely cautious and thus more conservative in patients in settings with no or limited access to vasopressors and mechanical ventilation, where consideration should be given to stopping fluid administration if the patient develops signs of respiratory distress or lung crepitations on chest auscultation (1A). This also applies for fluid resuscitation in children (1A). Patients with severe malaria or severe dengue without hypotension should not receive fluid bolus therapy

(continued)

Table 7.1 (continued)

5	Vasopressors and inotropes	We recommend against the start of a vasopressor before initial fluid resuscitation, especially when a central line cannot be used (1C). We suggest starting a vasopressor in patients with persistent arterial hypotension (2C) and recommend targeting a mean arterial blood pressure ≥65 mmHg (1B). We recommend using norepinephrine (noradrenaline) as first-line vasopressor (1B) and suggest using dopamine if norepinephrine is not available (2B). The target for titration of inotropic drugs could be normalization of plasma lactate levels (<2 mmol/L) or normalization of capillary refill time (<3 s) or reduction in skin mottling (UG) if plasma lactate levels cannot be measured. We suggest using dobutamine as first-line inotrope (2B) and epinephrine (adrenaline) if dobutamine is not available (2B). We recommend administering vasopressors via a central venous line (1C) and suggest titrations of vasopressors and inotropes using a syringe or infusion pump when available (2D)

Abbreviation: *UG* ungraded

Table 7.2 Different methods of measuring and interpreting capillary refill time in children

Method	Interpretation
Apply pressure to the nail bed or other area with visible circulation; measure the length of time it takes for blanching to disappear	A capillary refill time <2 s is normal; >4 s is abnormal; a capillary refill time between 2 and 4 s should prompt further consideration of the presence of shock
The preferred location to test capillary refill time is sternum; if finger or toe is used, leg or arm must be elevated; press firmly for 5 s	A capillary refill time >5 s indicates an inadequate cardiac output
After fingertip pressure to a distal extremity, blood should refill the area within less than 2 s after release	A capillary refill time >2 s in the setting of other signs of shock indicates a compensated shock state
Press on sternum or digit at the level of the heart for 5 s	A capillary refill time > 2 s is a clinical feature of shock
Cutaneous pressure on the sternum or on a digit for 5 s	A slower refill than 2 s can indicate poor skin perfusion, a sign which may be helpful in early septic shock
Grasp the child's thumb or big toe between the finger and thumb and look at the pink of the nail bed; apply minimal pressure necessary for 3 s to produce blanching of the nail bed; time the capillary refill from the moment of release until total return of the pink color	Capillary refill time should be <3 s; if >3 s the child may have a problem with shock

Adapted and modified from Pandey et al. [37]

well to plasma lactate levels, urine output, degree of organ dysfunctions, and even mortality in patients with septic shock [13]. Patients whose mottling score decreased during the resuscitation period had a better prognosis [13]. The prognostic value of this score was confirmed in other cohorts of critically ill patients [14, 15]. The mottling score had a good reproducibility and did not suffer from interobserver variability [13].

Table 7.3 Skin mottling score after initial fluid resuscitation

Score		Description
0	No	No mottling
1	Modest	Coin size—localized to the center of the knee
2	Moderate	Mottling does not exceed the superior edge of the kneecap
3	Mild	Mottling does not exceed the middle thigh
4	Severe	Mottling does not exceed beyond the fold of the groin
5	Grave	Mottling exceeds beyond the fold of the groin

Adapted from Ait-Oufella et al. [13]

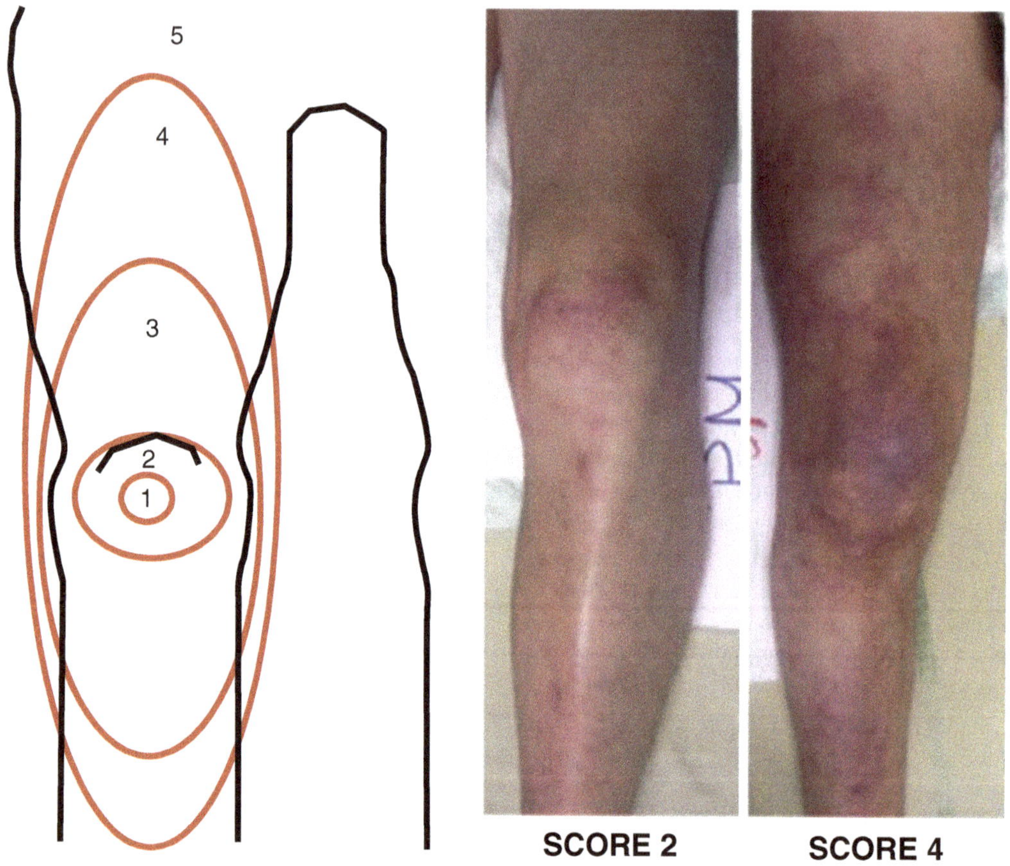

Fig. 7.1 Skin mottling score; from Ait-Oufella et al. [13]

Skin temperature gradients, the difference between two different measurement points, such as between the forearm and fingertip, or the central and toe, could be useful in detecting changes in skin perfusions in sepsis and septic shock [16, 17]. The advantage of using skin temperature gradients between the forearm and fingertip, instead of a single skin temperature, is that both spots are similarly affected by ambient temperature. The normal skin temperature gradient between forearm and fingertip is 0 °C. Skin temperature gradients between the forearm and fingertip of >4 °C were associated with severe vasoconstriction. Increased skin temperature gradient was related to the outcome of sepsis [18].

We suggest using capillary refill time, skin mottling scores, and, if affordable, skin temperature gradients to assess adequacy of tissue perfusion in pediatric and adult sepsis and septic shock, either alone or in combination (UG). It remains uncertain whether these tools are effective in malaria. These tools are noninvasive and safe and come at no additional or low costs, though costs of temperature probes could still be too high for certain resource-limited settings. This recommendation remains weak, mainly because of the absence of evidence that these bedside tools can adequately guide important decisions in hemodynamic support.

7.3 The Passive Leg Raise Test and Other Simple Tools to Replace Direct Measurements of Cardiac Output

If it is decided that a patient is hypovolemic, it should also be determined whether that patients is "fluid responsive." The method for performing passive leg raise test is important because it fundamentally affects its hemodynamic effects and reliability [19]. The test needs to be executed so that it does not result in pain and anxiety as this may influence the results. Furthermore, a proper passive leg raise test consists lifting the bed at the foot end and not lifting the legs (Fig. 7.2). The latter could be a challenge in resource-limited settings where beds are usually not easy adjustable. While it is best to use a direct measure of cardiac output or stroke volume, this is frequently impossible in settings where resources are low. A less accurate but still acceptable approach is to detect changes in pulse pressure. The test then starts with an initial (noninvasive) blood pressure measurement—after 60–90 s of passively raising the legs, the blood pressure measurement is repeated—and a change in the difference between systolic and diastolic pressure >15% could indicate that the patient is "fluid responsive" [20].

It remains uncertain whether the passive leg raise test has comparable predictive values in various types of sepsis and septic shock, e.g., in severe malaria or severe dengue, as literature is lacking. This could actually be seen as one major objection against widespread use of passive leg raise tests in resource-limited settings. This is also true for young children. So far, only one preliminary study suggests that a

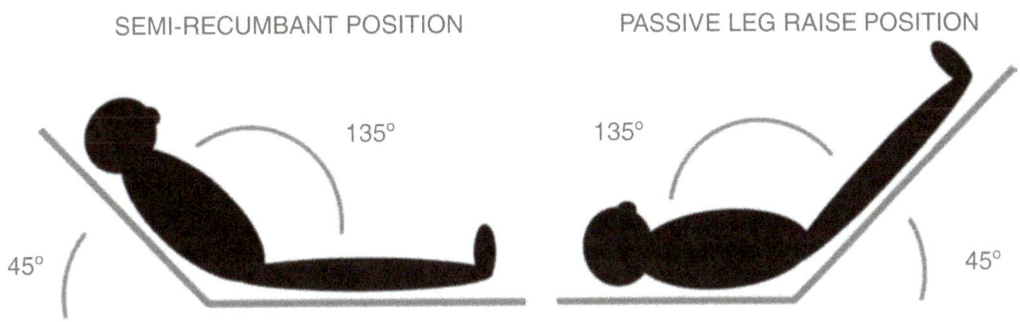

Fig. 7.2 For maximal reliability, a passive leg raise test should be performed following some rules. One possible variation of test starts from the semi-recumbent position. The second step comprises to go down the trunk and raise legs maintaining the angle between them using the automatic motion of the bed for avoiding artifacts. Finally the third step goes back to the semi-recumbent position to ensure that the subject recovers the previous hemodynamic parameters

passive leg raise test is helpful in predicting fluid responsiveness in children but not in those under 5 years of age [21].

We *suggest* using the passive leg raise test to guide fluid resuscitation in sepsis or septic shock in resource-limited settings (2A). It is uncertain whether the passive leg raise test has predictive values in all types of sepsis and septic shock, like in severe malaria or severe dengue. We *suggest* using the passive leg raise test and in children but only in those above the age of 5 (2C). We *recommend* direct measurement of changes in cardiac output when performing a passive leg raise test (1C) and *suggest* using changes in pulse pressure if the former is not possible (2C).

7.4 Fluid Strategies

There is a large body of literature from resource-rich settings on the choice of fluids in severe sepsis and septic shock, with a strong focus on sepsis caused by bacterial pathogens. The theoretical benefits of colloid solutions over crystalloids, with better retention in the intravascular compartment, have not translated to better outcomes with colloids for the treatment of severe sepsis of septic shock in randomized clinical trials performed in resource-rich settings. In addition, synthetic colloid solutions have shown important adverse effects, in particular nephrotoxicity with the use of starch solutions. Consequently, the Surviving Sepsis Campaign makes a strong recommendation for the use of crystalloid solutions over colloids for fluid resuscitation [1].

The "Fluid Expansion as Supportive Therapy" trial in children in sub-Saharan Africa with compensated septic shock, of which 57% had severe falciparum malaria, showed a detrimental effect of saline bolus as well as albumin bolus therapy compared to a more conservative fluid therapy [22]. The study supersedes earlier small studies suggesting a survival benefit of albumin infusion over crystalloids in children with severe falciparum malaria and severe sepsis [23, 24].

Three randomized trials in patients with dengue shock syndrome did not show better outcome parameters with (more expensive) colloids over crystalloid fluids [25–27]. A quasi-randomized study from the Philippines alternating allocation of colloids with crystalloids also did not show an additional benefit of colloids [28].

From the task force members' experience, it is important that in wards caring for critically ill patients, intravenous fluids are stockpiled so that they are immediately available for emergency treatment, to save time and to prevent incurring additional costs for the patient's family.

We *recommend* crystalloid solutions as the initial fluid of choice in patients with bacterial severe sepsis or septic shock (1B) and *recommend* against the use of synthetic colloid solutions (1B). We *recommend* the same for patients with severe falciparum malaria (1B). We also *recommend* using crystalloids and not colloids in severe dengue with compensated shock for initial fluid resuscitation (1B), but there is insufficient evidence to recommend fluid choices in severe dengue with hypotensive shock. In order to avoid delays in initial resuscitation, it is advisable that wards carrying for patients with sepsis or septic shock stockpile crystalloid solutions for their immediate availability, to avoid delaying initial fluid resuscitation (UG).

7.5 Amounts and Timing of IV Fluids

A landmark study from an emergency department in a resource-rich setting found that so-called early goal-directed therapy, in which intravenous fluids were given to swiftly have physiological parameters return to pre-defined levels, reduced mortality by as much as a third [29]. Early goal-directed therapy has since become mainstream practice in the treatment of critically ill patients. The Surviving Sepsis Campaign recommends that, in the resuscitation from sepsis-induced hypoperfusion, at least 30 ml/kg of intravenous crystalloid fluid be given within the first 3 h [1].

The largest fluid trial performed in resource-limited settings is the above-cited FEAST trial in children [22]. This trial showed an alarming increase in mortality with bolus intravenous infusion in critically ill children. There is an ongoing debate whether mortality increased because of development of pulmonary fluid overload, which could not be compensated for by mechanical ventilation; a secondary analysis of FEAST exploring whether boluses may have caused excess deaths from fluid overload actually suggested cardiovascular collapse rather than fluid overload appeared to contribute most to excess deaths with rapid fluid resuscitation [30]. Nevertheless, similar alarming findings come from several studies in adult patients in resource-limited settings [31–34]. The most recent trial clearly showed a protocol for early resuscitation with administration of intravenous fluids and vasopressors to increase mortality [34]. The absolute or relative absence of vasopressors and maybe mechanical ventilation could make fluid loading too dangerous.

We *recommend* that fluid resuscitation is initiated in patients with sepsis and suspected hypovolemia as early as possible, ideally within the first 30 min after recognition, and to start with 30 ml/kg over the first 3 h (1A). Larger amounts of fluid may be needed in patient that remains fluid responsive (e.g., according to the results of a passive leg raise test) and still shows signs of tissue hypoperfusion (e.g., according to the capillary refill time, the skin mottling score, or skin temperature gradients) (1C). We *recommend* being extremely cautious and thus more conservative in patients in settings with no or limited access to vasopressors and mechanical ventilation, where consideration should be given to stopping fluid administration if the patient develops signs of respiratory distress or lung crepitations on chest auscultation (1A). This also applies for fluid resuscitation in children (1A). Patients with severe malaria or severe dengue without hypotension should not receive fluid bolus therapy (see Chap. 9).

7.6 Vasopressors and Inotropes

The Surviving Sepsis Campaign recommends norepinephrine as the first-choice vasopressor and adding epinephrine to norepinephrine with the intent of raising MAP to target, to decrease norepinephrine dosage. The Surviving Sepsis Campaign also suggests using dopamine as an alternative vasopressor only in selected patients and using dobutamine in patients who show evidence of persistent hypoperfusion despite adequate fluid loading and the use of vasopressors [1].

Extravasation of vasopressors causes skin necrosis, and extravasation is more likely with administration through a peripheral infusion line compared to central venous administration. Central venous catheters, however, are frequently not available, expensive, and inserted too late and frequently require extra payments by family members of the patient further delaying its use. Administration of vasopressors is thus frequently done through a peripheral line. We consider it reasonable to await the effect of initial fluid resuscitation before starting infusion of vasopressors through a peripheral infusion line, but in patients with extreme low blood pressure, and in those not immediately responding to initial fluid loading, it could be necessary to continue without a central venous catheter. Additional advantages of a central venous line are that it can also be used for repeated blood sampling, measurement of static hemodynamic measures, and where possible follow-up of central venous oxygenation.

Vasopressors and inotropes have a narrow therapeutic window, necessitating accurate dosing. Continuous administration at exact doses is safeguarded preferably by automatic infusion with a syringe or infusion pump. Although less accurate, when syringe pumps are not available, these drugs can be diluted in normal saline and administered using a mechanical drop counter.

Norepinephrine is not generally available in hospitals with limited resources. Dopamine is more widely available, but reported best access in resource-limited settings is to epinephrine. We prefer dopamine to epinephrine as the latter may cause lactate acidosis [35, 36]. In resource-limited settings, dobutamine is only available in selected regions, and stockouts of the drug are very common.

Titration of inotropes in resource-limited ICUs is a challenge, as assessed by means of plasma lactate levels is expensive and frequently not possible. Capillary refill time (<3 s) and the skin mottling score can be used to evaluate the effect of infusion of vasopressors and inotropes, but there is no documented evidence regarding efficacy or safety. Of note, vasopressors can affect capillary refill time and skin mottling scores.

We *recommend* against the start of a vasopressor before initial fluid resuscitation, especially when a central line cannot be used (1C). We *suggest* starting a vasopressor in patients with persistent arterial hypotension (2C) and *recommend* targeting a mean arterial blood pressure ≥65 mmHg (1B). We *recommend* using norepinephrine (noradrenaline) as first-line vasopressor (1B) and *suggest* using dopamine if norepinephrine is not available (2B). The target for titration of inotropic drugs could be normalization of plasma lactate levels (<2 mmol/L) or normalization of capillary refill time (<3 s) or reduction in skin mottling (UG) if plasma lactate levels cannot be measured. We *suggest* using dobutamine as first-line inotrope (2B) and epinephrine (adrenaline) if dobutamine is not available (2B). We *recommend* administering vasopressors via a central venous line (1C) and *suggest* titrations of vasopressors and inotropes using a syringe or infusion pump when available (2D).

7.7 Conclusions

The paucity of evidence from resource-limited settings and in specific types of sepsis and septic shock underscores the urgent need for rigorous trials, since efficacy and effectiveness of commonly used interventions in resource-rich settings could differ importantly in resource-limited settings.

References

1. Rhodes A, Evans LE, Alhazzani W, Levy MM, Antonelli M, Ferrer R, Kumar A, Sevransky JE, Sprung CL, Nunnally ME, Rochwerg B, Rubenfeld GD, Angus DC, Annane D, Beale RJ, Bellinghan GJ, Bernard GR, Chiche JD, Coopersmith C, De Backer DP, French CJ, Fujishima S, Gerlach H, Hidalgo JL, Hollenberg SM, Jones AE, Karnad DR, Kleinpell RM, Koh Y, Lisboa TC, Machado FR, Marini JJ, Marshall JC, Mazuski JE, McIntyre LA, McLean AS, Mehta S, Moreno RP, Myburgh J, Navalesi P, Nishida O, Osborn TM, Perner A, Plunkett CM, Ranieri M, Schorr CA, Seckel MA, Seymour CW, Shieh L, Shukri KA, Simpson SQ, Singer M, Thompson BT, Townsend SR, Van der Poll T, Vincent JL, Wiersinga WJ, Zimmerman JL, Dellinger RP. Surviving Sepsis Campaign: International Guidelines for Management of Sepsis and Septic Shock: 2016. Crit Care Med. 2017;45:486–552.
2. Arabi YM, Schultz MJ, Salluh JIF. Intensive Care Medicine in 2050: global perspectives. Intensive Care Med. 2017;43:1695–9.
3. Schultz MJ, Dunser MW, Dondorp AM, Adhikari NK, Iyer S, Kwizera A, Lubell Y, Papali A, Pisani L, Riviello BD, Angus DC, Azevedo LC, Baker T, Diaz JV, Festic E, Haniffa R, Jawa R, Jacob ST, Kissoon N, Lodha R, Martin-Loeches I, Lundeg G, Misango D, Mer M, Mohanty S, Murthy S, Musa N, Nakibuuka J, Serpa Neto A, Nguyen Thi Hoang M, Nguyen Thien B, Pattnaik R, Phua J, Preller J, Povoa P, Ranjit S, Talmor D, Thevanayagam J, Thwaites CL, Global Intensive Care Working Group of the European Society of Intensive Care Medicine. Current challenges in the management of sepsis in ICUs in resource-poor settings and suggestions for the future. Intensive Care Med. 2017;43:612–24.
4. Hernandez G, Pedreros C, Veas E, Bruhn A, Romero C, Rovegno M, Neira R, Bravo S, Castro R, Kattan E, Ince C. Evolution of peripheral vs metabolic perfusion parameters during septic shock resuscitation. A clinical-physiologic study. J Crit Care. 2012;27:283–8.
5. Lima A, Jansen TC, van Bommel J, Ince C, Bakker J. The prognostic value of the subjective assessment of peripheral perfusion in critically ill patients. Crit Care Med. 2009;37:934–8.
6. van Genderen ME, Lima A, Akkerhuis M, Bakker J, van Bommel J. Persistent peripheral and microcirculatory perfusion alterations after out-of-hospital cardiac arrest are associated with poor survival. Crit Care Med. 2012;40:2287–94.
7. Hernandez G, Luengo C, Bruhn A, Kattan E, Friedman G, Ospina-Tascon GA, Fuentealba A, Castro R, Regueira T, Romero C, Ince C, Bakker J. When to stop septic shock resuscitation: clues from a dynamic perfusion monitoring. Ann Intensive Care. 2014;4:30.
8. Ait-Oufella H, Bige N, Boelle PY, Pichereau C, Alves M, Bertinchamp R, Baudel JL, Galbois A, Maury E, Guidet B. Capillary refill time exploration during septic shock. Intensive Care Med. 2014;40:958–64.
9. Brunauer A, Kokofer A, Bataar O, Gradwohl-Matis I, Dankl D, Bakker J, Dunser MW. Changes in peripheral perfusion relate to visceral organ perfusion in early septic shock: a pilot study. J Crit Care. 2016;35:105–9.
10. King D, Morton R, Bevan C. How to use capillary refill time. Arch Dis Child Educ Pract Ed. 2014;99:111–6.
11. Postelnicu R, Evans L. Monitoring of the physical exam in sepsis. Curr Opin Crit Care. 2017;23:232–6.

12. Hanson J, Lam SW, Alam S, Pattnaik R, Mahanta KC, Uddin Hasan M, Mohanty S, Mishra S, Cohen S, Day N, White N, Dondorp A. The reliability of the physical examination to guide fluid therapy in adults with severe falciparum malaria: an observational study. Malar J. 2013;12:348.
13. Ait-Oufella H, Lemoinne S, Boelle PY, Galbois A, Baudel JL, Lemant J, Joffre J, Margetis D, Guidet B, Maury E, Offenstadt G. Mottling score predicts survival in septic shock. Intensive Care Med. 2011;37:801–7.
14. Ait-Oufella H, Joffre J, Boelle PY, Galbois A, Bourcier S, Baudel JL, Margetis D, Alves M, Offenstadt G, Guidet B, Maury E. Knee area tissue oxygen saturation is predictive of 14-day mortality in septic shock. Intensive Care Med. 2012;38:976–83.
15. Coudroy R, Jamet A, Frat JP, Veinstein A, Chatellier D, Goudet V, Cabasson S, Thille AW, Robert R. Incidence and impact of skin mottling over the knee and its duration on outcome in critically ill patients. Intensive Care Med. 2015;41:452–9.
16. Akata T, Kanna T, Yoshino J, Higashi M, Fukui K, Takahashi S. Reliability of fingertip skin-surface temperature and its related thermal measures as indices of peripheral perfusion in the clinical setting of the operating theatre. Anaesth Intensive Care. 2004;32:519–29.
17. Rubinstein EH, Sessler DI. Skin-surface temperature gradients correlate with fingertip blood flow in humans. Anesthesiology. 1990;73:541–5.
18. Thompson MJ, Ninis N, Perera R, Mayon-White R, Phillips C, Bailey L, Harnden A, Mant D, Levin M. Clinical recognition of meningococcal disease in children and adolescents. Lancet. 2006;367:397–403.
19. Monnet X, Teboul JL. Passive leg raising: five rules, not a drop of fluid! Crit Care. 2015;19:18.
20. Cherpanath TG, Hirsch A, Geerts BF, Lagrand WK, Leeflang MM, Schultz MJ, Groeneveld AB. Predicting fluid responsiveness by passive leg raising: a systematic review and meta-analysis of 23 clinical trials. Crit Care Med. 2016;44:981–91.
21. Lu GP, Yan G, Chen Y, Lu ZJ, Zhang LE, Kissoon N. The passive leg raise test to predict fluid responsiveness in children—preliminary observations. Indian J Pediatr. 2015;82:5–12.
22. Maitland K, Kiguli S, Opoka RO, Engoru C, Olupot-Olupot P, Akech SO, Nyeko R, Mtove G, Reyburn H, Lang T, Brent B, Evans JA, Tibenderana JK, Crawley J, Russell EC, Levin M, Babiker AG, Gibb DM, Group FT. Mortality after fluid bolus in African children with severe infection. N Engl J Med. 2011;364:2483–95.
23. Maitland K, Pamba A, English M, Peshu N, Marsh K, Newton C, Levin M. Randomized trial of volume expansion with albumin or saline in children with severe malaria: preliminary evidence of albumin benefit. Clin Infect Dis. 2005;40:538–45.
24. Akech S, Ledermann H, Maitland K. Choice of fluids for resuscitation in children with severe infection and shock: systematic review. BMJ. 2010;341:c4416.
25. Wills BA, Nguyen MD, Ha TL, Dong TH, Tran TN, Le TT, Tran VD, Nguyen TH, Nguyen VC, Stepniewska K, White NJ, Farrar JJ. Comparison of three fluid solutions for resuscitation in dengue shock syndrome. N Engl J Med. 2005;353:877–89.
26. Dung NM, Day NP, Tam DT, Loan HT, Chau HT, Minh LN, Diet TV, Bethell DB, Kneen R, Hien TT, White NJ, Farrar JJ. Fluid replacement in dengue shock syndrome: a randomized, double-blind comparison of four intravenous-fluid regimens. Clin Infect Dis. 1999;29:787–94.
27. Ngo NT, Cao XT, Kneen R, Wills B, Nguyen VM, Nguyen TQ, Chu VT, Nguyen TT, Simpson JA, Solomon T, White NJ, Farrar J. Acute management of dengue shock syndrome: a randomized double-blind comparison of 4 intravenous fluid regimens in the first hour. Clin Infect Dis. 2001;32:204–13.
28. Cifra HL, Velasco JN. A comparative study of the efficacy of 6%. Haes-Steril and Ringer's lactate in the management of dengue shock syndrome 555. Crit Care Shock. 2003;6:95–100.
29. Rivers E, Nguyen B, Havstad S, Ressler J, Muzzin A, Knoblich B, Peterson E, Tomlanovich M, Early Goal-Directed Therapy Collaborative Group. Early goal-directed therapy in the treatment of severe sepsis and septic shock. N Engl J Med. 2001;345:1368–77.
30. Maitland K, George EC, Evans JA, Kiguli S, Olupot-Olupot P, Akech SO, Opoka RO, Engoru C, Nyeko R, Mtove G, Reyburn H, Brent B, Nteziyaremye J, Mpoya A, Prevatt N, Dambisya CM, Semakula D, Ddungu A, Okuuny V, Wokulira R, Timbwa M, Otii B, Levin M, Crawley J,

Babiker AG, Gibb DM. Exploring mechanisms of excess mortality with early fluid resuscitation: insights from the FEAST trial. BMC Med. 2013;11:68.
31. Andrews B, Muchemwa L, Kelly P, Lakhi S, Heimburger DC, Bernard GR. Simplified severe sepsis protocol: a randomized controlled trial of modified early goal-directed therapy in Zambia. Crit Care Med. 2014;42:2315–24.
32. Baker T, Schell CO, Lugazia E, Blixt J, Mulungu M, Castegren M, Eriksen J, Konrad D. Vital signs directed therapy: improving care in an intensive care unit in a low-income country. PLoS One. 2015;10:e0144801.
33. Jacob ST, Banura P, Baeten JM, Moore CC, Meya D, Nakiyingi L, Burke R, Horton CL, Iga B, Wald A, Reynolds SJ, Mayanja-Kizza H, Scheld WM, Promoting Resource-Limited Interventions for Sepsis Management in Uganda Study Group. The impact of early monitored management on survival in hospitalized adult Ugandan patients with severe sepsis: a prospective intervention study. Crit Care Med. 2012;40:2050–8.
34. Andrews B, Semler MW, Muchemwa L, Kelly P, Lakhi S, Heimburger DC, Mabula C, Bwalya M, Bernard GR. Effect of an early resuscitation protocol on in-hospital mortality among adults with sepsis and hypotension: a randomized clinical trial. JAMA. 2017;318:1233–40.
35. Day NP, Phu NH, Bethell DP, Mai NT, Chau TT, Hien TT, White NJ. The effects of dopamine and adrenaline infusions on acid-base balance and systemic haemodynamics in severe infection. Lancet. 1996;348:219–23.
36. Mahmoud KM, Ammar AS. Norepinephrine supplemented with dobutamine or epinephrine for the cardiovascular support of patients with septic shock. Indian J Crit Care Med. 2012;16:75–80.
37. Pandey A, John BM. Capillary refill time. Is it time to fill the gaps? Med J Armed Forces India. 2013;69:97–8.

Open Access This chapter is licensed under the terms of the Creative Commons Attribution 4.0 International License (http://creativecommons.org/licenses/by/4.0/), which permits use, sharing, adaptation, distribution and reproduction in any medium or format, as long as you give appropriate credit to the original author(s) and the source, provide a link to the Creative Commons license and indicate if changes were made.

The images or other third party material in this chapter are included in the chapter's Creative Commons license, unless indicated otherwise in a credit line to the material. If material is not included in the chapter's Creative Commons license and your intended use is not permitted by statutory regulation or exceeds the permitted use, you will need to obtain permission directly from the copyright holder.

Infection Management in Patients with Sepsis and Septic Shock in Resource-Limited Settings

8

C. Louise Thwaites, Ganbold Lundeg, Arjen M. Dondorp, Neill K. J. Adhikari, Jane Nakibuuka, Randeep Jawa, Mervyn Mer, Srinivas Murthy, Marcus J. Schultz, Binh Nguyen Thien, and Arthur Kwizera

C. L. Thwaites (✉)
Oxford University Clinical Research Unit, Hospital for Tropical Diseases, Ho Chi Minh City, Vietnam

Nuffield Department of Clinical Medicine, Oxford Centre for Tropical Medicine and Global Health, Oxford, UK
e-mail: lthwaites@oucru.org

G. Lundeg
Department of Critical Care Medicine, Mongolian National University of Medical Sciences, Ulaanbaatar, Mongolia

A. M. Dondorp · M. J. Schultz
Mahidol-Oxford Tropical Medicine Research Unit (MORU), Faculty of Tropical Medicine, Mahidol University, Bangkok, Thailand

Department of Intensive Care, Academic Medical Center, University of Amsterdam, Amsterdam, The Netherlands

N. K. J. Adhikari
Department of Intensive Care, Sunnybrook Health Sciences Centre, University of Toronto, Toronto, Canada

J. Nakibuuka
Department of Intensive Care, Mulago National Referral and University Teaching Hospital, Kampala, Uganda

R. Jawa
Department of Intensive Care, Stony Brook University Medical Center, Stony Brook, NY, USA

M. Mer
Department of Intensive Care, Johannesburg Hospital, University of the Witwatersrand, Johannesburg, South Africa

S. Murthy
Department of Intensive Care, BC Children's Hospital, University of British Columbia, Vancouver, Canada

© The Author(s) 2019
A. M. Dondorp et al. (eds.), *Sepsis Management in Resource-limited Settings*,
https://doi.org/10.1007/978-3-030-03143-5_8

B. N. Thien
Department of Intensive Care, Trung Vuong Hospital, Ho Chi Minh City, Viet Nam

A. Kwizera
Department of Anesthesia and Intensive Care, Mulago National Referral Hospital, Kampala, Uganda

8.1 Introduction and Definitions

Although there are only limited data available, studies indicate that sepsis and septic shock in resource-limited settings are at least as common as in resource-rich settings. There are important differences in the causative pathogens of sepsis and septic shock between resource-rich and resource-limited settings. Staffing, diagnostic facilities, therapeutic options, and other factors also differ in resource-limited settings, which makes that the Surviving Sepsis Campaign (SSC) guidelines on sepsis management derived from high-income settings are not necessarily directly applicable to these settings [1]. In this chapter, SSC recommendations that were deemed warranting additional evaluation for their use in resource-limited settings were reviewed specifically relevant evidence generated in resource-limited settings. During this exercise the European Society of Intensive Care Medicine's and the Society of Critical Care Medicine's Consensus Definitions for Sepsis and Septic Shock (Sepsis-3) were published [2]. For the purposes of this article, where published studies have used former definitions of severe sepsis and septic shock to characterize patients, these have been left as originally published. For further clarification, we refer readers to the SSC guidelines and the article in this series examining sepsis recognition [3, 4]. Resource-limited settings were defined as those within low- or middle-income countries according to the World Bank [5] or described as "resource-limited" or "developing countries" by authors of the referenced studies. A flowchart summarizing the approach to the management of patients with sepsis or septic shock in resource-limited setting is provided in Fig. 8.1.

8.2 Factors Guiding the Choice of Empiric Antibiotic Choice in Sepsis and Septic Shock in Resource-Limited Settings

Hospital- and especially ICU-related infections are more likely to be caused by multidrug-resistant organisms, and previous antibiotic use is a risk factor for antibiotic resistance. Misdirected initial antibiotic therapy is associated with poor outcome [6, 7], but there is a paucity of epidemiological data in most resource-limited settings. The aim of empirical antibiotic therapy is to treat the causative pathogen in the septic patient before definitive microbiological results are available. General principles guiding the choice of initial empirical antibiotic therapy apply to both resource-rich and resource-limited settings [8, 9] and should take into consideration the pathogens and resistance patterns most likely to be encountered. This will depend on the suspected site and focus of the infection as well as healthcare setting

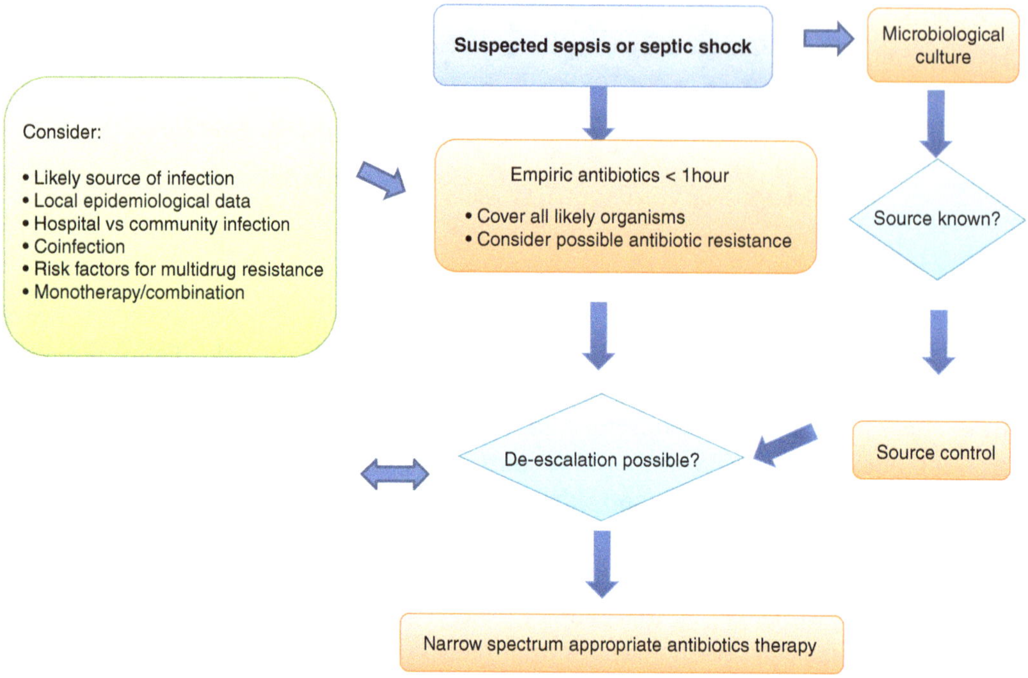

Fig. 8.1 Flowchart showing infection management in patients with sepsis or septic shock in resource-limited setting

and geographical location. Increasing evidence in both resource-rich settings and resource-limited settings shows that inappropriate initial antibiotics are associated with worse outcome [10].

Specific issues to consider in resource-limited settings include the different causative microorganisms in these often tropical countries, sparse epidemiological data because of limited microbiological laboratory capacity, and a greater degree of antimicrobial resistance, driven by poor stewardship especially in the private health and agricultural sectors. In some settings the range of available antibiotics may be reduced, and, compared to resource-rich settings, cost of treatment plays a larger role in the choice of the empirical drug as antibiotic costs are often disproportionately high compared to other therapies [11].

We found only three studies from resource-limited settings that specifically examined the causative organisms of severe sepsis and septic shock (using previous SSC definitions [12]) [9, 13, 14]. We therefore included other studies describing causes of sepsis in resource-limited settings, which were thought representative of potential pathogens encountered. The collected evidence is presented below.

8.2.1 Bacterial Pathogens

A retrospective study from a tertiary referral hospital in Turkey described pathogens and likely sources of infection from all cases of sepsis, including patients with severe sepsis and septic shock, between 2002 and 2003. Gram-negative bacteria, particularly *Klebsiella* spp. and *Escherichia coli*, were the most commonly isolated organisms from blood cultures (27 out of 41 isolates) and *E. coli* from urine culture (14 out of 63 samples). The respiratory tract was most frequently identified as the likely source of sepsis [9]. Similar results were reported from a prospective study of severe sepsis and septic shock in ICU patients in Thailand conducted between 2004 and 2006. Out of 390 patients, 241 patients had microorganisms isolated from any site, and 106 had positive blood cultures [14]. The main pathogens were *Klebsiella pneumoniae* (19.9%) and *E. coli* (14%). Again, the respiratory tract was the most common source of infection. In surgical ICUs in China, 381 cases of severe sepsis and septic shock in 10 units across 6 provinces were studied prospectively between 2004 and 2005. The majority (53.8%) of cases were caused by Gram-negative bacteria, but in a significant proportion of cases (28.3%), fungi were isolated. In this series, the commonest organisms isolated were *Acinetobacter baumannii* and *Candida albicans*, with the abdomen being the most frequent site of infection [13].

In addition to these studies, several other authors have reported the causes of bacteremia in resource-limited settings. Causative organisms varied according to location and between environments. Compared to many high-income settings, Gram-negative organisms were identified as particularly important causes of community-acquired bacteremia with distinct geographical differences, for example, non-typhoid *Salmonella* in sub-Saharan Africa, *Salmonellae typhi* and *paratyphi* in South and Southeast Asia, and *Burkholderia pseudomallei* in Southeast Asia [14–16]. The Gram-positive *Streptococcus suis* was reported to be a relatively common cause of sepsis in Southeast Asia [17].

A meta-analysis of community-acquired bloodstream infections across Africa involving 58,296 patients showed that in non-malarial bloodstream infections, the commonest isolate was *Salmonella enterica* (mainly non-typhoidal species), although among the five studies in adults that used mycobacterial culture techniques, *Mycobacterium tuberculosis* was the commonest pathogen isolated, in 33.8% of isolates.

Coexisting infection is an important factor in resource-limited settings. In the study above, HIV prevalence was 24% and was associated with increased likelihood of *M. tuberculosis* or non-typhoidal *Salmonella* bloodstream infection (OR 23.4 and 8.2, respectively) [15]. Malaria predisposes infected individuals to invasive bacterial infection, and in areas with high-malarial burden, it is a significant risk factor for bacteremia. In a case-control study of childhood bacteremia in Kenya, underlying malaria occurred in 62% of cases of bacteremia [18]. Secondary invasive bacterial infection is also a common complication of late-stage visceral leishmaniasis but is also associated with geographical variation. In one series of sepsis associated with visceral leishmaniasis in Ethiopia, 69% of cases were due to *Staphylococcus aureus* in contrast to elsewhere in Africa where Gram-negative bacteria were more commonly reported [15, 19].

The distinction between community- and healthcare-associated infection is, as expected, also an important determinant of the predicted causative organism. In the study from Turkey described above [9], blood culture isolates from community-acquired infection were more likely to be Gram-positive organisms (56% cases), whereas Gram-negative organisms accounted for 80% of cases of hospital-acquired isolates. In a study of bloodstream infections in South Africa [20], non-fermenting Gram-negative bacteria and *Enterobacteriaceae* were the most commonly isolated organisms from hospital-acquired bloodstream infections, whereas Gram-positive bacteria were most common in community-associated infections. Within the health-care environment, *A. baumannii* was almost exclusively associated with ICU infection, but *S. aureus*, *E. coli*, and *K. pneumoniae* were associated with infections from other healthcare settings. Similar differences were shown in the prospective studies in Thailand and China described above [13, 14].

8.2.2 Antimicrobial Resistance

In a review of 83 studies examining antibiotic susceptibility of bacteria causing infections in sub-Saharan Africa and Asia, the authors concluded that only limited data were available to guide antibiotic treatment which show considerable variation in resistance patterns, both regionally and locally [21].

In the study from South Africa, described above, all community isolates of *S. aureus* were cloxacillin-sensitive compared to only 52% of hospital isolates. Increased antibiotic resistance was also noted in hospital isolates of *Enterobacteriaceae* compared to community isolates. Similarly, in 98 patients with *S. aureus* bloodstream infections in Thailand, community isolates were all methicillin-sensitive. Methicillin-resistant *S. aureus* (MRSA) was only associated with hospital-associated infection, particularly in ICU [22]. However, in a different series of Thai ICU patients with severe sepsis and septic shock due to respiratory infection, 22% community-acquired *S. aureus* infections were found to be methicillin-resistant [14]. Across 55 ICUs in 8 developing settings, 84% of *S. aureus* intravascular device-associated nosocomial infections were due to MRSA [23]. In a review of *S. aureus* epidemiology across Asia, hospital-acquired MRSA rates in general clinical samples collected between 1993 and 2011 were usually in excess of 20% (Vietnam, Thailand, Indonesia, Malaysia, China) and in some instances over 80% (India, Sri Lanka) [24]. In samples from community-acquired infection, MRSA rates were also variable, ranging from 3.2% (Malaysia 2009) to 39% (Sri Lanka 2004–2006) [24]. Most studies were laboratory-based surveillance studies lacking clinical data, and many of the community isolates were from superficial skin infections; thus, the relationship to organisms causing sepsis and septic shock was not clear.

Levels of Gram-negative bacterial resistance in resource-limited settings are often high and increasing, particularly in Asia, but there remain significant geographical variations [25, 26]. Extended-spectrum beta-lactamase (ESBL)-producing *E. coli* were reported in 9% of *E. coli* isolates from blood cultures in Laos between 2004 and 2009 [27]. In Cambodia between 2007 and 2010, ESBL rates were 49% in *Enterobacteriaceae* causing bloodstream infections in adults (mostly *E. coli*) [28]. 2008 data showed rates of ESBL-producing bacteria causing significant abdominal infections to be 2.9% in Malaysia compared to 59% and 61% in China and India, respectively [25]. More recently, nosocomial-acquired ESBL rates above 80% in India and more than 60% in China have been reported [29]. Between 2011 and 2012,

51.6% of ICU patients with bacterial sepsis in Mongolia were infected by at least one resistant bacterium, the majority of which were Gram-negative organisms [30].

In Asia and the Middle East, increased carbapenem use due to high-ESBL rates has resulted in the appearance of carbapenem resistance. While community-acquired infection data are limited, data from hospitals show that carbapenem-resistant organisms causing hospital-acquired infection are an increasing concern. In Asia *K. pneumoniae* carbapenemase (KPC)-related resistance was first noted in China in 2004. New Delhi metallo-β-lactamase-1 (NDM-1)-associated resistance was first reported in 2008 in a patient initially treated in India [26]. In India data indicate that 5–8% of hospital-related *Enterobacteriaceae* infections are carbapenem-resistant organisms [31]. In one neonatal intensive care unit in Pakistan, rates of imipenem-resistant *K. pneumoniae* causing late-onset sepsis increased from 0% to 72% of isolates over a 2-year period between 2009 and 2011 [32].

The situation in Africa has been described in a recent systematic review [33]. This describes a recent rapid emergence of carbapenem resistance throughout the region, although data are more limited. Of note is that even in countries without access to carbapenems, resistance has still emerged due to use of other antibiotic classes, as shown by the emergence of OXA-23 carbapenemase-resistant *A. baumannii* in Madagascar [34].

Several authors examined risk factors for antimicrobial resistance in resource-limited settings. A study of patients with *Klebsiella* spp. and *E. coli* bloodstream infections in India identified previous antibiotic use and transfer from other healthcare settings as risk factors for ESBL production [35]. In patients with febrile neutropenia in Lebanon, previous broad-spectrum antibiotic use was a risk factor for bacteremia with multidrug-resistant organisms [36]. Previous use of carbapenems was found to be the sole risk factor for adult patients with pan-resistant *Pseudomonas aeruginosa* bacteremia in Brazil [37].

8.2.3 Appropriateness of Antibiotic Choices

Two studies [6, 7] assessed the impact of inappropriate antibiotic use on outcome. In a single-center study in Brazil [6], prescription of appropriate empiric antibiotics was associated with survival benefit (odds ratio (OR) for death = 0.536 (95%) confidence interval [0.314–0.916]; $p = 0.023$). In a study of nosocomial infections in Thailand comparing combination therapy to monotherapy, combination therapy was more successful, in part due to increasing the chances of the bacteria being susceptible to the antibiotics [7].

8.2.4 Costs

Since antibiotic therapy is usually paid out of pocket by the patient or their relatives, cost is an important factor guiding antibiotic choice. For many antibiotics, generic products are available at a much lower price; however, the quality of these drugs is not always guaranteed [38]. In a study in India where ciprofloxacin, artesunate, and rifampicin were purchased from 100 different outlets, 43% samples fell below the 90% of stated content [39]. A review of published and unpublished studies of antimalarial drugs across sites in Southeast Asia and Africa showed 35% of samples failed chemical analysis [40]. In a systematic review of 66 studies of substandard pharmaceuticals (mainly antibiotics) conducted in Africa and Southeast Asia, 91% of studies found products to be substandard, and 44% showed evidence of counterfeiting [38].

8.2.5 Availability, Feasibility, Affordability, and Safety

There are significant differences in likely pathogenic organisms in resource-limited settings compared to resource-rich settings but also a high degree of variation between and within resource-limited settings. Hospital- and particularly ICU-related infections are more likely to be caused by multidrug-resistant organisms, and previous antibiotic use is a significant risk factor for resistance. Inappropriate antibiotic treatment is associated with worse outcome.

Ideally local epidemiological data should be used when choosing empiric therapy as large variations exist within regions. Establishment of well-chosen sentinel sites for monitoring of prevailing pathogens and their resistance patterns is suggested. The choice of empiric treatment is evidently dependent on the common causative pathogens and the resistance patterns of that area or hospital. Examples for community-acquired infections include Northeast Thailand, where 20% of sepsis is caused by *B. pseudomallei*, and therefore ceftazidime or a carbapenem should be included. In areas in Asia where scrub typhus is a common cause of severe fever and sepsis, doxycycline should be added to the empirical antibiotic regimen. Local resistance patterns should inform whether in areas with a high incidence of *S. typhi* bacteremia, fluoroquinolones are still usable. For hospital-acquired infections, examples include the current concerning spread beyond India of carbapenemase-producing Gram-negative bacteria. A policy used in some hospitals is to avoid carbapenems as empirical treatment when prevalence increases above 20% of Gram-negative bacteria. However, in most resource-limited settings, there is limited microbiological data to guide therapy, and the microbiological laboratory capacity of most resource-limited settings is unlikely to improve soon.

Based on the presented evidence, the following recommendations were derived. As poor outcome is associated with inappropriate initial antibiotic therapy, we *recommend* that empirical antibiotic therapy should cover all expected pathogens and likely resistance patterns (1C) based on locally acquired epidemiological data, as large regional variations exist (ungraded). We recognize that in settings with a limited range of antibiotics, this may be challenging. We *suggest* that research groups in collaboration with stakeholders provide microbiological data from sentinel sites throughout resource-limited settings to guide empirical antibiotic treatment (ungraded) (Table 8.1).

Table 8.1 Recommendations and suggestions on infection control in patients with sepsis or septic shock in resource-limited settings

1. Choice of empiric therapy As poor outcome is associated with inappropriate antibiotic therapy, empirical therapy should aim to cover all expected pathogens and likely resistance patterns (1C). We suggested that research groups in close collaboration with stakeholders provide microbiological data from sentinel sites throughout LMICs to guide empirical antibiotic treatment (ungraded)	
2. Timing of antibiotics	We recommend that appropriate antibiotics should be given within the first hour in severe sepsis and septic shock (1C)
3. Taking blood cultures	We recommend that blood cultures should be taken before the administration of antibiotics (1B). It is realized that in many hospitals in resource-limited countries, routine blood culture in sepsis is not feasible
4. Source control	We suggest source control is carried out within 12 h of admission to hospital except in the specific case of pancreatic necrosis (ungraded). Radiography and ultrasound are good first-line imaging techniques. If an intravascular device is suspected, this should be removed (ungraded)
5. Combination antibiotics	Where the possibility of multidrug-resistant microorganisms is high, we suggest that combination antibiotics should be used (2D). In settings with facilities for blood culture and antibiotic resistance testing, antimicrobial therapy should be de-escalated when culture results are available (ungraded). We suggest that choice of combination therapy should be guided by local epidemiology and known effective combinations (ungraded)
6. Biomarkers	Use of biomarkers like procalcitonin and C-reactive protein for de-escalation of antimicrobial therapy needs further study in resource-limited settings before a recommendation can be made

8.3 Timing of Antibiotic Treatment

Rapid elimination of causative microorganisms should help to prevent further pathological injury in severe sepsis and septic shock. Several, mainly retrospective, studies from resource-rich settings have shown an association between delay in antibiotic administration and worse outcome in sepsis and septic shock [41–43]. However, retrospective designs and the confounding effects of variable fluid resuscitation and assessment of appropriateness of antibiotics mean that interpretation of results is complex. A recent meta-analysis examining both prospective and retrospective studies failed to show significant benefit of antibiotic administration within 3 h of emergency department triage or 1 h of shock recognition [41]. Against a background of increasingly rapid antibiotic administration, recent discussion has focused on whether delaying treatment to ensure appropriate antibiotics are administered is beneficial.

In resource-limited settings, it may be more difficult to administer appropriate antibiotics within the first hour of sepsis recognition as limited staff have to prioritize multiple tasks. The subgroup members therefore wanted to consider whether antibiotic administration within the first hour was an important and feasible goal in resource-limited settings.

Reviewing the literature, we identified two studies involving patients from mixed-resource settings and three studies from resource-limited settings. A retrospective study included patients from both high- and middle-income countries (total 17,990 patients, with approximately 12% from South American ICUs) and examined the time from sepsis recognition to antibiotics in patients with severe sepsis and septic shock [44]. After adjustment for sepsis severity, geographical location, and admission source of sepsis, delay in antibiotic administration at hourly intervals up to 6 h was associated with increased mortality for both severe sepsis and septic shock.

A survey of SSC resuscitation and management bundle compliance across 150 ICUs in Asia (approximately 56% patients from resource-limited settings) reported that antibiotic administration <1 h (or <3 h from emergency department arrival) was associated with significant survival benefit (OR for death 0.76 [0.58–0.99]; $p = 0.02$) [45].

Another study compared outcome and timing of antibiotic therapy in a single center in Brazil [6]. This retrospective study of 1279 patients with severe sepsis and septic shock, where mean time to antibiotics was 2.5 h, showed broad-spectrum antibiotic administration within 1 h was not associated with improved outcome compared to >1 h in multivariate analysis (OR for death 0.77 [0.59–1.01]; $p = 0.06$). In the 358 patients with positive blood cultures, appropriate antibiotic therapy was an independent predictor of mortality, whereas antibiotic administration <1 h was not.

A prospective cohort study of 145 patients with sepsis in Iran evaluated the effect on outcome of time from arrival in the emergency department to administration of antibiotics and showed a significant relationship between mortality and hourly delay in antibiotic administration up to >2 h. Subgroup analysis showed that this relationship was strongest in patients with APACHE II scores >20 [46].

In a study of 104 patients with typhoidal ileal perforation in Tanzania, inadequate antibiotic therapy prior to admission was associated with increased mortality (OR 3.1 [1.45–7.86]; $p = 0.006$) [47].

8.3.1 Availability, Feasibility, and Affordability

The SSC states that the administration of appropriate antibiotics within an hour of severe sepsis or shock recognition is a goal rather than standard of care. Observational data from resource-limited settings suggests that in many settings, the administration of antibiotics to the majority of patients within 1 h is feasible, for example, in China 98% of patients received antibiotics within 1 h, and in Brazil 68% patients received the antibiotics within 1 h of sepsis recognition [48]. In Iran, 18% received antibiotics within 1 h of arrival at the emergency department, but 74% were treated within 2 h [46]. We found weak evidence from resource-limited settings suggesting timely administration of antibiotics is beneficial. Nevertheless, in one study that evaluated timely administration and appropriateness of antibiotics, appropriate initial antibiotic therapy was the only independent predictor of outcome [6]. Based on the provided evidence, we *recommend* appropriate antibiotics should be given within the first hour following recognition of sepsis and septic shock (1C).

8.4 Importance of Blood Cultures Before Initiation of Empirical Antibiotic Treatment

Definitive identification and sensitivity testing of causative organisms of sepsis and septic shock allow de-escalation of treatment and ensure that appropriate antibiotic therapy is given. Currently it is recommended that, if this does not delay administration of antibiotics, two sets of blood cultures should be taken, one of which should be drawn through an intravascular device (if one has been present for more than 48 h), as this may help determine the origin of the infection. Obtaining blood cultures is strongly recommended to aid microbiological identification, also in resource-limited settings [4]. However, setting specific evidence on the added value of blood cultures on patient outcome is important, since in resource-limited settings laboratory access may be restricted and additional costs of tests must be justified. Cultures taken before antibiotic administration are more sensitive, but in settings with limited numbers of staff, the benefits must be weighed against time diverted from performing other initial resuscitation measures.

In the literature search, we identified two relevant studies from resource-limited settings and one from mixed-resource settings assessing blood cultures and outcome in severe sepsis or septic shock. A prospective study from China in 212 patients with severe sepsis or septic shock and community-acquired pneumonia reported that obtaining blood cultures before antibiotic treatment was associated with a reduced risk of mortality (OR for death 0.46, [0.211–0.997]; $p = 0.039$) [48].

A large retrospective study from Brazil of 1279 patients with severe sepsis and septic shock reported that taking blood cultures was associated with lower mortality (OR 0.38, 95% CI [0.265–0.546]; $p < 0.001$), whereas antibiotic administration within 1 h was not [6].

A study examining compliance with SSC bundles in Asian ICUs found that taking of blood cultures before antibiotics was associated with improved survival (OR death 0.72, [0.54–0.95]; $p = 0.02$) [45].

8.4.1 Availability, Feasibility, and Affordability

We found evidence from resource-limited settings that taking blood cultures was associated with improved outcome in sepsis and septic shock, although observational data cannot exclude confounding by better prognosis due to a less cryptic presentation of sepsis as an explanation for this finding. Definitive microbiological diagnosis allows the administration of appropriate antibiotics. A prospective survey of 72 adults with severe sepsis or septic shock with *S. aureus* bacteremia in Thailand reported 78% patients were empirically treated with appropriate antibiotics, but after culture result, 98% were given effective antibiotic therapy [49]. In addition, as discussed above, by detecting infections such as tuberculosis or melioidosis, the necessary treatment to prevent relapse or resistance can be given.

In resource-limited settings, there may be no facilities for blood culture analysis. In other locations where there is some laboratory capability, manual methods using self-made broth and manual inoculation of plates are an alternative to more expensive-automated culture systems. Delay in sample processing may occur due to distance from laboratory facilities or lack of trained staff. There is no definitive data to guide temporary storage, but if it is not possible to process samples straightaway, then bottles should be stored at ambient temperature, not refrigerated (expert opinion).

We could not identify studies addressing the economic aspects of costs of implementation of microbiological capacity, versus the gains in disability-adjusted life years (DALYs), or restriction of antibiotic use. We also did not find any evidence to quantify the additional benefit of taking a second set of blood cultures.

Based on the presented evidence, we *recommend* that blood cultures should be taken before the administration of antibiotics in locations where this is possible (1B). Ideally two sets of blood cultures should be obtained. It is realized that in many hospitals, routine blood culture is unfeasible, but a recommendation of expanding microbiological laboratory capacity is beyond the scope of this article.

8.5 Source Control

Source control is generally understood as including "all physical measures taken to control a focus and modify factors in the infectious milieu that promote microbiological growth or impair host antimicrobial defenses" [50]. Initial identification of a focus of infection requires a combination of clinical examination and specialist investigations. Source control methods should have maximum efficacy and cause minimum physiological upset. In resource-rich settings, inadequate source control has been shown to be an independent predictor of mortality in patients with sepsis or septic shock [51–53]. However in some situations, e.g., peripancreatic necrosis, there is moderate evidence suggesting delay in surgical source control is more appropriate [54].

In resource-limited settings, source control may be affected by the different infections encountered as well as limited access to specific diagnostic or surgical modalities. When considering source control, the subgroup wished to particularly focus on evidence for conditions commonly encountered in resource-limited settings and not considered in current guidelines.

We searched the literature and identified seven papers from resource-limited settings regarding source control. We also included one study from a resource-rich setting that was specifically concerned with an important cause of sepsis and septic shock in resource-limited countries. Six of the studies concerned source identification. Three studies reported the use of chest radiography and ultrasound in source diagnosis of typhoid or tuberculoid gastrointestinal perforations, reporting the presence of pneumoperitoneum in 70–75% of cases on chest radiography and fluid collections in 70–97% of cases on abdominal ultrasound [47, 55–57]. In a retrospective Australian study of 78 cases of prostatic abscesses due to melioidosis, 85% of cases were detectable with ultrasound compared to a "gold standard" of computerized tomography (CT) [58]. In a prospective cohort study of 230 patients in Thailand, ultrasonography identified abdominal abscesses in 33% of patients (and 38% or those with positive blood cultures) although no comparison was made with CT [59].

Three studies examined timing of source control in typhoid gastrointestinal perforation. An early series in India reported an increased mortality rate associated with delay in surgery in a series of 100 consecutive cases of typhoidal ileac perforation [60]. Another study from India reported a nonsignificant reduction in mortality (19 vs. 32%) in those whose operation was performed within 48 h of perforation [61]. More recently, a retrospective case series in Tanzania reported that delay in surgery over 24 h was associated with higher mortality (24 vs. 14%) [47].

With respect to melioidosis, in the Australian series of prostatic abscesses, it was noted that only small abscesses (<1 cm) resolved with antibiotic therapy alone and drainage (either ultrasound- or CT-guided) was required in larger abscesses. Pus drained from the majority of abscesses showed viable bacteria despite supervised adequate and prolonged antibiotic therapy [58].

8.5.1 Availability, Affordability, and Feasibility

Removing the focus of infection in the septic patient is equally important in resource-limited settings as in high-income settings. However, source control and identification are challenging in resource-limited settings; poor investigative facilities limit diagnostic capability, and less invasive measures for control often require expensive equipment and expertise. Some conditions such as mycotic aneurysms in non-typhoidal salmonellae infections are reported to be invariably lethal without surgical resection [62]. Current SSC guidelines recommend source control within 12 h except in the case of pancreatic necrosis when delay appears to be beneficial. We found weak evidence from resource-limited settings to support timely source control (<24 h) in typhoidal perforations, although no studies specifically examined control <12 h. In view of the lack of evidence for other situations, we felt unable to apply a graded recommendation. There was no evidence of situations where delay in source control seemed beneficial.

Ultrasound and X-ray are the most available and inexpensive investigations to aid the anatomical infection site, and we found low-grade evidence of both investigations showing reasonable sensitivity in abdominal perforation and melioidosis. Radiological examination was available in 86% of patients with severe sepsis and septic shock associated with *S. aureus* bacteremia in Thailand [49], and in 15 out of 46 cases where an anatomical site of infection was identified, appropriate source control procedures occurred, although in five further cases, the patient was deemed unfit for the appropriate surgical procedure.

Based on the presented evidence, we suggest the infection source control is carried out within 12 h of admission to hospital (ungraded) except in the specific case of pancreatic necrosis. Radiography and ultrasound are good first-line imaging techniques (ungraded).

8.6 Use of Combination Antibiotic Therapy in Specific Situations

Although some data exist supporting combination therapy in all patients with sepsis or septic shock, particularly those with most severe disease [63–66], there are few randomized controlled trials examining this. Lack of good evidence and concerns over antimicrobial resistance and toxicity has meant that monotherapy is recommended in most instances. Notable exceptions are neutropenia and sepsis with Gram-negative multidrug-resistant bacteria or *S. pneumoniae* bacteremia. If combination therapy is used empirically, it is recommended that it is used for less than 3–5 days. Although there are often biologically plausible mechanisms of additive or synergistic action, success of combination therapy also appears to be related to the increased likelihood of the causative bacteria being susceptible to at least one antibiotic [67, 68]. In addition to multidrug-resistant infections, the subgroup wanted to assess evidence for benefit or combination therapy in specific diseases common to resource-limited settings.

We identified a total of nine relevant studies examining combination antibiotic therapy in patients in resource-limited settings: one meta-analysis of two randomized controlled trials in melioidosis, five studies examining combination therapy in multidrug-resistant (MDR) or extensively drug-resistant (XDR) *A. baumannii* infections (only one of which specifically addressed infections in patients with severe sepsis or septic shock), and one study of febrile neutropenia.

In a meta-analysis of two randomized clinical trials of additional cotrimoxazole to ceftazidime in the early phase of acute severe melioidosis in Thailand involving a total of 449 patients, no difference in mortality or recurrent disease was noted between the two treatment groups [69, 70]. Similarly, no difference was noted with combination therapy in the later eradication phase of treatment [71].

A retrospective study in Turkey investigated single agent (colistin) versus combination therapy (colistin/sulbactam) in 89 ICU patients with MDR *A. baumannii* ventilator-associated pneumonia, 80% of whom had severe sepsis or septic shock. After adjustment for APACHE II score, there was no difference in the mortality rate between groups. Clinical and bacteriological responses were higher in the combination group although not statistically significant [72].

A retrospective analysis of 110 nosocomial infections due to *A. baumannii* associated with systemic inflammatory response syndrome in Thailand found that there was improved clinical cure rate and outcome in patients treated with combination therapy and that combination therapy increased the chance of appropriate antibiotics [7].

A multicenter retrospective study of 214 patients in Turkey with XDR *A. baumannii* bloodstream infections found improved mortality and clinical and microbiological cure when colistin was used in combination compared to colistin alone [73].

Two hospital-wide studies of resistant *A. baumannii* isolates were identified: one of colistin-only susceptible strains and the other of multidrug-resistant strains (49 and 51 patients, respectively) reported to have nonsignificant reductions in mortality with combination treatment [74, 75].

One study compared combination therapy in 151 cases of febrile neutropenia in Turkey, analyzing response rates between non-carbapenem monotherapy or combination therapy and combination carbapenem therapy in 88 adults [76]. Similar rates of response were seen in all patients.

8.6.1 Availability, Affordability, and Feasibility

In many resource-limited settings, community infections are more likely to be caused by resistant organisms than in resource-rich settings [77]. Prior antibiotic use is known to affect the gut microflora which is the main source of pathogens for ICU-acquired infection; thus widespread unregulated community use of antibiotics is likely to lead to increased resistance, and this is reflected in the resistance profiles of organisms causing healthcare-associated infection in resource-limited settings [30, 78–80]. Limitation of laboratory and diagnostic facilities prevents definitive diagnosis or de-escalation of antibiotic treatment, and empiric therapy may remain the only therapeutic option. As antibiotics are often the most significant expenditure for patients with sepsis and septic shock in resource-limited settings, prolonged courses of combination therapy significantly increases healthcare costs [81]. A consensus paper from resource-rich settings concluded that the evidence is insufficient to warrant a general recommendation for combination antibiotic treatment [8], and we did not find any studies examining the benefit of combination therapy in situations where currently only monotherapy is advised in the current SSC guidelines. In studies of MDR or XDR *A. baumannii* infection, combination therapy appeared to be beneficial. In cases of XDR bacterial infection, some authors have argued that monotherapy should be avoided due to the risk of developing resistance. In addition combination therapy may be more efficient at killing bacteria and thus enable shorter courses of antibiotic therapy [67].

In the case of melioidosis, no evidence was found that initial combination treatment was superior although some have argued that combination therapy should be used for patients with deep-seated abscesses and focuses of infection [82].

Based on this we suggest that where the possibility of multidrug resistance is high, combination antibiotics should be used (2D). Choice of combination therapy should be guided by local epidemiology and known effective combinations (ungraded). Antimicrobial therapy should be de-escalated whenever possible (ungraded). We recognize that without microbiological information, de-escalation is difficult.

8.7 Use of Procalcitonin (PCT), C-Reactive Protein (CRP), or Other Biomarkers for De-escalation of Antibiotics

Reducing global antibiotic use is a major part of antibiotic stewardship programs aiming to reduce global spread of antimicrobial resistance. De-escalating treatment to narrow-spectrum agents and reducing the duration of antibiotic treatment are key elements in this approach. Since facilities for blood culture are often absent, the clinician often lacks guidance to de-escalate empirical-started antibiotic treatment. Semiquantitative CRP or PCT point-of-care tests have become increasingly available and could be a potential tool to guide de-escalation.

There are limited randomized controlled trial data concerning outcome following de-escalation of empiric antibiotic therapy [83]. There is more evidence on the use of biomarkers to de-escalate or terminate antibiotic therapy in severe sepsis and septic shock, but this comes mainly from resource-rich settings in Europe. The most widely available biomarkers studied for this purpose are PCT and CRP. PCT is generally more specific for bacterial sepsis but costlier compared to CRP. Results of several meta-analyses involving up to seven randomized controlled trials (total 1075 patients) have shown PCT can be used safely to reduce length of antibiotic treatment and may be cost-effective [84–89].

In resource-limited countries with high levels of antimicrobial resistance, strategies to reduce use of broad-spectrum agents are important. While we specifically searched for evidence of biomarkers in resource-limited settings, we also included studies from resource-rich settings that covered other biomarkers that would be potentially useful in resource-limited settings.

We identified two studies from resource-limited countries and also included one recent study from a resource-rich country on procalcitonin and one on fever course and white blood cell counts to guide antibiotic therapy [90] [91].

Eighty-one patients with a proven bacterial infection and sepsis, severe sepsis, or septic shock admitted to an ICU in Brazil were randomized to PCT-guided treatment or normal treatment. In the 51 patients per protocol analysis, median duration of antibiotic therapy was significantly lower in the PCT group, which was not at the expense of a worse treatment outcome. However, intention-to-treat analysis showed no difference. Reduced antibiotic costs led to significant cost savings in the PCT group, offsetting the increased cost of testing [91]. CRP levels were also measured in the PCT group, but these remained elevated until the end of antibiotic treatment.

A randomized clinical trial in China studied the use of PCT-guided initiation and termination of antibiotic therapy in 35 patients with severe acute pancreatitis compared to 36 patients who received a standard 14-day course of prophylactic antibiotics [92]. Average duration of antibiotic use, length of hospitalization, and costs of hospitalization were shorter in the PCT-guided group.

A more recent large multicenter randomized clinical trial from the Netherlands in 1575 critically ill patients showed that an antibiotic-stopping rule based on a reduction in plasma procalcitonin concentrations of >80% from its peak value (or an absolute decrease below 0·5 μg/L) resulted in a reduction of duration of antibiotic treatment and was associated with a significant decrease in mortality [93].

In a multicenter randomized clinical trial of 518 patients with complicated abdominal sepsis and adequate source control in the USA, patients were randomized to a white blood count/fever-guided cessation of antibiotics or a fixed 4-day course. In the white blood count/fever-guided group, antibiotic duration was significantly longer. There were no differences in outcome [90].

8.7.1 Availability, Affordability, and Feasibility

We found evidence from resource-limited settings that PCT-guided antibiotic policies can be cost-effective as cost of tests is offset by antibiotic cost savings [91, 92]. Two studies from resource-limited settings have shown benefit of PCT guidance in antibiotic de-escalation in sepsis and septic shock [91, 94]. CRP could be used as a cheaper alternative, but this will need additional evaluation. We did not find evidence of low-cost alternatives, including fever or white blood cell counts, being beneficial when compared to short-fixed durations of therapy.

Based on this we conclude that the use of biomarkers, in particular PCT and CRP, for de-escalation of antimicrobial therapy needs further study in resource-limited settings before a recommendation can be made.

8.8 Outstanding Questions for Future Research

In addition to reviewing the literature concerning the above questions, we also discussed areas currently lacking in evidence in resource-limited settings and where resource-rich country evidence may not be applicable.

Reducing duration of antibiotic use can reduce side effects, treatment costs, and antimicrobial resistance. Studies in resource-rich settings have shown that in general shortened courses of antibiotics do not appear to be harmful and may be associated with reduced antimicrobial resistance [66, 95]. Others, however, have argued that longer durations of treatment may be required in cases of immune deficiency, inadequate source control, MDR and XDR infections, poor tissue penetration of drugs, the presence of foreign materials, or inadequate initial antibiotics [95, 96]. Although reduced duration of antibiotic treatment would be particularly attractive in resource-limited settings, it remains unclear whether this can be safely adopted in places where definitive microbiological diagnosis is challenging and when there are high-prevalence rates of non-fermenting Gram-negative bacteria.

The recommendations for prevention of nosocomial infections in the current SSC guideline include a Grade 2B recommendation in favor of chlorhexidine mouthwash and selective digestive decontamination. These measures have been used in resource-rich settings [97], and the subgroup initially intended to discuss their use in resource-limited settings. However, they are yet to be tested in resource-limited settings, and as there are important differences in epidemiology of nosocomial infection and capacity for infection control, the subgroup felt that applying evidence from resource-rich settings was not appropriate. The efficacy and safety of these interventions in resource-limited settings therefore require further study.

Finally, the advent of new technologies with the ability to type and characterize microorganisms without the need for conventional culture techniques may negate the requirement for highly specialized microbiology staff and facilities. There is currently one ongoing study of their use in a resource-limited setting. However, careful cost-benefit analysis is required. These methods could eventually contribute significantly to improved management of patients with sepsis and septic shock as well as antibiotic stewardship programs.

References

1. Dondorp AM, Iyer SS, Schultz MJ. Critical care in resource-restricted settings. JAMA. 2016;315:753–4.
2. Singer M, Deutschman CS, Seymour CW, Shankar-Hari M, Annane D, Bauer M, Bellomo R, Bernard G, Chiche JD, Coppersmith CM, Hitchkiss RS, Rubenfeld GD, Poll TVD, J-l V, Angus DC. The third international consensus definitions for sepsis and septic shock (sepsis-3). JAMA. 2016;315:801–10.
3. Campaign SS surviving sepsis campaign responds to sepsis-3. In: Book surviving sepsis campaign responds to sepsis-3. http://www.survivingsepsis.org/SiteCollectionDocuments/SSC-Statements-Sepsis-Definitions-3-2016.pdf.
4. Kwizera A, Festic E, Dünser MW. What's new in sepsis recognition in resource-limited settings? Intensive Care Med. 2016;42(12):2030–3.
5. World B country and lending groups. In: Book country and lending groups. http://data.worldbank.org/about/country-and-lending-groups.
6. Yokota PK, Marra AR, Martino MD, Victor ES, Durao MS, Edmond MB, dos Santos OF. Impact of appropriate antimicrobial therapy for patients with severe sepsis and septic shock—a quality improvement study. PLoS One. 2014;9:e104475.
7. Santimaleeworagun W, Wongpoowarak P, Chayakul P, Pattharachayakul S, Tansakul P, Garey KW. Clinical outcomes of patients infected with carbapenem-resistant acinetobacter baumannii treated with single or combination antibiotic therapy. J Med Assoc Thail. 2011;94:863–70.
8. Bochud P-Y, Bonten M, Marchetti O, Calandra T. Antimicrobial therapy for patients with severe sepsis and septic shock: an evidence-based review. Crit Care Med. 2004;32:S495–510.
9. Tanriover MD, Guven GS, Sen D, Unal S, Uzun O. Epidemiology and outcome of sepsis in a tertiary-care hospital in a developing country. Epidemiol Infect. 2006;134:315–22.
10. Hranjec T, Rosenberger LH, Swenson B, Metzger R, Flohr TR, Politano AD, Riccio LM, Popovsky KA, Sawyer RG. Aggressive versus conservative initiation of antimicrobial treatment in critically ill surgical patients with suspected intensive-care-unit-acquired infection: a quasi-experimental, before and after observational cohort study. Lancet Infect Dis. 2012;12:774–80.
11. Fadare JO, Adeoti AO, Aina F, Solomon OA, Ijalana JO. The influence of health insurance scheme on the drug prescribing pattern in a Nigerian tertiary healthcare facility. Niger Med J. 2015;56:344–8.
12. Dellinger RP, Levy MM, Rhodes A, Annane D, Gerlach H, Opal SM, Sevransky JE, Sprung CL, Douglas IS, Jaeschke R, Osborn TM, Nunnally ME, Townsend SR, Reinhart K, Kleinpell RM, Angus DC, Deutschman CS, Machado FR, Rubenfeld GD, Webb SA, Beale RJ, Vincent JL, Moreno R, Surviving Sepsis Campaign Guidelines Committee including the Pediatric Subgroup. Surviving sepsis campaign: international guidelines for management of severe sepsis and septic shock: 2012. Crit Care Med. 2013;41:580–637.
13. Cheng B, Xie G, Yao S, Wu X, Guo Q, Gu M, Fang Q, Xu Q, Wang D, Jin Y, Yuan S, Wang J, Du Z, Sun Y, Fang X. Epidemiology of severe sepsis in critically ill surgical patients in ten university hospitals in China. Crit Care Med. 2007;35:2538–46.
14. Khwannimit B, Bhurayanontachai R. The epidemiology of, and risk factors for, mortality from severe sepsis and septic shock in a tertiary-care university hospital setting. Epidemiol Infect. 2009;137:1333–41.
15. Reddy EA, Shaw AV, Crump JA. Community-acquired bloodstream infections in Africa : a systematic review and meta-analysis. Lancet Infect Dis. 2010;10:417–32.
16. Murdoch DR. Microbiological patterns in sepsis: what happened in the last 20 years? Int J Antimicrob Agents. 2009;34(Suppl 4):S5–8.
17. Goyette-Desjardins G, Auger J-P, Xu J, Segura M, Gottschalk M. Streptococcus suis, an important pig pathogen and emerging zoonotic agent-an update on the worldwide distribution based on serotyping and sequence typing. Emerg Microbes Infect. 2014;3:e45.
18. Scott JAG, Berkley JA, Mwangi I, Ochola L, Uyoga S, MacHaria A, Ndila C, Lowe BS, Mwarumba S, Bauni E, Marsh K, Williams TN. Relation between falciparum malaria and bac-

teraemia in Kenyan children: a population-based, case-control study and a longitudinal study. Lancet. 2011;378:1316–23.
19. Endris M, Takele Y, Woldeyohannes D, Tiruneh M, Mohammed R, Moges F, Lynen L, Jacobs J, van Griensven J, Diro E. Bacterial sepsis in patients with visceral leishmaniasis in Northwest Ethiopia. Biomed Res Int. 2014;2014:361058.
20. McKay R, Bamford C. Community- versus healthcare-acquired bloodstream infections at Groote Schuur Hospital, Cape Town, South Africa. S Afr Med J. 2015;105:363.
21. Ashley EA, Lubell Y, White NJ, Turner P. Antimicrobial susceptibility of bacterial isolates from community acquired infections in Sub-Saharan Africa and Asian low and middle income countries. Trop Med Int Health. 2011;16:1167–79.
22. Nickerson EK, Hongsuwan M, Limmathurotsakul D, Wuthiekanun V, Shah KR, Srisomang P, Mahavanakul W, Wacharaprechasgul T, Fowler VG, West TE, Teerawatanasuk N, Becher H, White NJ, Chierakul W, Day NP, Peacock SJ. Staphylococcus aureus bacteraemia in a tropical setting: patient outcome and impact of antibiotic resistance. PLoS One. 2009;4:e4308.
23. Rosenthal VD, Maki DG, Salomao R, Moreno CA, Mehta Y, Higuera F, Cuellar LE, Arikan OA, Abouqal R, Leblebicioglu H. Device-associated nosocomial infections in 55 intensive care units of 8 developing countries. Ann Intern Med. 2006;145:582–91.
24. Chen CJ, Huang YC. New epidemiology of Staphylococcus aureus infection in Asia. Clin Microbiol Infect. 2014;20:605–23.
25. Hawkey PM. Multidrug-resistant Gram-negative bacteria: a product of globalization. J Hosp Infect. 2015;89:241–7.
26. Molton JS, Tambyah PA, Ang BSP, Ling ML, Fisher DA. The global spread of healthcare-associated multidrug-resistant bacteria: a perspective from Asia. Clin Infect Dis. 2013;56:1310–8.
27. Stoesser N, Crook DW, Moore CE, Phetsouvanh R, Chansamouth V, Newton PN, Jones N. Characteristics of CTX-M ESBL-producing Escherichia coli isolates from the lao people's democratic republic, 2004-09. In: Book characteristics of CTX-M ESBL-producing Escherichia coli isolates from the lao people's democratic republic, 2004-09. 2012.
28. Vlieghe ER, Huang TD, Phe T, Bogaerts P, Berhin C, De Smet B, Peetermans WE, Jacobs JA, Glupczynski Y. Prevalence and distribution of beta-lactamase coding genes in third-generation cephalosporin-resistant Enterobacteriaceae from bloodstream infections in Cambodia. Eur J Clin Microbiol Infect Dis. 2015;34:1223–9.
29. Livermore DM. Fourteen years in resistance. Int J Antimicrob Agents. 2012;39:283–94.
30. Bataar O, Khuderchuluun C, Lundeg G, Chimeddorj S, Brunauer A, Gradwohl-Matis I, Duenser MW. Rate and pattern of antibiotic resistance in microbiological cultures of sepsis patients in a low-middle-income country's ICU. Middle East J Anesthesiol. 2013;22:293–300.
31. Deshpande P, Shetty A, Kapadia F, Hedge A, Somon R, Rodrigues C. New Delhi Metallo 1: have carbapenems met their doom? Clin Infect Dis. 2010;51:1222–3.
32. Saleem AF, Qamar FN, Shahzad H, Qadir M, Zaidi AKM. Trends in antibiotic susceptibility and incidence of late-onset Klebsiella pneumoniae neonatal sepsis over a six-year period in a neonatal intensive care unit in Karachi, Pakistan. Int J Infect Dis. 2013;17:e961–5.
33. Manenzhe RI, Zar HJ, Nicol MP, Kaba M. The spread of carbapenemase-producing bacteria in Africa: a systematic review. J Antimicrob Chemother. 2015;70:23–40.
34. Andriamanantena TS, Ratsima E, Rakotonirina HC, Randrianirina F, Ramparany L, Carod J-F, Richard V, Talarmin A. Dissemination of multidrug resistant Acinetobacter baumannii in various hospitals of Antananarivo Madagascar. Ann Clin Microbiol Antimicrob. 2010;9:17.
35. Nasa P, Juneja D, Singh O, Dang R, Singh A. An observational study on bloodstream extended-spectrum beta-lactamase infection in critical care unit: Incidence, risk factors and its impact on outcome. Eur J Intern Med. 2012;23:192–5.
36. Moghnieh R, Estaitieh N, Mugharbil A, Jisr T, Abdallah DI, Ziade F, Sinno L, Ibrahim A. Third generation cephalosporin resistant Enterobacteriaceae and multidrug resistant gram-negative bacteria causing bacteremia in febrile neutropenia adult cancer patients in Lebanon, broad spectrum antibiotics use as a major risk factor, and correlation with poor prognosis. Front Cell Infect Microbiol. 2015;5:1–9.

37. Tuon FF, Gortz LW, Rocha JL. Risk factors for pan-resistant Pseudomonas aeruginosa bacteremia and the adequacy of antibiotic therapy. Braz J Infect Dis. 2012;16:351–6.
38. Fahad A, Alghannam A, Aslanpour Z, Evans S, Schifano F. A systematic review of counterfeit and substandard medicines in field quality surveys. Integr Pharm Res Pract. 2014;3:71–88.
39. Seear M, Gandhi D, Carr R, Dayal A, Raghavan D, Sharma N. The need for better data about counterfeit drugs in developing countries: a proposed standard research methodology tested in Chennai, India. J Clin Pharm Ther. 2011;36:488–95.
40. Nayyar GML, Breman JG, Newton PN, Herrington J. Poor-quality antimalarial drugs in southeast Asia and sub-Saharan Africa. In: Book poor-quality antimalarial drugs in southeast Asia and sub-Saharan Africa. 2012. p. 488–496.
41. Sterling SA, Miller WR, Pryor J, Puskarich MA, Jones AE. The impact of timing of antibiotics on outcomes in severe sepsis and septic shock. Crit Care Med. 2015;43:1.
42. Garnacho-Montero J, Gutiérrez-Pizarraya A, Escoresca-Ortega A, Fernández-Delgado E, López-Sánchez JM. Adequate antibiotic therapy prior to ICU admission in patients with severe sepsis and septic shock reduces hospital mortality. Crit Care. 2015;19:302.
43. Cañas B, Jáuregui R, Ballesteros M, Leizaola O, González-Castro A, Castellanos-Ortega A. Effects of antibiotic administration delay and inadequacy upon the survival of septic shock patients. Med Intensiva. 2015;39(8):459–66.
44. Ferrer R, Martin-Loeches I, Phillips G, Osborn TM, Townsend S, Dellinger RP, Artigas A, Schorr C, Levy MM. Empiric antibiotic treatment reduces mortality in severe sepsis and septic shock from the first hour: results from a guideline-based performance improvement program. Crit Care Med. 2014;42:1749–55.
45. Phua J, Koh Y, Du B, Tang YQ, Divatia JV, Tan CC, Gomersall CD, Faruq MO, Shrestha BR, Gia Binh N, Arabi YM, Salahuddin N, Wahyuprajitno B, Tu ML, Wahab AY, Hameed AA, Nishimura M, Procyshyn M, Chan YH, MOSAICS Study Group. Management of severe sepsis in patients admitted to Asian intensive care units: prospective cohort study. BMJ. 2011;342:d3245.
46. Jalili M, Barzegari H, Pourtabatabaei N, Honarmand AR, Boreiri M, Mehrvarz A, Ahmadinejad Z. Effect of door-to-antibiotic time on mortality of patients with sepsis in emergency department: a prospective cohort study. Acta Med Iran. 2013;51:454–60.
47. Chalya PL, Mabula JB, Koy M, Kataraihya JB, Jaka H, Mshana SE, Mirambo M, McHembe MD, Giiti G, Gilyoma JM. Typhoid intestinal perforations at a University teaching hospital in Northwestern Tanzania: a surgical experience of 104 cases in a resource-limited setting. World J Emerg Surg. 2012;7:4–4.
48. Guo Q, Li HY, Li YM, Nong LB, Xu YD, He GQ, Liu XQ, Jiang M, Xiao ZI, Zhong NS. Compliance with severe sepsis bundles and its effect on patient outcomes of severe community-acquired pneumonia in a limited resources country. Arch Med Sci. 2014;10:970–8.
49. Mahavanakul W, Nickerson EK, Srisomang P, Teparrukkul P, Lorvinitnun P, Wongyingsinn M, Chierakul W, Hongsuwan M, West TE, Day NP, Limmathurotsakul D, Peacock SJ. Feasibility of modified surviving sepsis campaign guidelines in a resource-restricted setting based on a cohort study of severe S. aureus sepsis. PLoS One. 2012;7:e29858.
50. Marshall JC, Maier RV, Jimenez M, Dellinger EP. Source control in the management of severe sepsis and septic shock: an evidence-based review. Crit Care Med. 2004;32:S513–26.
51. Kollef M, Micek S, Hampton N, Doherty JA, Kumar A. Septic shock attributed to Candida infection: importance of empiric therapy and source control. Clin Infect Dis. 2012;54:1739–46.
52. Tellor B, Skrupky LP, Symons W, High E, Micek ST, Mazuski JE. Inadequate source control and inappropriate antibiotics are key determinants of mortality in patients with intra-abdominal sepsis and associated bacteremia. Surg Infect (Larchmt). 2015;16:1–9.
53. Bloos F, Thomas-Rüddel D, Rüddel H, Engel C, Schwarzkopf D, Marshall JC, Harbarth S, Simon P, Riessen R, Keh D, Dey K, Weiß M, Toussaint S, Schädler D, Weyland A, Ragaller M, Schwarzkopf K, Eiche J, Kuhnle G, Hoyer H, Hartog C, Kaisers U, Reinhart K. Impact of compliance with infection management guidelines on outcome in patients with severe sepsis: a prospective observational multi-center study. Crit Care. 2014;18:R42.

54. Marshall JC, Al Naqbi A. Principles of source control in the management of sepsis. Crit Care Nurs Clin North Am. 2011;23:99–114.
55. Ansari AG, Naqvi QS, Naqvi H, et al. Management of typhoid ilial perforation: a surgical experience of 44 cases. Gomal J Med Sci. 2009;7:27–8.
56. Patil V, Vijayakumar A, Ajitha MB, Kumar LS. Comparison between tube ileostomy and loop ileostomy as a diversion procedure. ISRN Surg. 2012;2012:547523.
57. Ugochukwu AI, Amu OC, Nzegwu MA. Ileal perforation due to typhoid fever—review of operative management and outcome in an urban centre in Nigeria. Int J Surg. 2013;11:218–22.
58. Morse LP, Moller CC, Harvey E, Ward L, Cheng AC, Carson PJ, Currie BJ. Prostatic abscess due to Burkholderia pseudomallei: 81 cases from a 19-year prospective melioidosis study. J Urol. 2009;182:542–7. discussion 547
59. Maude RR, Teerapon I, Ariyaprasert P, Maude R, Hongsuwan M, Yuentrakul P, Limmathurotsakul D, Koh G, Chaowagul W, Day NPJ, Peacocka SJ. Maude meliodosis thailand. Trans R Soc Trop Med Hyg. 2012;106:629–31.
60. Khanna A, Misra MK. Typhoid perforation of the gut. Postgrad Med J. 1984;60:523–5.
61. Sitaram V, Moses BV, Fenn AS, Khanduri P. Typhoid ileal perforations: a retrospective study. Ann R Coll Surg Engl. 1990;72:347–9.
62. Wang JH, Liu YC, Yen MY, Wang JH, Chen YS, Wann SR, Cheng DL. Mycotic aneurysm due to non-typhi salmonella : report of 16 cases. Clin Infect Dis. 1996;23:743–7.
63. Kumar A, Safdar N, Kethireddy S, Chateau D. A survival benefit of combination antibiotic therapy for serious infections associated with sepsis and septic shock is contingent only on the risk of death: a meta-analytic/meta-regression study. Crit Care Med. 2010;38:1651–64.
64. Díaz-Martín A, Martínez-González ML, Ferrer R, Ortiz-Leyba C, Piacentini E, Lopez-Pueyo MJ, Martín-Loeches I, Levy MM, Artigas A, Garnacho-Montero J. Antibiotic prescription patterns in the empiric therapy of severe sepsis: combination of antimicrobials with different mechanisms of action reduces mortality. Crit Care. 2012;16:R223.
65. Gattarello S. What is new in antibiotic therapy in community-acquired pneumonia? An evidence-based approach focusing on combined therapy. Curr Infect Dis Rep. 2015;17:45.
66. Barrett J, Edgeworth J, Wyncoll D. Shortening the course of antibiotic treatment in the intensive care unit. Expert Rev Anti-Infect Ther. 2015;13:463–71.
67. Baker S, Thieu Nga TV, Thi Loan H, Campbell JI, Le Minh V, Van Hao N, Trung Nghia HD, Vinh Phat V, Minh Yen L, Hien TT, Thi Khanh Nhu N, Thwaites L, Van Vinh Chau N, Huong Lan NP, Hoang Nhu TD, Thwaites G, Thanh Tam PT, Thompson C, Tuyen HT, Parry CM. In vitro activity of colistin in antimicrobial combination against carbapenem-resistant Acinetobacter baumannii isolated from patients with ventilator-associated pneumonia in Vietnam. J Med Microbiol. 2015;64:1162–9.
68. Dinc G, Demiraslan H, Elmali F, Ahmed SS, Alp E, Doganay M. Antimicrobial efficacy of doripenem and its combinations with sulbactam, amikacin, colistin, tigecycline in experimental sepsis of carbapenem-resistant Acinetobacter baumannii. New Microbiol. 2015;38:67–73.
69. Chierakul W, Anunnatsiri S, Short JM, Maharjan B, Mootsikapun P, Simpson AJH, Limmathurotsakul D, Cheng AC, Stepniewska K, Newton PN, Chaowagul W, White NJ, Peacock SJ, Day NP, Chetchotisakd P. Two randomized controlled trials of ceftazidime alone versus ceftazidime in combination with trimethoprim-sulfamethoxazole for the treatment of severe melioidosis. Clin Infect Dis. 2005;41:1105–13.
70. Chierakul WAS, Chaowagul W, Peacock SJ, Chetchotisakd P, Day NPJ. Addition of Trimethoprim-sulfamethoxazole to ceftazidime during parenteral treatment of meliodosis is not associated with a long-term outcome benefit. Clin Infect Dis. 2007;45:521–3.
71. Chetchotisakd P, Chierakul W, Chaowagul W, Anunnatsiri S, Phimda K, Mootsikapun P, Chaisuksant S, Pilaikul J, Thinkhamrop B, Phiphitaporn S, Susaengrat W, Toondee C, Wongrattanacheewin S, Wuthiekanun V, Chantratita N, Thaipadungpanit J, Day NP, Limmathurotsakul D, Peacock SJ. Trimethoprim-sulfamethoxazole versus trimethoprim-sulfamethoxazole plus doxycycline as oral eradicative treatment for melioidosis (MERTH):

a multicentre, double-blind, non-inferiority, randomised controlled trial. Lancet. 2014;383:807–14.

72. Kalin G, Alp E, Akin A, Coskun R, Doganay M. Comparison of colistin and colistin/sulbactam for the treatment of multidrug resistant Acinetobacter baumannii ventilator-associated pneumonia. Infection. 2013;42:37–42.
73. Batirel A, Balkan II, Karabay O, Agalar C, Akalin S, Alici O, Alp E, Altay FA, Altin N, Arslan F, Aslan T, Bekiroglu N, Cesur S, Celik AD, Dogan M, Durdu B, Duygu F, Engin A, Engin DO, Gonen I, Guclu E, Guven T, Hatipoglu CA, Hosoglu S, Karahocagil MK, Kilic AU, Ormen B, Ozdemir D, Ozer S, Oztoprak N, Sezak N, Turhan V, Turker N, Yilmaz H. Comparison of colistin–carbapenem, colistin–sulbactam, and colistin plus other antibacterial agents for the treatment of extremely drug-resistant Acinetobacter baumannii bloodstream infections. Eur J Clin Microbiol Infect Dis. 2014;33:1311–22.
74. Zhou Q, Lee SK, Jiang SY, Chen C, Kamaluddeen M, Hu XJ, Wang CQ, Cao Y. Efficacy of an infection control program in reducing ventilator-associated pneumonia in a Chinese neonatal intensive care unit. Am J Infect Control. 2013;41:1059–64.
75. Simsek F, Gedik H, Yildirmak MT, Iris NT, Türkmen A, Ersoy A, Ersöz M, Gücüyener A. Colistin against colistin-only-susceptible Acinetobacter baumannii-related infections: monotherapy or combination therapy. Indian J Med Microbiol. 2012;30:448–52.
76. Gedik H, Yildirmak T, Simsek F, Kanturk A, Aydýn D, Anca D, Yokus O, Demirel N. The outcome of non-carbapenem-based empirical antibacterial therapy and VRE colonisation in patients with hematological malignancies. Afr Health Sci. 2013;13:363–8.
77. Kimang'a AN. A situational analysis of antimicrobial drug resistance in Africa: are we losing the battle? Ethiop J Health Sci. 2012;22:135–43.
78. Inchai J, Pothirat C, Liwsrisakun C, Deesomchok A, Kositsakulchai W, Chalermpanchai N. Ventilator-associated pneumonia: epidemiology and prognostic indicators of 30-day mortality. Jpn J Infect Dis. 2015;68:181–6.
79. Werarak P, Waiwarawut J, Tharavichitkul P, Pothirat C, Rungruanghiranya S, Geater SL, Chongthaleong A, Sittipunt C, Horsin P, Chalermskulrat W, Wiwatworapan T, Thummakul T, Mootsikapun P, Rungsrithong N, Supawita S, Chuchotthavorn C, Tongsai S, Thamlikitkul V. Acinetobacter baumannii nosocomial pneumonia in tertiary care hospitals in Thailand. J Med Assoc Thail. 2012;95(Suppl 2):S23–33.
80. Nhu NT, Lan NP, Campbell JI, Parry CM, Thompson C, Tuyen HT, Hoang NV, Tam PT, Le VM, Nga TV, Nhu Tdo H, Van Minh P, Nga NT, Thuy CT, Dung le T, Yen NT, Van Hao N, Loan HT, Yen LM, Nghia HD, Hien TT, Thwaites L, Thwaites G, Chau NV, Baker S. Emergence of carbapenem-resistant Acinetobacter baumannii as the major cause of ventilator-associated pneumonia in intensive care unit patients at an infectious disease hospital in southern Vietnam. J Med Microbiol. 2014;63:1386–94.
81. Hantrakun V, Chierakul W, Chetchotisakd P, Anunnatsiri S, Currie BJ, Peacock SJ, Day NPJ, Cheah P, Limmathurotsakul D, Lubell Y. Cost-effectiveness analysis of parenteral antimicrobials for acute melioidosis in Thailand. Trans R Soc Trop Med Hyg. 2015;109:416–8.
82. Dance D. Treatment and prophylaxis of melioidosis. Int J Antimicrob Agents. 2014;43:310–8.
83. Leone M, Bechis C, Baumstarck K, Lefrant JY, Albanèse J, Jaber S, Lepape A, Constantin JM, Papazian L, Bruder N, Allaouchiche B, Bézulier K, Antonini F, Textoris J, Martin C. De-escalation versus continuation of empirical antimicrobial treatment in severe sepsis: a multicenter non-blinded randomized noninferiority trial. Intensive Care Med. 2014;40:1399–408.
84. Nobre V, Harbarth S, Graf J-D, Rohner P, Pugin J. Use of procalcitonin to shorten antibiotic treatment duration in septic patients: a randomized trial. Am J Respir Crit Care Med. 2008;177:498–505.
85. Stolz D, Smyrnios N, Eggimann P, Pargger H, Thakkar N, Siegemund M, Marsch S, Azzola A, Rakic J, Mueller B, Tamm M. Procalcitonin for reduced antibiotic exposure in ventilator-associated pneumonia: a randomised study. Eur Respir J. 2009;34:1364–75.
86. Hochreiter M, Köhler T, Schweiger A, Keck F, Bein B, von Spiegel T, Schroeder S. Procalcitonin to guide duration of antibiotic therapy in intensive care patients: a randomized prospective controlled trial. Crit Care. 2009;13:R83.

87. Schroeder S, Hochreiter M, Koehler T, Schweiger AM, Bein B, Keck FS, Von Spiegel T. Procalcitonin (PCT)-guided algorithm reduces length of antibiotic treatment in surgical intensive care patients with severe sepsis: Results of a prospective randomized study. Langenbeck's Arch Surg. 2009;394:221–6.
88. Bouadma L, Luyt C-E, Tubach F, Cracco C, Alvarez A, Schwebel C, Schortgen F, Lasocki S, Veber B, Dehoux M, Bernard M, Pasquet B, Régnier B, Brun-Buisson C, Chastre J, Wolff M. Use of procalcitonin to reduce patients' exposure to antibiotics in intensive care units (PRORATA trial): a multicentre randomised controlled trial. Lancet. 2010;375:463–74.
89. Harrison M, Collins CD. Is procalcitonin-guided antimicrobial use cost-effective in adult patients with suspected bacterial infection and sepsis? Infect Control Hosp Epidemiol. 2015;36:265–72.
90. Sawyer RG, Claridge JA, Nathens AB, Rotstein OD, Duane TM, Evans HL, Cook CH, O'Neill PJ, Mazuski JE, Askari R, Wilson MA, Napolitano LM, Namias N, Miller PR, Dellinger EP, Watson CM, Coimbra R, Dent DL, Lowry SF, Cocanour CS, West MA, Banton KL, Cheadle WG, Lipsett PA, Guidry CA, Popovsky K. Trial of short-course antimicrobial therapy for intraabdominal infection. N Engl J Med. 2015;372:1996–2005.
91. Deliberato RO, Marra AR, Sanches PR, Martino MDV, Ferreira CEDS, Pasternak J, Paes AT, Pinto LM, dos Santos OFP, Edmond MB. Clinical and economic impact of procalcitonin to shorten antimicrobial therapy in septic patients with proven bacterial infection in an intensive care setting. Diagn Microbiol Infect Dis. 2013;76:266–71.
92. Qu R, Ji Y, Ling Y, Ye C-Y, Yang S-M, Liu Y-Y, Yang R-Y, Luo Y-F, Guo Z. Procalcitonin is a good tool to guide therapy in patients with severe acute pancreatitis. Saudi Med J. 2012;33:382–7.
93. de Jong E, van Oers JA, Beishuizen A, Vos P, Vermeijden WJ, Haas LE, Loef BG, Dormans T, van Melsen GC, Kluiters YC, Kemperman H, van den Elsen MJ, Schouten JA, Streefkerk JO, Krabbe HG, Kieft H, Kluge GH, van Dam VC, van Pelt J, Bormans L, Otten MB, Reidinga AC, Endeman H, Twisk JW, van de Garde EMW, de Smet A, Kesecioglu J, Girbes AR, Nijsten MW, de Lange DW. Efficacy and safety of procalcitonin guidance in reducing the duration of antibiotic treatment in critically ill patients: a randomised, controlled, open-label trial. Lancet Infect Dis. 2016;16:819–27.
94. Nargis W, Ibrahim M, Ahamed BU. Procalcitonin versus C-reactive protein: usefulness as biomarker of sepsis in ICU patient. Int J Crit Illn Inj Sci. 2014;4:195–9.
95. Pugh R, Grant C, Cooke RP, Dempsey G. Short-course versus prolonged-course antibiotic therapy for hospital-acquired pneumonia in critically ill adults (Review). Summary of findings for the main comparison. 2011.
96. Timsit J-F, Soubirou J-F, Voiriot G, Chemam S, Neuville M, Mourvillier B, Sonneville R, Mariotte E, Bouadma L, Wolff M. Treatment of bloodstream infections in ICUs. BMC Infect Dis. 2014;14:1–11.
97. Klompas M, Speck K, Howell MD, Greene LR, Berenholtz SM. Reappraisal of routine oral care with chlorhexidine gluconate for patients receiving mechanical ventilation systematic review and meta-analysis. JAMA Intern Med. 2014;174(5):751–61.

Open Access This chapter is licensed under the terms of the Creative Commons Attribution 4.0 International License (http://creativecommons.org/licenses/by/4.0/), which permits use, sharing, adaptation, distribution and reproduction in any medium or format, as long as you give appropriate credit to the original author(s) and the source, provide a link to the Creative Commons license and indicate if changes were made.

The images or other third party material in this chapter are included in the chapter's Creative Commons license, unless indicated otherwise in a credit line to the material. If material is not included in the chapter's Creative Commons license and your intended use is not permitted by statutory regulation or exceeds the permitted use, you will need to obtain permission directly from the copyright holder.

Management of Severe Malaria and Severe Dengue in Resource-Limited Settings

9

Arjen M. Dondorp, Mai Nguyen Thi Hoang, Mervyn Mer, Martin W. Dünser, Sanjib Mohanty, Jane Nakibuuka, Marcus J. Schultz, C. Louise Thwaites, and Bridget Wills

A. M. Dondorp (✉)
Mahidol–Oxford Research Unit (MORU), Faculty of Tropical Medicine, Mahidol University, Bangkok, Thailand

Oxford Centre for Tropical Medicine and Global Health, Nuffield Department of Clinical Medicine, University of Oxford, Oxford, UK

Department of Intensive Care, Academic Medical Center, University of Amsterdam, Amsterdam, The Netherlands

M. N. T. Hoang
Oxford University Clinical Research Unit, Hospital for Tropical Diseases, Ho Chi Minh City, Vietnam

M. Mer
Department of Critical Care, Johannesburg Hospital and University of the Witwatersrand, Johannesburg, South Africa

M. W. Dünser
Department of Anesthesiology and Intensive Care Medicine, Kepler University Hospital, Linz, Austria

S. Mohanty
Department of Medicine, Ispat Hospital, Rourkela, Rourkela, Odisha, India

J. Nakibuuka
Department of Paediatrics, Mulago National Referral and University Teaching Hospital, Kampala, Uganda

M. J. Schultz
Mahidol–Oxford Research Unit (MORU), Faculty of Tropical Medicine, Mahidol University, Bangkok, Thailand

Department of Intensive Care, Academic Medical Center, University of Amsterdam, Amsterdam, The Netherlands

C. L. Thwaites · B. Wills
Oxford Centre for Tropical Medicine and Global Health, Nuffield Department of Clinical Medicine, University of Oxford, Oxford, UK

Oxford University Clinical Research Unit, Hospital for Tropical Diseases, Ho Chi Minh City, Vietnam

© The Author(s) 2019
A. M. Dondorp et al. (eds.), *Sepsis Management in Resource-limited Settings*,
https://doi.org/10.1007/978-3-030-03143-5_9

9.1 Introduction

Sepsis in resource-limited settings will often have different etiologies to those in Western settings, including severe malaria, severe dengue, viral hemorrhagic fevers, melioidosis, typhus, and leptospirosis. The Surviving Sepsis Campaign (SSC) guidelines [1] are mainly based on evidence from studies on bacterial sepsis. These guidelines are widely applicable, but there are also exceptions. We here focus on disease-specific recommendations for the management of severe falciparum malaria and severe dengue. An international team with extensive practical experience in resource-limited intensive care units (ICUs) identified key questions concerning the SSC's management recommendations on these diseases. Pertinent evidence from resource-limited settings was evaluated using the Grading of Recommendations Assessment, Development, and Evaluation (GRADE) tools.

Severe falciparum malaria is a multiorgan disease caused by *Plasmodium falciparum* transmitted by *Anopheles* mosquitoes. The highest transmission and disease burden is in sub-Saharan Africa, where severe malaria is largely a pediatric disease, as older children and adults become partly immune. In Asia and South America, all age groups may be affected. Independent of age, the presenting symptoms with the strongest prognostic significance are coma (cerebral malaria), metabolic (lactic) acidosis, and renal dysfunction. Acute respiratory distress syndrome is a common and often fatal complication in adult patients with severe malaria. Hypotension occurs infrequently (~12% of cases), and should raise a suspicion of concomitant bacterial sepsis. One of the main pathophysiologic differences of severe falciparum malaria compared to bacterial sepsis is microcirculatory impairment caused by sequestration of parasite-infected erythrocytes, red cell rigidity, and red cell clumping.

Severe dengue is caused by dengue virus transmitted by *Aedes* mosquitoes. Approximately 1–5% of patients will develop severe manifestations. The defining feature is a vasculopathy with increased capillary permeability, causing plasma leakage, reduced intravascular volume, and if severe life-threatening hypovolemic shock [2]. This "critical phase" typically starts during the period of defervescence and lasts for approximately 48 h. Bleeding complications and organ involvement of the brain, liver, kidney, and heart may be additional features and occur more frequently in adult cases [3]. Recommendations and suggestions are summarized in Table 9.1.

9.2 Fluid Management in Severe Malaria

Severe malaria is an old disease, and historically, the guidance for fluid management has been to "keep them dry." This approach was subsequently challenged when it was recognized that severe malaria is a severe sepsis syndrome with signs of tissue hypoperfusion and thus might benefit from fluid bolus therapy. The SSC guidelines recommend in patients with sepsis-induced tissue hypoperfusion and suspicion of hypovolemia an initial fluid challenge of minimal 30 mL/kg of crystalloids, to be completed within 3 h, of which a portion may be albumin equivalent;

Table 9.1 Recommendations and suggestions for the management of patients with severe malaria and severe dengue in resource-limited settings (with grading)

Fluid management of severe malaria	We recommend not to use fluid bolus therapy in normotensive patients with severe falciparum malaria (1A). We suggest that patients receive maintenance isotonic crystalloid fluid therapy (2–4 mL/kg/h), which may subsequently be reduced to 1 mL/kg/h in patients receiving additional fluids, e.g., through enteral tube feeding (2D). We suggest that in patients with hypotensive shock, fluid bolus therapy (30 mL/kg) with isotonic crystalloids be commenced (ungraded) and, if available, early initiation of vasopressor medication (ungraded)
Timing of enteral feeding in cerebral malaria	We suggest initiating enteral feeding in non-intubated adult patients with cerebral malaria after 60 h, in order to limit the possibility of aspiration pneumonia (2B). There are insufficient data to make this recommendation for children with cerebral malaria
Permissive hypercapnia in ventilated cerebral malaria	We suggest not to use a strategy of permissive hypercapnia to achieve ventilation with low tidal volumes in patients with cerebral malaria, because of the high incidence of brain swelling in these patients (ungraded)
Fluid management in severe dengue	We recommend that fluid resuscitation in severe dengue is executed promptly and guided by pulse pressure, capillary refill time, hematocrit, and urine output according to WHO guidelines and that fluid therapy should be restricted as soon as the critical phase of the disease is over to avoid pulmonary edema (1C). We recommend that rapid administration of large fluid boluses should be avoided, unless the patient is hypotensive (1D). We recommend that in dengue patients with compensated shock, colloid fluids are not used (1A)
Use of corticosteroids in severe dengue	We recommend not to use corticosteroids in the treatment of severe dengue (1B)
Use of prophylactic platelet transfusion in severe dengue	We recommend not to use prophylactic platelet transfusion for thrombocytopenia in the absence of active bleeding complications or other risk factors (uncontrolled arterial hypertension, recent stroke, head trauma or surgery, continuation of an anticoagulant treatment, existing hemorrhagic diathesis) (1B)

this applies to patients with hypotension or a plasma lactate ≥4 mmol/L [1]. It was shown by various techniques that both children and adults with severe falciparum malaria are intravascular dehydrated [4–6] although this was debated by some [7]. Small trials in African children with severe malaria suggested a benefit from fluid bolus therapy, in particular with albumin [8–11], as recently reviewed [12]. However, a subsequent large trial on fluid bolus therapy in 3138 African children with severe infections and compensated shock, of which 57% had falciparum malaria, showed overall a 40% increase in mortality with fluid bolus therapy (20 mL/kg or 40 mL/kg with either saline or albumin). In the 1793 children with severe *P. falciparum* malaria, mortality in the bolus groups was 51% higher (RR 1.51 [1.17–1.95]) than without fluid bolus therapy [13]. In the same study, febrile patients with hypotensive ("decompensated") shock were randomized between 20 and 40 mL/kg fluid bolus therapy with either saline or albumin; 69% of the children (9 of 13) in the albumin bolus group and 56% (9 of 16) in the saline-bolus group died ($P = 0.45$). In Asian studies in adult severe malaria, rapid fluid resuscitation did not improve metabolic acidosis [14, 15], and transpulmonary thermodilution-guided rapid fluid resuscitation resulted in pulmonary edema in 8/28 (29%) patients [15]. One observational study showed no deterioration in renal function or plasma lactate with maintenance fluid therapy between 1.3 and 2.2 mL/kg/h [16]. A recent systematic review concluded that fluid bolus therapy with either crystalloid or albumen is not beneficial in severe falciparum malaria [17].

We *recommend* not to use fluid bolus therapy in normotensive patients with severe falciparum malaria (1A). We *suggest* not to use colloid therapy, including albumin 5% (2C). In normotensive patients, we *suggest* initial crystalloid fluid therapy of 2–4 mL/kg/h (2D). In patients receiving enteral fluids, e.g., through enteral tube feeding, we suggest that this can be reduced to 1 mL/kg/h (2D). This is slightly more conservative than the recommendation in the management guidelines for severe malaria issued by the World Health Organization, recommending 3–5 mL/kg/h [18]. There are no data on the benefit of balanced fluids over normal saline. We suggest fluid bolus therapy (30 mL/kg) with an isotonic crystalline in patients with hypotensive shock and, if available, early start of vasopressive medication (ungraded). Hypotensive shock in a patient with severe malaria could indicate concomitant bacterial sepsis, and be evaluated and treated accordingly.

9.3 Timing of Enteral Nasogastric Tube Feeding in Cerebral Malaria

The SSC guidelines suggest administering oral or enteral (if necessary) feeds, as tolerated, rather than either complete fasting or provision of only intravenous glucose within the first 48 h after a diagnosis of severe sepsis/septic shock (grade 2C) [1]. Early enteral feeding is thought to preserve gut integrity and function, maintain bile secretion and secretory IgA, maintain gut-associated lymphoid tissue (GALT) resulting in reduced translocation, improve splanchnic blood flow, and act prophylactically against stress ulceration. In patients with severe malaria, malnutrition is common, as is concomitant invasive bacterial infection [19]. Therefore, the recommendation for early start of enteral feeding seems valid for patients with severe malaria, including intubated patients with cerebral malaria. However, in resource-limited settings, endotracheal intubation of comatose patient is often not practiced, and there might be an increased risk of aspiration pneumonia.

We could identify one randomized clinical trial on the timing of enteral feeding in patients with cerebral malaria [20]. This trial in (mainly) adult Bangladeshi patients with cerebral malaria who were not on mechanical ventilation, and thus had an unprotected airway, showed that early (<60 h) enteral feeding was associated with aspiration pneumonia in 9/27 (33%) versus 0/29 with late start after 60 h ($p = 0.001$). This despite proper positioning of patients, and pre-feed inspection of gastric retention. No difference in the incidence of hypoglycemia was observed.

We *suggest* starting enteral feeding in non-intubated adult patients with cerebral malaria after 60 h (2B). There are insufficient data on pediatric patients with cerebral malaria from African settings.

9.4 Mechanical Ventilation in Patients with Severe Malaria and Acute Respiratory Distress Syndrome

Acute respiratory distress syndrome (ARDS), or pulmonary malaria, is a feared complication of severe falciparum malaria and can also complicate the course of vivax malaria [21]. The incidence of ARDS in adult patients with severe malaria is estimated 5 to 25% and up to 29% in pregnant women; ARDS is thought to be rare in pediatric severe malaria [22]. To protect the lung from the damaging effects of mechanical ventilation, the SSC recommends targeting a tidal volume of 6 mL/kg predicted body weight in patients with sepsis-induced acute respiratory distress syndrome (ARDS), that plateau pressures be measured in patients with ARDS and that the initial upper limit goal for plateau pressures in a passively inflated lung be <30 cm H_2O [1]. There are no randomized clinical trials to evaluate this recommendation specifically for ARDS in the context of severe malaria. However, given the large benefit of this ventilation strategy in patients with other causes of ARDS, this recommendation should also be valid in severe malaria. The SSC guidelines also suggest that to facilitate the use of a lung protective ventilatory strategy, permissive hypercapnia can be used. It should be noted that availability of blood gas or end-tidal CO_2 monitoring is limited in resource-limited settings, compromising its safe implementation.

There are no randomized clinical trials on the use of permissive hypercapnia in mechanically ventilated patients with severe falciparum malaria. However, in cerebral malaria, brain swelling is common, caused by an increase in intracerebral blood volume including the sequestered parasitized red blood cell mass, vasogenic edema, and cytotoxic edema, and is more prominent in pediatric cases [23–26]. Because hypercapnia will further increase intracranial pressure, we *suggest* against the use of permissive hypercapnia to achieve the goal of low tidal volume ventilation in patients with cerebral malaria, as cerebral malaria is associated with brain swelling and variably increased intracranial pressure (ungraded).

9.5 Fluid Management in Severe Dengue

Severe dengue can be defined as a sepsis syndrome. Yet, important aspects of the pathophysiology of the circulatory changes are distinct from bacterial sepsis. Dengue shock syndrome is characterized by a vasculopathy during the critical phase of the disease, with a plasma leak and hemoconcentration, causing important intravascular volume depletion [3]. This initially leads to a compensated shock with signs of tissue hypoperfusion and a decreased pulse pressure with preserved systolic blood pressure. This can be followed by life-threatening hypotensive shock. Hemorrhage, in particular from the gastrointestinal tract, and more rarely myocarditis, can contribute to circulatory shock. The onset is usually more gradual than with bacterial sepsis. Management of patients with severe dengue relies largely on careful monitoring, including early recognition of vascular leakage and proper fluid replacement, combined with prompt but carefully guided volume resuscitation for patients who develop dengue shock syndrome. The SSC guidelines advocate fluid bolus therapy for patients with sepsis-induced tissue hypoperfusion and suspicion of hypovolemia [1], which might not be appropriate for patients with severe dengue and compensated shock. In addition, because of the prominent plasma leak, the use of colloids might be beneficial in dengue with hypotensive shock, as opposed to its use in patients with bacterial sepsis. The WHO guidelines for the management of patients with severe dengue distinguish patients with compensated shock from those with decompensated (hypotensive) shock [2, 27]. In compensated shock, recommended initial fluid therapy is with isotonic crystalloid solutions at 5–10 mL/kg over 1 h, which can be tapered every few hours if the patient improves guided by the pulse pressure, capillary refill time, hematocrit, and urine output. Prudential fluid therapy is important throughout the disease, but in particular fluid administration should be restricted as soon as the critical phase of the disease is over to avoid pulmonary edema. In the same guidelines, it is recommended in patients with hypotensive shock, to resuscitate with crystalloid or colloid solution at 20 mL/kg as a bolus given over 15 min.

No randomized clinical trials to support the WHO fluid resuscitation recommendations could be identified. Fluid bolus therapy, and liberal fluid management more in general, was a risk factor for respiratory distress in a large prospective observational study in Latin American and Asian patients with dengue [28]. A large prospective observational study in 1719 Vietnamese children with laboratory-confirmed dengue shock syndrome practiced an initial fluid regimen of Ringer's lactate solution at 25 mL/kg over 2 h, with colloid solutions reserved for children presenting with decompensated shock [29]. The observed case fatality rate with this approach was 8/1719 children (0.5%).

We *recommend* to follow the current WHO guidelines on fluid management in severe dengue/dengue shock syndrome (1C). We *recommend* that rapid (<30 min) administration of large (>15 mL/kg) fluid boluses should be avoided, unless the patient is hypotensive (1D).

There are several randomized clinical trials comparing crystalloid with colloid fluid management for the treatment of patients with severe dengue and compensated shock. In a Vietnamese trial, 383 children with moderately severe dengue shock syndrome were randomized to fluid therapy with either Ringer's lactate, 6% dextrose, or 6% hydroxyethyl starch in a 1:1:1 ratio [30]. The need for rescue resuscitation with a colloid or the proportion of children with shock recurrence (which carries a worse prognosis) was similar between treatment arms. An additional two other randomized trials did not show better outcome parameters with (more expensive) colloids over crystalloid fluids [31, 32]. A quasi-randomized study from the Philippines with alternate allocation of starch versus crystalloid fluids also did not show an additional benefit of colloid therapy [33].

We *recommend* that in dengue patients with compensated shock, colloids are not used for initial resuscitation (1A). There is insufficient evidence to recommend fluid choice in severe dengue with hypotensive shock, but there is discussion among experts whether there is a role for colloids in severe dengue patients with hypotension, given the prominent role of capillary leak it its pathogenesis. Since current evidence strongly suggests that all hydroxyethyl starches (HES) increase the risk of acute kidney injury and renal replacement therapy [34], we *suggest* not to use HES for fluid resuscitation in patients with severe dengue (ungraded).

9.6 Use of Corticosteroids in Severe Dengue

Both humoral and cellular immune responses are thought to be implicated in the pathogenesis of vasculopathy, which is central in the pathogenesis of dengue shock syndrome [35]. The risk for developing severe disease is increased in secondary heterotypic infections, in which antibody-dependent enhancement (ADE) of infection and cross-reactive memory T cells are thought to play a role. These insights have led to the use of immunomodulatory therapy with corticosteroids in severe dengue infection.

A Cochrane review on patients with dengue shock syndrome identified four randomized or quasi-randomized trials comparing corticosteroids with no corticosteroids or placebo involving 284 participants with dengue shock syndrome [36]. Corticosteroids did not reduce the number of deaths (RR 0.68, 95% CI 0.42–1.11; 284 participants, 4 trials), the need for blood transfusion (RR 1.08, 0.52–2.24; 89 participants, 2 trials), or the number of serious complications (convulsions and pulmonary hemorrhage, 1 trial). The evidence was rated low quality as most studies were underpowered or lacked stringent randomization or allocation concealment. Corticosteroids were administered after the onset of shock. A more recent Vietnamese randomized trial in 225 children with dengue fever evaluated early oral prednisolone therapy (2 mg/kg versus 0.5 mg/kg versus placebo for 3 days) [37]. The use of oral prednisolone was not associated with prolongation of viremia and was considered safe. However, no reduction in the development of dengue shock syndrome or other complications was observed with early prednisolone therapy, although the trial was not sufficiently powered to assess efficacy. An additional analysis of the same trial focusing on immunological endpoints did not show an important attenuation of the host immune response with prednisolone treatment [38]. An additional Cochrane review of trials on the early use of corticosteroids in patients with dengue fever identified four studies (including the study discussed above), enrolling a total of 664 children and adults, showing no benefit of corticosteroids regarding mortality or dengue complications, although the evidence was considered low to very low quality [39].

With the current level of evidence, the use of corticosteroids is not recommended in the treatment of severe dengue (1B).

9.7 Preventive Platelet Transfusion in Patients with Severe Dengue

Bleeding is a feared complication of severe dengue infection. Thrombocytopenia with a thrombocytopathy is invariably present in patients with severe dengue infection. However, vasculopathy is a central and important additional contributor to the bleeding risk [3]. Prophylactic transfusion of platelets is a common practice in dengue-endemic countries [40]. Platelet transfusion is not without risks, since it can cause allergic reactions and transmission of blood-borne pathogens.

An open-label randomized study in 87 patients with dengue and a platelet count below 30,000/μL did not show decreased incidence of severe bleeding with prophylactic platelet transfusion [41]. A non-randomized Singaporean study in 256 dengue patients with thrombocytopenia <20,000/μL, of whom 188 were given prophylactic platelet transfusion, also did not show decreased bleeding episodes in the treatment group [42]. An observational study from Martinique during a dengue outbreak evaluated a conservative strategy to prophylactic platelet transfusion (only if platelets count <5000/μL, or in case of additional risk factors). A poor correlation between thrombocytopenia and the occurrence of severe bleeding during admission was observed, and the followed conservative transfusion strategy was considered safe [43]. The WHO guidelines do not recommend prophylactic platelet transfusion in severe dengue. The results of the Adult Dengue Platelet Study (ADEPT, ClinicalTrials.gov: NCT01030211), a prospective randomized open-label trial to examine the safety and efficacy of prophylactic platelet transfusion in Singaporean adults with severe dengue-related thrombocytopenia (platelet count below 20,000/μL but no bleeding), are pending. In resource-limited settings, the availability of safe pathogens vs. screened blood products can be limited, and platelet transfusion can have important cost implications, supporting restrictive use of platelet transfusion.

We do *not recommend* platelet transfusion for thrombocytopenia in the absence of active bleeding complications or other risk factors such as the use of anticoagulants, existing hemorrhagic diathesis, uncontrolled arterial hypertension, recent stroke, head trauma or surgery (1C). In case of bleeding complications, we *suggest* transfusion of fresh-frozen plasma (or cryoprecipitate) and platelet concentrate (ungraded).

9.8 Conclusions

Although most recommendations in the SSC guidelines are also applicable for the management of severe malaria and severe dengue, there are some important exceptions, in particular regarding fluid management.

References

1. Dellinger RP, Levy MM, Rhodes A, Annane D, Gerlach H, Opal SM, Sevransky JE, Sprung CL, Douglas IS, Jaeschke R, Osborn TM, Nunnally ME, Townsend SR, Reinhart K, Kleinpell RM, Angus DC, Deutschman CS, Machado FR, Rubenfeld GD, Webb S, Beale RJ, Vincent JL, Moreno R. Surviving Sepsis Campaign: international guidelines for management of severe sepsis and septic shock, 2012. Intensive Care Med. 2013;39:165–228.
2. WHO. Dengue: guidelines for treatment, prev control. In: Book dengue: guidelines for treatment, prev control. Geneva: World Health Organization; 2009.
3. Simmons CP, Farrar JJ, Nguyen v V, Wills B. Dengue. N Engl J Med. 2012;366:1423–32.

4. Yacoub S, Lang HJ, Shebbe M, Timbwa M, Ohuma E, Tulloh R, Maitland K. Cardiac function and hemodynamics in Kenyan children with severe malaria. Crit Care Med. 2010;38:940–5.
5. Maitland K, Levin M, English M, Mithwani S, Peshu N, Marsh K, Newton CR. Severe P. falciparum malaria in Kenyan children: evidence for hypovolaemia. QJM. 2003;96:427–34.
6. Hanson JP, Lam SW, Mohanty S, Alam S, Pattnaik R, Mahanta KC, Hasan MU, Charunwatthana P, Mishra SK, Day NP, White NJ, Dondorp AM. Fluid resuscitation of adults with severe falciparum malaria: effects on acid-base status, renal function, and extravascular lung water. Crit Care Med. 2013;41:972–81.
7. Planche T, Onanga M, Schwenk A, Dzeing A, Borrmann S, Faucher JF, Wright A, Bluck L, Ward L, Kombila M, Kremsner PG, Krishna S. Assessment of volume depletion in children with malaria. PLoS Med. 2004;1:e18.
8. Maitland K, Pamba A, English M, Peshu N, Levin M, Marsh K, Newton CR. Pre-transfusion management of children with severe malarial anaemia: a randomised controlled trial of intravascular volume expansion. Br J Haematol. 2005;128:393–400.
9. Maitland K, Pamba A, English M, Peshu N, Marsh K, Newton C, Levin M. Randomized trial of volume expansion with albumin or saline in children with severe malaria: preliminary evidence of albumin benefit. Clin Infect Dis. 2005;40:538–45.
10. Akech S, Gwer S, Idro R, Fegan G, Eziefula AC, Newton CR, Levin M, Maitland K. Volume expansion with albumin compared to gelofusine in children with severe malaria: results of a controlled trial. PLoS Clin Trials. 2006;1:e21.
11. Maitland K, Pamba A, Newton CR, Levin M. Response to volume resuscitation in children with severe malaria. Pediatr Crit Care Med. 2003;4:426–31.
12. Akech S, Ledermann H, Maitland K. Choice of fluids for resuscitation in children with severe infection and shock: systematic review. BMJ. 2010;341:c4416.
13. Maitland K, Kiguli S, Opoka RO, Engoru C, Olupot-Olupot P, Akech SO, Nyeko R, Mtove G, Reyburn H, Lang T, Brent B, Evans JA, Tibenderana JK, Crawley J, Russell EC, Levin M, Babiker AG, Gibb DM. Mortality after fluid bolus in African children with severe infection. N Engl J Med. 2011;364:2483–95.
14. Nguyen HP, Hanson J, Bethell D, Nguyen TH, Tran TH, Ly VC, Pham PL, Dinh XS, Dondorp A, White N, Day N. A retrospective analysis of the haemodynamic and metabolic effects of fluid resuscitation in Vietnamese adults with severe falciparum malaria. PLoS One. 2011;6:e25523.
15. Hanson J. Fluid resuscitation of adults with severe falciparum malaria: effects on acid-base status, renal function, and extravascular lung water. Crit Care Med. 2013;41(4):972–81.
16. Aung NM, Kaung M, Kyi TT, Kyaw MP, Min M, Htet ZW, Anstey NM, Kyi MM, Hanson J. The safety of a conservative fluid replacement strategy in adults hospitalised with malaria. PLoS One. 2015;10:e0143062.
17. Hodgson SH, Angus BJ. Malaria: fluid therapy in severe disease. BMJ Clin Evid. 2016;2016:pii: 0913.
18. WHO. Severe malaria. Tropical Med Int Health. 2014;19:7–131.
19. Berkley JA, Bejon P, Mwangi T, Gwer S, Maitland K, Williams TN, Mohammed S, Osier F, Kinyanjui S, Fegan G, Lowe BS, English M, Peshu N, Marsh K, Newton CR. HIV infection, malnutrition, and invasive bacterial infection among children with severe malaria. Clin Infect Dis. 2009;49:336–43.
20. Maude RJ, Hoque G, Hasan MU, Sayeed A, Akter S, Samad R, Alam B, Yunus EB, Rahman R, Rahman W, Chowdhury R, Seal T, Charunwatthana P, Chang CC, White NJ, Faiz MA, Day NP, Dondorp AM, Hossain A. Timing of enteral feeding in cerebral malaria in resource-poor settings: a randomized trial. PLoS One. 2011;6:e27273.
21. White NJ, Pukrittayakamee S, Hien TT, Faiz MA, Mokuolu OA, Dondorp AM. Malaria. Lancet. 2014;383:723–35.
22. Taylor WR, Hanson J, Turner GD, White NJ, Dondorp AM. Respiratory manifestations of malaria. Chest. 2012;142:492–505.

23. Warrell DA, Looareesuwan S, Phillips RE, White NJ, Warrell MJ, Chapel HM, Areekul S, Tharavanij S. Function of the blood-cerebrospinal fluid barrier in human cerebral malaria: rejection of the permeability hypothesis. Am J Trop Med Hyg. 1986;35:882–9.
24. Brown H, Rogerson S, Taylor T, Tembo M, Mwenechanya J, Molyneux M, Turner G. Blood-brain barrier function in cerebral malaria in Malawian children. Am J Trop Med Hyg. 2001;64:207–13.
25. Mohanty S, Mishra SK, Patnaik R, Dutt AK, Pradhan S, Das B, Patnaik J, Mohanty AK, Lee SJ, Dondorp AM. Brain swelling and mannitol therapy in adult cerebral malaria: a randomized trial. Clin Infect Dis. 2011;53:349–55.
26. Seydel KB, Kampondeni SD, Valim C, Potchen MJ, Milner DA, Muwalo FW, Birbeck GL, Bradley WG, Fox LL, Glover SJ, Hammond CA, Heyderman RS, Chilingulo CA, Molyneux ME, Taylor TE. Brain swelling and death in children with cerebral malaria. N Engl J Med. 2015;372:1126–37.
27. WHO. Handbook for clinical management of dengue. Geneva: WHO; 2012.
28. Rosenberger KD, Lum L, Alexander N, Junghanss T, Wills B, Jaenisch T. Vascular leakage in dengue—clinical spectrum and influence of parenteral fluid therapy. Tropical Med Int Health. 2016;21:445–53.
29. Lam PK, Tam DT, Diet TV, Tam CT, Tien NT, Kieu NT, Simmons C, Farrar J, Nga NT, Qui PT, Dung NM, Wolbers M, Wills B. Clinical characteristics of Dengue shock syndrome in Vietnamese children: a 10-year prospective study in a single hospital. Clin Infect Dis. 2013;57:1577–86.
30. Wills BA, Nguyen MD, Ha TL, Dong TH, Tran TN, Le TT, Tran VD, Nguyen TH, Nguyen VC, Stepniewska K, White NJ, Farrar JJ. Comparison of three fluid solutions for resuscitation in dengue shock syndrome. N Engl J Med. 2005;353:877–89.
31. Dung NM, Day NP, Tam DT, Loan HT, Chau HT, Minh LN, Diet TV, Bethell DB, Kneen R, Hien TT, White NJ, Farrar JJ. Fluid replacement in dengue shock syndrome: a randomized, double-blind comparison of four intravenous-fluid regimens. Clin Infect Dis. 1999;29:787–94.
32. Ngo NT, Cao XT, Kneen R, Wills B, Nguyen VM, Nguyen TQ, Chu VT, Nguyen TT, Simpson JA, Solomon T, White NJ, Farrar J. Acute management of dengue shock syndrome: a randomized double-blind comparison of 4 intravenous fluid regimens in the first hour. Clin Infect Dis. 2001;32:204–13.
33. Cifra HL, Velasco NJJ. A comparative study of the efficacy of 6% Haes-Steril and Ringer's lactate in the management of dengue shock syndrome. Crit Care Shock. 2003;6:95–100.
34. Mutter TC, Ruth CA, Dart AB. Hydroxyethyl starch (HES) versus other fluid therapies: effects on kidney function. Cochrane Database Syst Rev. 2013:CD007594.
35. Simmons CP, McPherson K, Van Vinh Chau N, Hoai Tam DT, Young P, Mackenzie J, Wills B. Recent advances in dengue pathogenesis and clinical management. Vaccine. 2015;33:7061–8.
36. Panpanich R, Sornchai P, Kanjanaratanakorn K. Corticosteroids for treating dengue shock syndrome. Cochrane Database Syst Rev. 2006:CD003488.
37. Tam DT, Ngoc TV, Tien NT, Kieu NT, Thuy TT, Thanh LT, Tam CT, Truong NT, Dung NT, Qui PT, Hien TT, Farrar JJ, Simmons CP, Wolbers M, Wills BA. Effects of short-course oral corticosteroid therapy in early dengue infection in Vietnamese patients: a randomized, placebo-controlled trial. Clin Infect Dis. 2012;55:1216–24.
38. Nguyen TH, Vu TT, Farrar J, Hoang TL, Dong TH, Ngoc Tran V, Phung KL, Wolbers M, Whitehead SS, Hibberd ML, Wills B, Simmons CP. Corticosteroids for dengue—why don't they work? PLoS Negl Trop Dis. 2013;7:e2592.
39. Zhang F, Kramer CV. Corticosteroids for dengue infection. Cochrane Database Syst Rev. 2014:CD003488.
40. Whitehorn J, Rodriguez Roche R, Guzman MG, Martinez E, Gomez WV, Nainggolan L, Laksono IS, Mishra A, Lum L, Faiz A, Sall A, Dawurung J, Borges A, Leo YS, Blumberg L, Bausch DG, Kroeger A, Horstick O, Thwaites G, Wertheim H, Larsson M, Hien TT, Peeling R, Wills B, Simmons C, Farrar J. Prophylactic platelets in dengue: survey responses highlight lack of an evidence base. PLoS Negl Trop Dis. 2012;6:e1716.

41. Khan Assir MZ, Kamran U, Ahmad HI, Bashir S, Mansoor H, Anees SB, Akram J. Effectiveness of platelet transfusion in dengue fever: a randomized controlled trial. Transfus Med Hemother. 2013;40:362–8.
42. Lye DC, Lee VJ, Sun Y, Leo YS. Lack of efficacy of prophylactic platelet transfusion for severe thrombocytopenia in adults with acute uncomplicated dengue infection. Clin Infect Dis. 2009;48:1262–5.
43. Thomas L, Kaidomar S, Kerob-Bauchet B, Moravie V, Brouste Y, King JP, Schmitt S, Besnier F, Abel S, Mehdaoui H, Plumelle Y, Najioullah F, Fonteau C, Richard P, Cesaire R, Cabie A. Prospective observational study of low thresholds for platelet transfusion in adult dengue patients. Transfusion. 2009;49:1400–11.

Open Access This chapter is licensed under the terms of the Creative Commons Attribution 4.0 International License (http://creativecommons.org/licenses/by/4.0/), which permits use, sharing, adaptation, distribution and reproduction in any medium or format, as long as you give appropriate credit to the original author(s) and the source, provide a link to the Creative Commons license and indicate if changes were made.

The images or other third party material in this chapter are included in the chapter's Creative Commons license, unless indicated otherwise in a credit line to the material. If material is not included in the chapter's Creative Commons license and your intended use is not permitted by statutory regulation or exceeds the permitted use, you will need to obtain permission directly from the copyright holder.

Pediatric Sepsis and Septic Shock Management in Resource-Limited Settings

10

Ndidiamaka Musa, Srinivas Murthy, Niranjan Kissoon, Rakesh Lodha, and Suchitra Ranjit

10.1 Introduction

Infectious diseases leading to septic shock remain a major cause of childhood mortality around the globe [1, 2]. Recommendations in the Surviving Sepsis Campaign (SSC) guidelines for pediatric patients rely on evidence from resource-rich settings [3]. However, recommendations are context dependent, and published guidelines deriving evidence primarily from resource-rich settings may be less relevant in areas where resources are minimal and the epidemiology is very different, given the differences in infection-related mortality between regions. Thus, recommendations for the treatment of septic shock in children in intensive care units (ICUs) in resource-limited settings are sorely needed.

There is no standardized definition of an ICU, but for the purposes of these recommendations, we are focusing on referral hospitals with the capability to intensively monitor critically ill children, ideally with the availability of some form of mechanical ventilation [4]. These ICUs may not exclusively care for children and are likely staffed by a variety of care providers, within a context of a resource-limited health system. The need for these recommendations is underlined by the surprising results from one large randomized controlled trial on fluid therapy in

N. Musa
Seattle Children's Hospital, University of Washington, Seattle, WA, USA

S. Murthy (✉) · N. Kissoon
BC Children's Hospital, University of British Columbia, Vancouver, BC, Canada

R. Lodha
All India Institute of Medical Sciences, New Delhi, India

S. Ranjit
Apollo Hospital, Chennai, India

© The Author(s) 2019

A. M. Dondorp et al. (eds.), *Sepsis Management in Resource-limited Settings*,
https://doi.org/10.1007/978-3-030-03143-5_10

African children [5], at least suggesting that not all evidence for benefit from certain interventions in resource-rich settings guarantees equal benefit in resource-limited settings. The World Health Organization (WHO) issues guidelines on emergency triage and treatment, which these recommendations aim to supplement by addressing ICU-specific contexts.

We provide a set of simple, readily available, and affordable recommendations based on management of pediatric patients with severe sepsis and septic shock in resource-limited settings. Recommendations and suggestions are summarized in Table 10.1.

Table 10.1 Recommendations and suggestions on pediatric sepsis or septic shock management in resource-limited settings (with grading)

1	Identification	Observe for a combination of danger signs of end-organ dysfunction and including lactic acid levels if affordable and available (1C)
2	Intraosseous access	Placement of an intraosseous line must be considered for vascular access after 3–5 min of intravenous access attempts (2B)
3	Resuscitation of malnourished children	Children with severe acute malnutrition without signs of severe shock should not receive rapid intravenous fluids as bolus therapy (2C); children with severe acute malnutrition and signs of septic shock have high levels of mortality, and we suggest that they should be given intravenous rehydration with either half-strength Darrow's solution with 5% dextrose or Ringer's lactate solution with 5% dextrose at a rate of 10–15 ml/kg/hour with avoidance of rapid bolus therapy (2C)
4	Bolus fluid resuscitation	Use a careful but foremost individualized approach to fluid administration in children with sepsis in resource-poor settings (1B); for those who do not have evidence for severely impaired circulation, administer maintenance fluids only (1B)—for those who do have evidence of severely impaired circulation, very carefully administer 10–20 mL/kg of crystalloids over 30 minutes, which may be repeated if there are no signs of improvement and no signs of fluid overload (2C)
5	Goal-directed fluid resuscitation	No recommendation can be made regarding incorporating early goal-directed therapy for children with septic shock in resource-limited ICUs, specifically pertaining to using central venous oxygen saturation, lactate, or central venous pressure to guide resuscitation (UG); incorporate quality assurance protocols for timely antibiotic administration, oxygen and respiratory support, and fluid management protocols into resource-limited settings for the management of pediatric sepsis (1D)
6	Transfusion in severe malaria and sepsis	Transfuse children with severe anemia and malaria only if there are signs of severe sepsis such as respiratory distress or shock (1C); transfuse children with severe anemia (hemoglobin level < 4 g/dL) (1D); there is no evidence to support a specific transfusion threshold for children with anemia and sepsis in resource-limited settings
7	Noninvasive ventilation	Children with severe respiratory distress and hypoxemia from sepsis related to pneumonia benefit from bubble CPAP (1B)
8	Low tidal volume ventilation	Use a tidal volume of 5 to 8 mL/kg predicted body weight in all mechanically ventilated children with sepsis-induced acute lung injury in resource-limited settings (1D)

10.2 Identification of Septic Shock in Children

The burden of septic shock in children admitted to ICUs in resource-limited settings is undoubtedly large, though difficult to define. The International Consensus Conference on Pediatric Sepsis [3] defines sepsis as the systemic inflammatory response syndrome (SIRS) plus suspected or proven infection, while septic shock incorporates cardiovascular dysfunction leading to hypotension. New adult definitions have yet to be validated in children or in low-resource settings [4]. From a clinician's viewpoint, a diagnosis of septic shock recognizes that children who die from infections, regardless of their source, develop various combinations of cardiac failure, acute respiratory distress syndrome, or other organ dysfunction. Indeed, the largest clinical trial of children with severe febrile illness and impaired perfusion in sub-Saharan Africa supports this contention, where the major cause of death in this population is cardiovascular collapse [5, 6]. It may be possible to identify children with septic shock, regardless of underlying etiology, relatively early in ICUs, where intensive monitoring is available and mechanical ventilation possible. Recognizing this complex syndrome (septic shock) rather than focusing on a single disease entity, i.e., pneumonia or diarrhea may be important, given that interventions must often be performed before a definitive diagnosis is available [7–11]. The WHO uses this approach by highlighting danger signs and therapies rather than individual diseases through their emergency triage and treatment (ETAT) [12]. Emergency signs of shock or severely impaired circulation, as outlined by ETAT, include cold extremities, weak pulse volume, and prolonged capillary refill, with a definition of shock constituting having *all* three of the above. These recommendations are supplemental to existing guidelines such as ETAT on the identification of severely ill children and are restricted to the context of intensive care units, where advanced monitoring is feasible.

A large number of studies examined various clinical tools in various settings in determining outcomes of children with severe infections in low-resource settings. The accuracy of International Consensus Conference definitions or other alternate definitions has not been prospectively validated in ICUs in resource-limited settings. A systematic review of sepsis definitions focusing upon low-resource settings in children was identified. Using data from the FEAST trial [13], the presence of a weak pulse, prolonged capillary refill time, a temperature gradient, and coma were all significantly associated with a higher rate of mortality in this large population with sepsis. Prolonged capillary refill time has been shown to be a predictor of outcomes in severely ill children with infection in other high- and low-resource settings, [13, 16–18], although poor inter-rater variability and reproducibility render its clinical utility by inexperienced clinicians suspect [19–22]. Weak pulse volume, declining mental status, and hypothermia are also all associated with worse outcomes in children with severe infections [13, 23–26]. Hypoxemia, as measured by pulse oximetry, is a consistent predictor of outcome in severely ill children with infections, though not consistently associated with elevated mortality [14, 15, 27, 28]. Also, consistent across the studies in low-middle-income countries is the role of lactate in predicting likelihood of mortality in children with severe infections

[16, 29–32]. The recent creation of a bedside clinical risk score, FEAST PET, for triage and identification of severely ill children in resource-limited settings shows great promise [13]. The role of the WHO criteria in defining shock, as outlined above, is unclear, given a relatively low incidence among studied cohorts in emergency room populations [5, 33, 34], and likely bears little relevance within any ICU context where more intensive monitoring is available.

The systematic review of definitions documented accuracy of modified definitions of SIRS and international consensus criteria, which deserves further validation in larger cohorts and vital sign changes with age [35–37]. An observational study of children in resource-limited ICUs to develop a score for early identification of children with nosocomial infections shows great promise [38]. Sepsis screening tools for inpatients using chart abstraction or electronic health record data have been used successfully in resource-rich contexts but are likely not feasible in resource-limited settings [39, 40].

The use of clinical skills, incorporating historical findings of poor feeding and declining mental status and physical findings of weak pulse volume, prolonged capillary refill time, and temperature abnormalities, can identify most patients with septic shock and can be easily taught in any context. Pulse oximetry is becoming more available and feasible, with low-cost devices being disseminated; given the prevalence of pneumonia, this could hold great use for further management and research, limiting the need for expensive blood-gas analysis. Point-of-care lactic acid determination is becoming more prevalent in all health settings and should be further studied as a management guide for severe sepsis in resource-limited settings. Emergency triage and treatment protocols from the World Health Organization have been disseminated widely in low-income settings for the identification of shock.

We recommend that severely ill children with signs of infection be identified by observing for a combination of danger signs of end-organ dysfunction, including lactic acid levels (1C). More studies are urgently required to determine accuracy of definitions and scoring systems for septic shock identification and mortality prediction in ICUs in resource-limited settings.

10.3 Intraosseous Access as Initial Vascular Access in Septic Children

Rapid vascular access is critical and usually a rate-limiting step in the resuscitation of children in shock. The International Liaison Committee on Resuscitation has recommended the placement of an intraosseous access if vascular access cannot be achieved in a timely manner [41]. Vascular access facilitates intravascular volume replacement as well as early antimicrobial administration, with a delay in rapid administration of antibiotics associated with higher mortality in critically ill adults as well as children [42, 43]. Intraosseous access is a rapid and safe alternative to peripheral and central venous access when time is of the essence [44]. Children in resource-limited settings sometimes present late in shock when peripheral veins may not be visible due to vascular collapse, thus making intravenous access challenging and time-consuming. In these settings, a rapidly placed intraosseous line can be lifesaving.

A search of the medical literature resulted in one clinical trial from India, a case series from Northern Iraq, and two systematic reviews. The clinical trial compared intraosseous and intravenous access in severely dehydrated children with hypovolemic shock from gastroenteritis [45]. Sixty children with severe dehydration according to WHO classification received 30 mL/kg of normal saline by either intravenous or intraosseous routes assigned alternately, followed by identical protocols regarding the reintroduction of oral fluids. The primary end point was time to placement, with secondary end points including stabilization of vital signs, correction of dehydration, and complications. There was no difference in efficacy of rehydration or correction of laboratory abnormalities between groups. Intraosseous placement was significantly faster (67 vs 129 s) and more reliable, with a 33% failure rate in intravenous placement and no failures in intraosseous placement at 5 min. There were no short-term complications, but long-term follow-up was not included. The study was not specific to sepsis, but it was context specific addressing intraosseous use in shock in LMICs.

The case series documented experiences with alternate modes of vascular access in dehydrated children at a military hospital in Iraq [46]. Intraosseous access was effective and timely in this context.

A systematic review addressed intraosseous access as an alternative route for rehydration in resource-limited settings by reviewing 16 articles: 1 clinical trial (described above), 12 case reports, and 3 case series [47]. Conclusions from this systematic review indicated that intraosseous access was easy to obtain and effective in rehydration and medication administration. A Cochrane review included the study from India as discussed above [45, 48]. This review looked at the comparison of routes for achieving parenteral access, with a focus on the management of patients with Ebola virus disease. The authors concluded that quality of the evidence based on GRADE criteria is limited because of lack of adequately powered trials [48]. All of these studies are downgraded for indirectness to children with septic shock and for bias.

All of the studies described above reported that the use of the intraosseous route was safe and associated with no major adverse events. Successful use of the intraosseous route relies on an initial outlay of resources for the device and training for placement. Intraosseous needles are inexpensive and can be readily available in appropriate settings. Non-disposable needles are available and can be sterilized and reused and hence further reduce their costs.

We suggest that in severely ill children with sepsis in resource-limited settings, the placement of an intraosseous line can be considered for vascular access after 3–5 min of intravenous access attempts (2B). Further studies are required to document its role in resource-limited settings, including maintaining training of practitioners.

10.4 Bolus Fluids or Blood to Malnourished Children with Signs of Severe Sepsis

Undernutrition is a major contributor to childhood mortality worldwide and renders children more vulnerable to contract infections as well as more commonly to suffer from severe sepsis and septic shock. The risk of overhydration in malnourished children leading to interstitial, pulmonary, and cerebral edema has resulted in recommendations of cautious fluid administration in modest amounts. Additionally, recommendations have favored hypotonic fluid administration and limiting sodium intake because of the concern of precipitating heart failure, under the premise that malnourished children, especially those with pitting edema, are sodium overloaded. The most recent guidelines from the WHO state that children with severe acute malnutrition should receive slow infusions of intravenous fluids at 15 mL/kg/h only in the setting of shock with one of half-strength Darrow's, Ringer's lactate, or half-normal saline, with 5% dextrose added to each [49]. WHO guidelines state that blood should be administered with similar indications for anemia due to malaria or if there is a failure to improve after 1 h of intravenous therapy [12].

Nine observational studies [26, 50–57], one randomized controlled trial [58], and a systematic review [59] were included in the final review. There were no randomized trials examining transfusion or fluids versus none in severely malnourished children with septic shock. Observational studies were of moderate quality and described clinical practice with transfusions and fluid administration. The one randomized trial that was identified compared half-strength Darrow's to Ringer's lactate solution in malnourished children with shock. The observational studies and the systematic review are consistent in describing that malnourished children who do not have signs of shock (of varying definitions) or do not have severe anemia should not receive intravenous fluids or blood which is associated with increased mortality in this group. This approach, however, must be tempered by the large risk of substantial selection bias in these studies. The randomized trial comparing half-strength Darrow's with 5% dextrose versus Ringer's lactate was stopped due to high levels of baseline mortality (51%) and inadequate correction of shock in all study arms, revealing no significant harm from isotonic fluid administration, compared to hypotonic fluids. A randomized trial looking at composition of an oral rehydration solution in children with severe malnourishment, severe dehydration, and cholera documented no adverse events from 100 mL/kg of intravenous fluid over 4–6 h [56]. There are no comparative data for blood transfusion thresholds or indications for this population.

Intravenous fluids are typically available in resource-limited settings; however, half-strength Darrow's is often unavailable in many regions. Blood is often unavailable or not readily accessible in many of these settings.

Based upon the available evidence, we suggest that children with severe acute malnutrition without signs of impaired circulation not receive rapid intravenous fluids as bolus therapy (2C). Children with severe acute malnutrition and signs of septic shock have high levels of mortality, and we suggest that they should be given intravenous rehydration with either half-strength Darrow's solution with 5%

dextrose or Ringer's lactate solution with 5% dextrose at a rate of 15 mL/kg/h, as per the WHO recommendations (2C). There is no evidence to support a specific blood transfusion threshold in this population, with consensus guidelines suggesting transfusion if the hemoglobin level is <4 g/dL or <6 g/dL in patients with signs of shock.

10.5 Bolus Fluid Resuscitation with 5% Albumin or Normal Saline, Compared to No Bolus Fluids, in Pediatric Sepsis

The major physiological abnormality in shock is hypovolemia, either due to fluid loss as in dehydration and hemorrhage (absolute hypovolemia) or due to redistribution of fluids as seen with capillary leaks in severe sepsis and septic shock (relative hypovolemia). This results in impaired cardiac filling, tissue perfusion, and oxygen delivery to the vital organs. Early intravascular fluid infusion to correct hypovolemia should improve this physiologic state, in principle. Fluid boluses include rapid administration of isotonic or colloid solutions; however, there is no clear consensus on whether to use crystalloids or colloids in early fluid resuscitation. In critically ill adults in high-income settings, outcome is largely dependent on the quantity rather than type of fluids used in the first hour [60]. The approach that is widely endorsed in pediatric life support training programs is to administer bolus resuscitation preferably within the first 15 min of diagnosing shock [61, 62]. As per these guidelines, rapid fluid boluses of 10–20 mL/kg should be administered, observing for improvement in perfusion as well as for markers of fluid overload—the development of rales, hepatomegaly, and increased work of breathing. Up to 60 mL/kg may be administered in the first hour, with a 2C recommendation per the Surviving Sepsis Campaign guidelines; however, no clear agreement exists supporting the present practice. The WHO advocates exercising caution in aggressive fluid administration, especially in children with shock in resource-limited conditions [12, 63].

We could identify only two randomized controlled trials that compared different rates of fluid administration in the first hour in children presenting with impaired circulation and were potentially relevant to these recommendations. After further screening, one trial had to be excluded as there was no comparator arm receiving maintenance fluid only or maintenance fluids plus a small bolus [64]. There were two recently published systematic reviews, which have data mostly derived from the one large randomized controlled trial [65, 66].

Only one study—the Fluid Expansion as Supportive Therapy (FEAST Trial)—compared bolus with maintenance fluid alone [5]. We also identified articles reporting the subgroup analysis of the data from this trial [6, 67]. In this randomized controlled trial performed in Uganda, Kenya, and Tanzania (n = 3141), children with severe febrile illness *and* clinical evidence of impaired perfusion (one or more of the following—capillary refill >2 s, lower limb temperature gradient, weak pulse volume, severe tachycardia) were randomized to fluid bolus therapy or maintenance fluids only. Major exclusion criteria were children with malnutrition and/or dehydration. The majority of children had malaria, and a third had a hemoglobin level of <5 g/dL. The 48-h mortality was 10.6%, 10.5%, and 7.3% in the albumin bolus, saline bolus, and control groups, respectively (relative risk for saline bolus vs. control, 1.44; 95% confidence interval [CI] 1.09 to 1.90; $p = 0.01$; relative risk for albumin bolus vs. saline bolus, 1.01; 95% CI 0.78 to 1.29; $p = 0.96$; and relative risk for any bolus vs. control, 1.45; 95% CI 1.13 to 1.86; $p = 0.003$). There was no difference in neurologic sequelae, pulmonary edema, or increased intracranial pressure between groups.

Interestingly, at 1 h, shock had resolved (responders) more frequently in the bolus versus the control groups (43% vs. 32%, $p < 0.001$), but excess mortality with boluses was reported in both responders (relative risk 1.98, 95% confidence interval 0.94 to 4.17, $p = 0.06$) and non-responders (relative risk 1.67, 95% confidence interval 1.23 to 2.28, $p = 0.001$). Only 65 children met the WHO criteria for shock, for which the children receiving boluses had a higher mortality than the no bolus arm [RR: 2.4; 95% CI 0.84, 6.88]. The systematic reviews largely support these findings, with the data for children with severely impaired circulation being less convincing and the data being driven primarily by the large FEAST study. Definitions for shock were variable, and determining fluid responsiveness by severity of illness was not performed.

Patients enrolled in the FEAST trial had no access to intensive care including respiratory support and ventilators. Saline is safe, inexpensive, and readily available as compared to 5% albumin, which may not be affordable in resource-poor areas. The availability of monitoring of shock with blood lactate levels, central venous pressure, central venous oxygen saturation levels, and other invasive monitoring is unavailable in the included studies.

Based upon the available evidence, we recommend a careful, individualized approach to fluid administration in children with sepsis in ICUs in resource-limited settings (1B). For those without evidence of severely impaired circulation in a resource-limited ICU, we recommend administration of maintenance fluids only (1B). For those with evidence of severely impaired circulation, we suggest very careful administration of 10–20 mL/kg of crystalloids over 30 min. This may be repeated if there are no signs of improvement and no signs of fluid overload (2C). Further studies incorporating goal-directed resuscitation in resource-limited settings are urgently required (See Sect. 10.6), as is standardization of the definitions of shock for clinical and research purposes.

10.6 Should Sepsis Management Be Guided by Goal-Directed Protocols of Care for Children in Resource-Limited Settings?

The implementation of "sepsis bundles" to enable rapid diagnosis and time-sensitive management based on protocols upon presentation has been adopted in numerous healthcare settings [68]. Diagnosis is facilitated through rapid triage and deployment of diagnostic tests, while management is ideally guided by a protocol based on local context and resources. Given the wide variability of available resources in low- and middle-income settings, there is a great need for contextual-based protocols for sepsis management for children in these settings. However evidence for generating these protocols is lacking because large randomized trials addressing the role of goal-directed protocols for sepsis management have only been studied in adults in high-income countries.

The search criteria identified a number of studies examining goal-directed sepsis protocols in children, six of which were conducted outside of high-income regions. There were two randomized controlled trials in low- and middle-income countries: one from Brazil examining early goal-directed therapy in children using central venous oxygen saturation-guided resuscitation versus usual care in children with septic shock [69] and the other from India examining different fluid protocols with early initiation of inotropic support [64]. There were three observational studies with significant bias, examining central venous oxygen saturation-guided resuscitation in children in India [70], a before-after study examining implementation of Surviving Sepsis Campaign guidelines, in India [71], and a retrospective study from Brazil examining time-to-fluid administration as it relates to clinical outcome [72]. There was also a before-after study for patient flow optimization in a Malawi hospital that included a number of children with presumed severe sepsis [73]. A worldwide quality assurance program assessed compliance with sepsis bundles in various pediatric settings [68]. There are four observational and retrospective studies examining sepsis protocols in children in high-income regions that were deemed relevant [74–77]. There are three major adult randomized trials recently published examining goal-directed therapy in adults in high-income countries, with an associated meta-analysis [78–81], one randomized study in adults in Zambia [82], and a before-after study in adults in Uganda [83]. There are no randomized studies examining goal-directed resuscitation or protocol-based sepsis care in children in high-income countries.

The randomized studies in adults with septic shock in high-income countries are consistent in showing no benefit from specific early goal-directed resuscitation protocols, when compared with usual care guided by current standards of care, but the evidence is downgraded for indirectness to our question. The randomized adult study performed in Zambia documented no difference in mortality in a management protocol guided by jugular venous pressure assessment, compared with usual care. The adult study performed in Uganda documented a 12% absolute risk reduction in mortality with early sepsis management guided by a dedicated study officer through a before-after design. Both are downgraded for indirectness to our population of interest.

The observational studies in children in high-income countries document improvement in the outcomes of duration of hospitalization, survival, and time to interventions but were downgraded for poor quality. The randomized study in Brazil revealed significant mortality benefits with early goal-directed therapy. The trial in India was downgraded for indirectness related to the question at hand. The observational studies document a mortality benefit for instituting a protocol for sepsis care for children in LMICs but were downgraded for bias. The quality assurance program documented improved survival with sepsis bundle compliance, but numbers from resource-limited settings were small.

Relevant resources including personnel, equipment, and supplies are less readily available for children in resource-limited settings as compared to adults, and hence protocols for children should be more modest in their scope and are less likely to be followed. Intuitively, it seems reasonable that early goal-directed protocols would be of benefit in guiding care in those who are unfamiliar in treating children with sepsis and septic shock. However, the availability of many of the tools for currently recommended early goal-directed protocols is poor in many LMICs [84], including monitoring capabilities such as frequent lactate monitoring and central venous oxygen saturation monitoring and management such as transfusions and inotrope administration.

Based upon the available evidence and resources, we can make no recommendation regarding incorporating early goal-directed therapy for children with septic shock in resource-limited settings, specifically pertaining to using central venous oxygen saturation, lactate, or central venous pressure to guide resuscitation. Further studies are required to determine the major differences between adults and children with regard to goal-directed resuscitation in septic shock.

We recommend incorporation of quality assurance protocols for timely antibiotic administration, oxygen and respiratory support, and fluid management protocols into resource-limited settings for the management of pediatric sepsis (1D). Resource capabilities for fluid resuscitation and monitoring should be expanded to allow for further study and implementation of resuscitation research in critically ill children admitted to resource-limited ICUs.

10.7 Is Transfusion Recommended for Children with Anemia and Sepsis Due to Severe Malaria in Resource-Limited Settings?

Severe anemia is a major contributor to child mortality worldwide. Administration of blood to children with severe anemia, malaria, and signs of severe illness such as respiratory distress or shock is essential. The balance of benefits and risks of blood transfusions is particularly important in settings where blood supply is limited. Given the risks associated with transfusion, transfusion practices must be evidence-based and associated with benefit in any setting. The current WHO recommendations suggest limiting transfusions to those with hemoglobin levels less than 4 g/dL or less than 6 g/dL with signs of severe disease [63]. However, clinical evidence for these thresholds is lacking.

The systematic search resulted in two randomized controlled trials from sub-Saharan Africa, one meta-analysis of the published randomized controlled trials, a subgroup analysis of another randomized controlled trial, and a number of observational and retrospective publications that directly or indirectly address the question.

The two randomized trials [85, 86] and the meta-analysis [87] report that there is insufficient evidence to routinely recommend giving blood to children with severe anemia due to malaria. The subgroup analysis of a large fluid resuscitation trial in children with signs of sepsis in sub-Saharan Africa documented a large burden of anemia and a significant delay in blood transfusions leading to an increased risk of associated mortality [88]. Nine observational or retrospective studies [50–52, 89–94] suggest a benefit to transfusing children with severe malaria and anemia, especially if accompanied by signs of severe sepsis such as shock and/or respiratory distress. A randomized trial of 20 mL/kg versus 30 mL/kg of blood transfused in children with severe anemia, including malaria, showed higher rates of anemia correction in the larger blood volume group [95].

We have the opinion that blood transfusions should be made more readily available for those in need. Observational and other data suggest that mortality is high in patients who meet the current WHO recommendations for receiving blood during the waiting period after recognition of the need for blood transfusion [88]. Ensuring safe and rapidly accessible blood supplies is an area of active investigation, as well as optimizing initial transfusion strategies in critically ill children in low-resource settings.

Based upon the available evidence, we recommend transfusing children with severe anemia and malaria only if there are signs of severity such as respiratory distress or shock (1C). We recommend that children with severe anemia (hemoglobin levels <4 g/dL) be transfused (1D). There is no evidence to support a specific transfusion threshold for children with severe anemia and sepsis in ICUs in resource-limited settings. Further evidence is needed to make a recommendation for children with severe anemia and malaria (hemoglobin levels <4–6 g/dL) without respiratory distress or shock.

10.8 Noninvasive Ventilation for Children with Acute Respiratory Distress from Sepsis in Resource-Limited Settings

Pneumonia is the leading cause of death in the under-five age group in resource-limited settings [96]. Reed and colleagues demonstrated that in children hospitalized with pneumonia, hypoxia and malnutrition were the strongest predictors of mortality [97]. The management of hypoxia continues to be a major challenge for clinicians in developing countries [98]. While about 10–20% of sick children will be referred to a hospital, the delay in recognition, late presentation, lack of resources, and illness severity make the first 24 h of hospitalization the most vulnerable period, with a third of patient deaths occurring during this time [73]. Improving oxygen therapy has been shown to reduce mortality from severe pneumonia in resource-limited settings [99]. However, observational studies from these settings have demonstrated that despite the provision of oxygen, antibiotics, and supportive care, case fatality rates for severe pneumonia and hypoxemia remain unacceptably high (5–15%) [100–108].

While mechanical ventilation may be of benefit in decreasing mortality, it is an expensive and complex respiratory support method that requires a high level of technical skill and maintenance for optimal benefit. Many countries do not have the funds, infrastructure, or expertise to provide such technology to all patients [109]. Therefore, noninvasive respiratory support technologies could be lifesaving in resource-limited settings.

Two randomized controlled trials were identified in children looking at the use of continuous positive airway pressure (CPAP) in children in resource-limited settings [110, 111]. There were three observational studies [112–114] and a systematic review primarily looking at neonates [109].

A randomized controlled trial in Bangladesh examined the role of bubble CPAP for children with severe pneumonia and hypoxemia. This open-label trial enrolled children under 5 years with severe pneumonia and hypoxemia to receive oxygen therapy by either bubble CPAP (5 L/min starting at a CPAP level of 5 cm H_2O), standard low-flow nasal cannula (2 L/min), or high-flow nasal cannula (2 L/kg per min up to the maximum of 12 L/min). The trial was stopped early for higher mortality in the low-flow oxygen group. For the composite primary outcome of treatment failure, the study concluded that bubble CPAP improved outcomes when compared with the low-flow group (RR 0.27, 99.7% CI 0.07–0.99: $p = 0.026$). There was no statistically significant difference between the bubble CPAP and high-flow nasal cannula group for the primary outcome (RR 0.50, 99.7% CI 0.11–2.29, $p = 0.175$). A randomized controlled trial in Ghana compared early CPAP for children with respiratory distress to delayed CPAP, documenting an improvement in the primary outcome of improved respiratory rate [111]. Two observational study in Malawi reported both improved respiratory physiology with the use of bubble CPAP in children up to age 14 years and a 70% survival in all children treated with bubble CPAP, with a strong ease of use reported [112, 114]. An observational study in India reported a decreased rate of need for intubation, compared with children started on nasal prong oxygen [113].

The systematic review study examining the efficacy and safety of bubble CPAP primarily in premature infants in LMICs included 19 studies. The three randomized controlled trials revealed a reduced need of mechanical ventilation of 30–50% for bubble CPAP compared with oxygen therapy, which was downgraded for indirectness to population.

Bubble CPAP is a relatively low-cost device, especially when compared with invasive mechanical ventilation. Its availability is increasing, with novel devices and strategies in place in various regions of the world. Training and device management are minimal for its dissemination, with minimal ICU staffing present in the documented studies. No significant safety issues from bubble CPAP are documented. Upper limits for age of bubble CPAP are unclear, with the previously mentioned study from Malawi documenting decreasing mask tolerance as age increases. Ventilator CPAP is available in certain ICUs in resource-limited settings and can be used as an alternative, where available. High-flow nasal cannulas are an increasingly used option in resource-rich settings, with limited studies in resource-limited settings currently available. The oxygen requirement for high-flow nasal cannula is often greater than with bubble CPAP, which may be a limitation in some settings. The recent ETAT guidelines review the full evidence for high-flow nasal cannula in resource-limited settings [12].

Based on the available evidence, we recommend that children with severe respiratory distress and hypoxemia from sepsis related to pneumonia benefit from bubble CPAP in resource-limited settings (1B). Further research needs to clarify upper age limits for effectiveness of bubble CPAP and the role of humidified high-flow nasal cannula.

10.9 Should Low Tidal Volume Ventilation Be Recommended for Children with Acute Lung Injury from Sepsis in Resource-Limited ICUs?

The data for the use of low tidal volumes (4–6 mL/kg) in children with acute lung injury have been extrapolated from adult data and adapted to children in resource-rich settings. There are no randomized controlled trials in children to date comparing low tidal volumes (4–6 mL/kg) to high tidal volumes (12 mL/kg). The Pediatric Acute Lung Injury Mechanical Ventilation (PALIVE) study demonstrated that children were generally ventilated with a mean tidal volume of 8 mL/kg in resource-rich settings [115]. Current guidelines in resource-rich settings recommend using tidal volumes of 5–8 mL/kg for any mechanically ventilated pediatric patient and using patient-specific tidal volumes according to disease severity [116]. The definitions of acute lung injury and the pediatric acute respiratory distress syndrome have recently incorporated pulse oximetry for contexts where blood-gas analysis is unavailable.

There was one observational study from a resource-limited setting, comparing historical controls in an era of high tidal volume to a group ventilated with low tidal volumes [117]. We identified a systematic review and meta-analysis that examined observational studies in children [118].

The meta-analysis demonstrated no association between tidal volume and mortality in ventilated children, with significant heterogeneity in the pooled analysis. This review included the one observational study from a resource-limited setting that demonstrated a mortality benefit to low tidal volume strategy [117]. This review is downgraded for quality and indirectness.

The availability of mechanical ventilation is limited in many resource-limited ICUs. Low tidal volume ventilation, where available, is likely to be safe, as documented in the adult studies. The diagnosis of the acute respiratory distress syndrome is often difficult in resource-limited settings, and specific criteria should be developed and implemented where the appropriate diagnostics are unavailable, including pulse oximetry [119]. Monitoring ventilated patients with blood-gas analysis to follow permissive hypercapnia is a challenge in resource-limited settings without access to blood-gas analyzers.

We recommend using a tidal volume of 5–8 mL/kg in all mechanically ventilated children with sepsis-induced acute lung injury in resource-limited settings (1D). Further research to better define and manage the acute respiratory distress syndrome in children in ICUs in resource-limited settings is urgently needed.

Acknowledgment All authors of this chapter are members of the 'European Society of Intensive Care Medicine (ESICM) Global Intensive Care' working group and the Mahidol-Oxford Research Unit (MORU) in Bangkok, Thailand.

References

1. GRADE handbook for grading quality of evidence and strength of recommendations. Updated October 2013. 2013.
2. Dellinger RP, Levy MM, Rhodes A, Annane D, Gerlach H, Opal SM, Sevransky JE, Sprung CL, Douglas IS, Jaeschke R, et al. Surviving sepsis campaign: international guidelines for management of severe sepsis and septic shock: 2012. Crit Care Med. 2013;41(2):580–637.
3. Goldstein B, Giroir B, Randolph A. International Consensus Conference on Pediatric S: International pediatric sepsis consensus conference: definitions for sepsis and organ dysfunction in pediatrics. Pediatr Crit Care Med. 2005;6(1):2–8.
4. Singer M, Deutschman CS, Seymour CW, Shankar-Hari M, Annane D, Bauer M, Bellomo R, Bernard GR, Chiche JD, Coopersmith CM, et al. The Third International Consensus Definitions for Sepsis and Septic Shock (Sepsis-3). JAMA. 2016;315(8):801–10.
5. Maitland K, Kiguli S, Opoka RO, Engoru C, Olupot-Olupot P, Akech SO, Nyeko R, Mtove G, Reyburn H, Lang T, et al. Mortality after fluid bolus in African children with severe infection. N Engl J Med. 2011;364(26):2483–95.
6. Maitland K, George EC, Evans JA, Kiguli S, Olupot-Olupot P, Akech SO, Opoka RO, Engoru C, Nyeko R, Mtove G, et al. Exploring mechanisms of excess mortality with early fluid resuscitation: insights from the FEAST trial. BMC Med. 2013;11:68.
7. Milner D Jr, Factor R, Whitten R, Carr RA, Kamiza S, Pinkus G, Molyneux M, Taylor T. Pulmonary pathology in pediatric cerebral malaria. Hum Pathol. 2013;44(12):2719–26.
8. Schmidt WP, Cairncross S, Barreto ML, Clasen T, Genser B. Recent diarrhoeal illness and risk of lower respiratory infections in children under the age of 5 years. Int J Epidemiol. 2009;38(3):766–72.
9. Azim T, Islam LN, Sarker MS, Ahmad SM, Hamadani JD, Faruque SM, Salam MA. Immune response of Bangladeshi children with acute diarrhea who subsequently have persistent diarrhea. J Pediatr Gastroenterol Nutr. 2000;31(5):528–35.
10. Sarmin M, Ahmed T, Bardhan PK, Chisti MJ. Specialist hospital study shows that septic shock and drowsiness predict mortality in children under five with diarrhoea. Acta Paediatr. 2014;103(7):e306–11.
11. Chan M, Lake A. Integrated action for the prevention and control of pneumonia and diarrhoea. Lancet. 2013;381(9876):1436–7.
12. World Health Organization. Paediatric emergency triage, assessment and treatment: care of critically-ill children. Geneva: WHO; 2016.
13. George EC, Walker AS, Kiguli S, Olupot-Olupot P, Opoka RO, Engoru C, Akech SO, Nyeko R, Mtove G, Reyburn H, et al. Predicting mortality in sick African children: the FEAST Paediatric Emergency Triage (PET) score. BMC Med. 2015;13(1):174.
14. Subhi R, Adamson M, Campbell H, Weber M, Smith K, Duke T. Hypoxaemia in Developing Countries Study G: the prevalence of hypoxaemia among ill children in developing countries: a systematic review. Lancet Infect Dis. 2009;9(4):219–27.
15. Mwaniki MK, Nokes DJ, Ignas J, Munywoki P, Ngama M, Newton CR, Maitland K, Berkley JA. Emergency triage assessment for hypoxaemia in neonates and young children in a Kenyan hospital: an observational study. Bull World Health Organ. 2009;87(4):263–70.
16. English M, Muambi B, Mithwani S, Marsh K. Lactic acidosis and oxygen debt in African children with severe anaemia. QJM. 1997;90(9):563–9.
17. Evans JA, May J, Ansong D, Antwi S, Asafo-Adjei E, Nguah SB, Osei-Kwakye K, Akoto AO, Ofori AO, Sambian D, et al. Capillary refill time as an independent prognostic indicator in severe and complicated malaria. J Pediatr. 2006;149(5):676–81.

18. Raimer PL, Han YY, Weber MS, Annich GM, Custer JR. A normal capillary refill time of </= 2 seconds is associated with superior vena cava oxygen saturations of >/= 70%. J Pediatr. 2011;158(6):968–72.
19. Leonard PA, Beattie TF. Is measurement of capillary refill time useful as part of the initial assessment of children? Eur J Emerg Med. 2004;11(3):158–63.
20. Otieno H, Were E, Ahmed I, Charo E, Brent A, Maitland K. Are bedside features of shock reproducible between different observers? Arch Dis Child. 2004;89(10):977–9.
21. Lobos AT, Lee S, Menon K. Capillary refill time and cardiac output in children undergoing cardiac catheterization. Pediatr Crit Care Med. 2012;13(2):136–40.
22. Tibby SM, Hatherill M, Murdoch IA. Capillary refill and core-peripheral temperature gap as indicators of haemodynamic status in paediatric intensive care patients. Arch Dis Child. 1999;80(2):163–6.
23. Tripathy R, Parida S, Das L, Mishra DP, Tripathy D, Das MC, Chen H, Maguire JH, Panigrahi P. Clinical manifestations and predictors of severe malaria in Indian children. Pediatrics. 2007;120(3):e454–60.
24. Jeena PM, Adhikari M, Carlin JB, Qazi S, Weber MW, Hamer DH. Clinical profile and predictors of severe illness in young South African infants (<60 days). S Afr Med J. 2008;98(11):883–8.
25. Norton EB, Archibald LK, Nwanyanwu OC, Kazembe PN, Dobbie H, Reller LB, Jarvis WR, Jason J. Clinical predictors of bloodstream infections and mortality in hospitalized Malawian children. Pediatr Infect Dis J. 2004;23(2):145–51. discussion 151-145
26. Maitland K, Berkley JA, Shebbe M, Peshu N, English M, Newton CR. Children with severe malnutrition: can those at highest risk of death be identified with the WHO protocol? PLoS Med. 2006;3(12):e500.
27. Orimadegun AE, Ogunbosi BO, Carson SS. Prevalence and predictors of hypoxaemia in respiratory and non-respiratory primary diagnoses among emergently ill children at a tertiary hospital in south western Nigeria. Trans R Soc Trop Med Hyg. 2013;107(11):699–705.
28. Orimadegun A, Ogunbosi B, Orimadegun B. Hypoxemia predicts death from severe falciparum malaria among children under 5 years of age in Nigeria: the need for pulse oximetry in case management. Afr Health Sci. 2014;14(2):397–407.
29. Hatherill M, Waggie Z, Purves L, Reynolds L, Argent A. Mortality and the nature of metabolic acidosis in children with shock. Intensive Care Med. 2003;29(2):286–91.
30. Hawkes M, Conroy AL, Opoka RO, Namasopo S, Liles WC, John CC, Kain KC. Performance of point-of-care diagnostics for glucose, lactate, and hemoglobin in the management of severe malaria in a resource-constrained hospital in Uganda. Am J Trop Med Hyg. 2014;90(4):605–8.
31. Jat KR, Jhamb U, Gupta VK. Serum lactate levels as the predictor of outcome in pediatric septic shock. Indian J Crit Care Med. 2011;15(2):102–7.
32. Ramakrishna B, Graham SM, Phiri A, Mankhambo L, Duke T. Lactate as a predictor of mortality in Malawian children with WHO-defined pneumonia. Arch Dis Child. 2012;97(4):336–42.
33. Tamburlini G, Di Mario S, Maggi RS, Vilarim JN, Gove S. Evaluation of guidelines for emergency triage assessment and treatment in developing countries. Arch Dis Child. 1999;81(6):478–82.
34. Robertson MA, Molyneux EM. Description of cause of serious illness and outcome in patients identified using ETAT guidelines in urban Malawi. Arch Dis Child. 2001;85(3):214–7.
35. Wiens MO, Kumbakumba E, Kissoon N, Ansermino JM, Ndamira A, Larson CP. Pediatric sepsis in the developing world: challenges in defining sepsis and issues in post-discharge mortality. Clin Epidemiol. 2012;4:319–25.
36. Berkley JA, Maitland K, Mwangi I, Ngetsa C, Mwarumba S, Lowe BS, Newton CR, Marsh K, Scott JA, English M. Use of clinical syndromes to target antibiotic prescribing in seriously ill children in malaria endemic area: observational study. BMJ. 2005;330(7498):995.
37. Bonafide CP, Brady PW, Keren R, Conway PH, Marsolo K, Daymont C. Development of heart and respiratory rate percentile curves for hospitalized children. Pediatrics. 2013;131(4):e1150–7.

38. Saptharishi LG, Jayashree M, Singhi S. Development and validation of the "Pediatric Risk of Nosocomial Sepsis (PRiNS)" score for health care-associated infections in a medical pediatric intensive care unit of a developing economy-a prospective observational cohort study. J Crit Care. 2016;32:152–8.
39. Sepanski RJ, Godambe SA, Mangum CD, Bovat CS, Zaritsky AL, Shah SH. Designing a pediatric severe sepsis screening tool. Front Pediatr. 2014;2:56.
40. Moore LJ, Jones SL, Kreiner LA, McKinley B, Sucher JF, Todd SR, Turner KL, Valdivia A, Moore FA. Validation of a screening tool for the early identification of sepsis. J Trauma. 2009;66(6):1539–46. discussion 1546-1537
41. International Liaison Committee on Resuscitation. The International Liaison Committee on Resuscitation (ILCOR) consensus on science with treatment recommendations for pediatric and neonatal patients: pediatric basic and advanced life support. Pediatrics. 2006;117(5):e955–77.
42. Gaieski DF, Mikkelsen ME, Band RA, Pines JM, Massone R, Furia FF, Shofer FS, Goyal M. Impact of time to antibiotics on survival in patients with severe sepsis or septic shock in whom early goal-directed therapy was initiated in the emergency department. Crit Care Med. 2010;38(4):1045–53.
43. Weiss SL, Fitzgerald JC, Balamuth F, Alpern ER, Lavelle J, Chilutti M, Grundmeier R, Nadkarni VM, Thomas NJ. Delayed antimicrobial therapy increases mortality and organ dysfunction duration in pediatric sepsis. Crit Care Med. 2014;42(11):2409–17.
44. Luck RP, Haines C, Mull CC. Intraosseous access. J Emerg Med. 2010;39(4):468–75.
45. Banerjee S, Singhi SC, Singh S, Singh M. The intraosseous route is a suitable alternative to intravenous route for fluid resuscitation in severely dehydrated children. Indian Pediatr. 1994;31(12):1511–20.
46. Tighe SQ, Rudland SV, Kemp PM, Kershaw CR. Paediatric resuscitation in adverse circumstances: a comparison of three routes of systemic access. J R Nav Med Serv. 1993;79(2):75–9.
47. Rouhani S, Meloney L, Ahn R, Nelson BD, Burke TF. Alternative rehydration methods: a systematic review and lessons for resource-limited care. Pediatrics. 2011;127(3):e748–57.
48. Ker K, Tansley G, Beecher D, Perner A, Shakur H, Harris T, Roberts I. Comparison of routes for achieving parenteral access with a focus on the management of patients with Ebola virus disease. Cochrane Database Syst Rev. 2015;2:CD011386.
49. World Health Organization. Updates on the management of severe acute malnutrition in infants and children. Geneva: WHO; 2013.
50. Lackritz EM, Campbell CC, Ruebush TK 2nd, Hightower AW, Wakube W, Steketee RW, Were JB. Effect of blood transfusion on survival among children in a Kenyan hospital. Lancet. 1992;340(8818):524–8.
51. English M, Ahmed M, Ngando C, Berkley J, Ross A. Blood transfusion for severe anaemia in children in a Kenyan hospital. Lancet. 2002;359(9305):494–5.
52. Cheema B, Molyneux EM, Emmanuel JC, M'Baya B, Esan M, Kamwendo H, Kalilani-Phiri L, Boele van Hensbroek M. Development and evaluation of a new paediatric blood transfusion protocol for Africa. Transfus Med. 2010;20(3):140–51.
53. Ahmed T, Ali M, Ullah MM, Choudhury IA, Haque ME, Salam MA, Rabbani GH, Suskind RM, Fuchs GJ. Mortality in severely malnourished children with diarrhoea and use of a standardised management protocol. Lancet. 1999;353(9168):1919–22.
54. Bachou H, Tumwine JK, Mwadime RK, Tylleskar T. Risk factors in hospital deaths in severely malnourished children in Kampala, Uganda. BMC Pediatr. 2006;6:7.
55. Chisti MJ, Salam MA, Ashraf H, Faruque AS, Bardhan PK, Hossain MI, Shahid AS, Shahunja KM, Das SK, Imran G, et al. Clinical risk factors of death from pneumonia in children with severe acute malnutrition in an urban critical care ward of Bangladesh. PLoS One. 2013;8(9):e73728.
56. Alam NH, Islam S, Sattar S, Monira S, Desjeux JF. Safety of rapid intravenous rehydration and comparative efficacy of 3 oral rehydration solutions in the treatment of severely malnourished children with dehydrating cholera. J Pediatr Gastroenterol Nutr. 2009;48(3):318–27.

57. Bachou H, Tumwine JK, Mwadime RK, Ahmed T, Tylleskar T. Reduction of unnecessary transfusion and intravenous fluids in severely malnourished children is not enough to reduce mortality. Ann Trop Paediatr. 2008;28(1):23–33.
58. Akech SO, Karisa J, Nakamya P, Boga M, Maitland K. Phase II trial of isotonic fluid resuscitation in Kenyan children with severe malnutrition and hypovolaemia. BMC Pediatr. 2010;10:71.
59. Akech S, Ledermann H, Maitland K. Choice of fluids for resuscitation in children with severe infection and shock: systematic review. BMJ. 2010;341:c4416.
60. Finfer S, Bellomo R, Boyce N, French J, Myburgh J, Norton R, Investigators SS. A comparison of albumin and saline for fluid resuscitation in the intensive care unit. N Engl J Med. 2004;350(22):2247–56.
61. Brierley J, Carcillo JA, Choong K, Cornell T, Decaen A, Deymann A, Doctor A, Davis A, Duff J, Dugas MA, et al. Clinical practice parameters for hemodynamic support of pediatric and neonatal septic shock: 2007 update from the American College of Critical Care Medicine. Crit Care Med. 2009;37(2):666–88.
62. de Caen AR, Berg MD, Chameides L, Gooden CK, Hickey RW, Scott HF, Sutton RM, Tijssen JA, Topjian A, van der Jagt EW, et al. Part 12: pediatric advanced life support: 2015 American Heart Association guidelines update for cardiopulmonary resuscitation and emergency cardiovascular care. Circulation. 2015;132(18 Suppl 2):S526–42.
63. World Health Organization. Pocket book of hospital care for children: guidelines for the management of common childhood illnesses. 2nd ed. Geneva: WHO; 2013.
64. Santhanam I, Sangareddi S, Venkataraman S, Kissoon N, Thiruvengadamudayan V, Kasthuri RK. A prospective randomized controlled study of two fluid regimens in the initial management of septic shock in the emergency department. Pediatr Emerg Care. 2008;24(10):647–55.
65. Ford N, Hargreaves S, Shanks L. Mortality after fluid bolus in children with shock due to sepsis or severe infection: a systematic review and meta-analysis. PLoS One. 2012;7(8):e43953.
66. Opiyo N, Molyneux E, Sinclair D, Garner P, English M. Immediate fluid management of children with severe febrile illness and signs of impaired circulation in low-income settings: a contextualised systematic review. BMJ Open. 2014;4(4):e004934.
67. Kiguli S, Akech SO, Mtove G, Opoka RO, Engoru C, Olupot-Olupot P, Nyeko R, Evans J, Crawley J, Prevatt N, et al. WHO guidelines on fluid resuscitation in children: missing the FEAST data. BMJ. 2014;348:f7003.
68. Kissoon N, Carcillo JA, Espinosa V, Argent A, Devictor D, Madden M, Singhi S, van der Voort E, Latour J. Global sepsis initiative vanguard center c: world federation of pediatric intensive care and critical care societies: global sepsis initiative. Pediatr Crit Care Med. 2011;12(5):494–503.
69. de Oliveira CF, de Oliveira DS, Gottschald AF, Moura JD, Costa GA, Ventura AC, Fernandes JC, Vaz FA, Carcillo JA, Rivers EP, et al. ACCM/PALS haemodynamic support guidelines for paediatric septic shock: an outcomes comparison with and without monitoring central venous oxygen saturation. Intensive Care Med. 2008;34(6):1065–75.
70. Sankar J, Sankar MJ, Suresh CP, Dubey NK, Singh A. Early goal-directed therapy in pediatric septic shock: comparison of outcomes "with" and "without" intermittent superior venacaval oxygen saturation monitoring: a prospective cohort study*. Pediatr Crit Care Med. 2014;15(4):e157–67.
71. Samransamruajkit R, Uppala R, Pongsanon K, Deelodejanawong J, Sritippayawan S, Prapphal N. Clinical outcomes after utilizing surviving sepsis campaign in children with septic shock and prognostic value of initial plasma NT-proBNP. Indian J Crit Care Med. 2014;18(2):70–6.
72. Oliveira CF, Nogueira de Sa FR, Oliveira DS, Gottschald AF, Moura JD, Shibata AR, Troster EJ, Vaz FA, Carcillo JA. Time- and fluid-sensitive resuscitation for hemodynamic support of children in septic shock: barriers to the implementation of the American College of Critical Care Medicine/Pediatric Advanced Life Support Guidelines in a pediatric intensive care unit in a developing world. Pediatr Emerg Care. 2008;24(12):810–5.

73. Molyneux E, Ahmad S, Robertson A. Improved triage and emergency care for children reduces inpatient mortality in a resource-constrained setting. Bull World Health Organ. 2006;84(4):314–9.
74. Paul R, Neuman MI, Monuteaux MC, Melendez E. Adherence to PALS sepsis guidelines and hospital length of stay. Pediatrics. 2012;130(2):e273–80.
75. Larsen GY, Mecham N, Greenberg R. An emergency department septic shock protocol and care guideline for children initiated at triage. Pediatrics. 2011;127(6):e1585–92.
76. Cruz AT, Perry AM, Williams EA, Graf JM, Wuestner ER, Patel B. Implementation of goal-directed therapy for children with suspected sepsis in the emergency department. Pediatrics. 2011;127(3):e758–66.
77. Han YY, Carcillo JA, Dragotta MA, Bills DM, Watson RS, Westerman ME, Orr RA. Early reversal of pediatric-neonatal septic shock by community physicians is associated with improved outcome. Pediatrics. 2003;112(4):793–9.
78. Mouncey PR, Osborn TM, Power GS, Harrison DA, Sadique MZ, Grieve RD, Jahan R, Harvey SE, Bell D, Bion JF, et al. Trial of early, goal-directed resuscitation for septic shock. N Engl J Med. 2015;372(14):1301–11.
79. Yealy DM, Kellum JA, Huang DT, Barnato AE, Weissfeld LA, Pike F, Terndrup T, Wang HE, Hou PC, et al. A randomized trial of protocol-based care for early septic shock. N Engl J Med. 2014;370(18):1683–93.
80. Peake SL, Delaney A, Bailey M, Bellomo R, Cameron PA, Cooper DJ, Higgins AM, Holdgate A, et al. Goal-directed resuscitation for patients with early septic shock. N Engl J Med. 2014;371(16):1496–506.
81. Angus DC, Barnato AE, Bell D, Bellomo R, Chong CR, Coats TJ, Davies A, Delaney A, Harrison DA, Holdgate A, et al. A systematic review and meta-analysis of early goal-directed therapy for septic shock: the ARISE, ProCESS and ProMISe Investigators. Intensive Care Med. 2015;41(9):1549–60.
82. Andrews B, Muchemwa L, Kelly P, Lakhi S, Heimburger DC, Bernard GR. Simplified severe sepsis protocol: a randomized controlled trial of modified early goal-directed therapy in Zambia. Crit Care Med. 2014;42(11):2315–24.
83. Jacob ST, Banura P, Baeten JM, Moore CC, Meya D, Nakiyingi L, Burke R, Horton CL, Iga B, Wald A, et al. The impact of early monitored management on survival in hospitalized adult Ugandan patients with severe sepsis: a prospective intervention study*. Crit Care Med. 2012;40(7):2050–8.
84. Baelani I, Jochberger S, Laimer T, Otieno D, Kabutu J, Wilson I, Baker T, Dunser MW. Availability of critical care resources to treat patients with severe sepsis or septic shock in Africa: a self-reported, continent-wide survey of anaesthesia providers. Crit Care. 2011;15(1):R10.
85. Bojang KA, Palmer A, Boele van Hensbroek M, Banya WA, Greenwood BM. Management of severe malarial anaemia in Gambian children. Trans R Soc Trop Med Hyg. 1997;91(5):557–61.
86. Holzer BR, Egger M, Teuscher T, Koch S, Mboya DM, Smith GD. Childhood anemia in Africa: to transfuse or not transfuse? Acta Trop. 1993;55(1–2):47–51.
87. Meremikwu M, Smith HJ. Blood transfusion for treating malarial anaemia. Cochrane Database Syst Rev. 2000(2):CD001475.
88. Kiguli S, Maitland K, George EC, Olupot-Olupot P, Opoka RO, Engoru C, Akech SO, Nyeko R, Mtove G, Reyburn H, et al. Anaemia and blood transfusion in African children presenting to hospital with severe febrile illness. BMC Med. 2015;13:21.
89. Dorward JA, Knowles JK, Dorward IM. Treatment of severe anaemia in children in a rural hospital. Trop Dr. 1989;19(4):155–8.
90. English M, Waruiru C, Marsh K. Transfusion for respiratory distress in life-threatening childhood malaria. Am J Trop Med Hyg. 1996;55(5):525–30.
91. Camacho LH, Gordeuk VR, Wilairatana P, Pootrakul P, Brittenham GM, Looareesuwan S. The course of anaemia after the treatment of acute, falciparum malaria. Ann Trop Med Parasitol. 1998;92(5):525–37.

92. Obonyo CO, Steyerberg EW, Oloo AJ, Habbema JD. Blood transfusions for severe malaria-related anemia in Africa: a decision analysis. Am J Trop Med Hyg. 1998;59(5):808–12.
93. Maitland K, Akech S, Gwer S, Idro R, Fegan G, Eziefula AC, Levin M, Newton CR. Phase III trials required to resolve clinical equipoise over optimal fluid management in children with severe malaria. PLoS Clin Trials. 2007;2(2):e2.
94. Mueller Y, Bastard M, Ehounou G, Itama J, Quere M, de la Tour R, Vala L, Etard JF, Bottineau MC. Effectiveness of blood transfusions and risk factors for mortality in children aged from 1 month to 4 years at the Bon Marche Hospital, Bunia, Democratic Republic of the Congo. Tropical Med Int Health. 2012;17(12):1457–64.
95. Olupot-Olupot P, Engoru C, Thompson J, Nteziyaremye J, Chebet M, Ssenyondo T, Dambisya CM, Okuuny V, Wokulira R, Amorut D, et al. Phase II trial of standard versus increased transfusion volume in Ugandan children with acute severe anemia. BMC Med. 2014;12:67.
96. Liu L, Johnson HL, Cousens S, Perin J, Scott S, Lawn JE, Rudan I, Campbell H, Cibulskis R, Li M, et al. Global, regional, and national causes of child mortality: an updated systematic analysis for 2010 with time trends since 2000. Lancet. 2012;379(9832):2151–61.
97. Reed C, Madhi SA, Klugman KP, Kuwanda L, Ortiz JR, Finelli L, Fry AM. Development of the Respiratory Index of Severity in Children (RISC) score among young children with respiratory infections in South Africa. PLoS One. 2012;7(1):e27793.
98. Graham SM, English M, Hazir T, Enarson P, Duke T. Challenges to improving case management of childhood pneumonia at health facilities in resource-limited settings. Bull World Health Organ. 2008;86(5):349–55.
99. Duke T, Wandi F, Jonathan M, Matai S, Kaupa M, Saavu M, Subhi R, Peel D. Improved oxygen systems for childhood pneumonia: a multihospital effectiveness study in Papua New Guinea. Lancet. 2008;372(9646):1328–33.
100. Tiewsoh K, Lodha R, Pandey RM, Broor S, Kalaivani M, Kabra SK. Factors determining the outcome of children hospitalized with severe pneumonia. BMC Pediatr. 2009;9:15.
101. Smyth A, Tong CY, Carty H, Hart CA. Impact of HIV on mortality from acute lower respiratory tract infection in rural Zambia. Arch Dis Child. 1997;77(3):227–30.
102. Shann F, Barker J, Poore P. Chloramphenicol alone versus chloramphenicol plus penicillin for severe pneumonia in children. Lancet. 1985;2(8457):684–6.
103. Sehgal V, Sethi GR, Sachdev HP, Satyanarayana L. Predictors of mortality in subjects hospitalized with acute lower respiratory tract infections. Indian Pediatr. 1997;34(3):213–9.
104. Mishra S, Kumar H, Anand VK, Patwari AK, Sharma D. ARI control programme: results in hospitalized children. J Trop Pediatr. 1993;39(5):288–92.
105. Duke T, Poka H, Dale F, Michael A, Mgone J, Wal T. Chloramphenicol versus benzylpenicillin and gentamicin for the treatment of severe pneumonia in children in Papua New Guinea: a randomised trial. Lancet. 2002;359(9305):474–80.
106. Duke T. CPAP: a guide for clinicians in developing countries. Paediatr Int Child Health. 2014;34(1):3–11.
107. Banajeh SM, Al-Sunbali NN, Al-Sanahani SH. Clinical characteristics and outcome of children aged under 5 years hospitalized with severe pneumonia in Yemen. Ann Trop Paediatr. 1997;17(4):321–6.
108. Bahl R, Mishra S, Sharma D, Singhal A, Kumari S. A bacteriological study in hospitalized children with pneumonia. Ann Trop Paediatr. 1995;15(2):173–7.
109. Martin S, Duke T, Davis P. Efficacy and safety of bubble CPAP in neonatal care in low and middle income countries: a systematic review. Arch Dis Child Fetal Neonatal Ed. 2014;99(6):F495–504.
110. Chisti MJ, Salam MA, Smith JH, Ahmed T, Pietroni MA, Shahunja KM, Shahid AS, Faruque AS, Ashraf H, Bardhan PK, et al. Bubble continuous positive airway pressure for children with severe pneumonia and hypoxaemia in Bangladesh: an open, randomised controlled trial. Lancet. 2015;386:1057–65.
111. Wilson PT, Morris MC, Biagas KV, Otupiri E, Moresky RT. A randomized clinical trial evaluating nasal continuous positive airway pressure for acute respiratory distress in a developing country. J Pediatr. 2013;162(5):988–92.

112. Walk J, Dinga P, Banda C, Msiska T, Chitsamba E, Chiwayula N, Lufesi N, Mlotha-Mitole R, Costello A, Phiri A, et al. Non-invasive ventilation with bubble CPAP is feasible and improves respiratory physiology in hospitalised Malawian children with acute respiratory failure. Paediatr Int Child Health. 2016;36(1):28–33.
113. Jayashree M, KiranBabu HB, Singhi S, Nallasamy K. Use of nasal bubble CPAP in children with hypoxemic clinical pneumonia-report from a resource limited set-up. J Trop Pediatr. 2016;62(1):69–74.
114. Machen HE, Mwanza ZV, Brown JK, Kawaza KM, Newberry L, Richards-Kortum RR, Oden ZM, Molyneux EM. Outcomes of patients with respiratory distress treated with bubble CPAP on a pediatric ward in Malawi. J Trop Pediatr. 2015;61(6):421–7.
115. Santschi M, Jouvet P, Leclerc F, Gauvin F, Newth CJ, Carroll CL, Flori H, Tasker RC, Rimensberger PC, Randolph AG, et al. Acute lung injury in children: therapeutic practice and feasibility of international clinical trials. Pediatr Crit Care Med. 2010;11(6):681–9.
116. Pediatric Acute Lung Injury Consensus Conference. Pediatric acute respiratory distress syndrome: consensus recommendations from the Pediatric Acute Lung Injury Consensus Conference. Pediatr Crit Care Med. 2015;16(5):428–39.
117. Khilnani P, Pao M, Singhal D, Jain R, Bakshi A, Uttam R. Effect of low tidal volumes vs conventional tidal volumes on outcomes of acute respiratory distress syndrome in critically ill children. Indian J Crit Care Med. 2005;9(4):195–9.
118. de Jager P, Burgerhof JG, van Heerde M, Albers MJ, Markhorst DG, Kneyber MC. Tidal volume and mortality in mechanically ventilated children: a systematic review and meta-analysis of observational studies*. Crit Care Med. 2014;42(12):2461–72.
119. Riviello ED, Kiviri W, Twagirumugabe T, Mueller A, Banner-Goodspeed VM, Officer L, Novack V, Mutumwinka M, Talmor DS, Fowler RA. Hospital incidence and outcomes of ARDS using the Kigali modification of the Berlin definition. Am J Respir Crit Care Med. 2016;193(1):52–9.

Open Access This chapter is licensed under the terms of the Creative Commons Attribution 4.0 International License (http://creativecommons.org/licenses/by/4.0/), which permits use, sharing, adaptation, distribution and reproduction in any medium or format, as long as you give appropriate credit to the original author(s) and the source, provide a link to the Creative Commons license and indicate if changes were made.

The images or other third party material in this chapter are included in the chapter's Creative Commons license, unless indicated otherwise in a credit line to the material. If material is not included in the chapter's Creative Commons license and your intended use is not permitted by statutory regulation or exceeds the permitted use, you will need to obtain permission directly from the copyright holder.

www.ingramcontent.com/pod-product-compliance
Lightning Source LLC
LaVergne TN
LVHW082225200926
848484LV00008B/2305